Professional Ethics in Obstetrics and Gynecology

Professional Ethics in Obstetrics and Gynecology

Laurence B. McCullough, PhD
Donald and Barbara Zucker School of Medicine at Hofstra/Northwell
and Lenox Hill Hospital

John H. Coverdale, MD, MEd
Baylor College of Medicine

Frank A. Chervenak, MD, MMM
Donald and Barbara Zucker School of Medicine at Hofstra/Northwell
and Lenox Hill Hospital

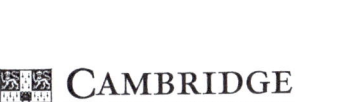

CAMBRIDGE
UNIVERSITY PRESS

University Printing House, Cambridge CB2 8BS, United Kingdom

One Liberty Plaza, 20th Floor, New York, NY 10006, USA

477 Williamstown Road, Port Melbourne, VIC 3207, Australia

314–321, 3rd Floor, Plot 3, Splendor Forum, Jasola District Centre,
New Delhi – 110025, India

79 Anson Road, #06–04/06, Singapore 079906

Cambridge University Press is part of the University of Cambridge.

It furthers the University's mission by disseminating knowledge in the pursuit of education, learning, and research at the highest international levels of excellence.

www.cambridge.org
Information on this title: www.cambridge.org/9781316631492
DOI: 10.1017/9781316841037

© 2020 Laurence B. McCullough, John H. Coverdale, and Frank A. Chervenak

This publication is in copyright. Subject to statutory exception and to the provisions of relevant collective licensing agreements, no reproduction of any part may take place without the written permission of Cambridge University Press.

First published 2020

Printed and bound in Great Britain by Clays Ltd, Elcograf S.p.A.

A catalogue record for this publication is available from the British Library.

Library of Congress Cataloging-in-Publication Data
Names: McCullough, Laurence B., author. | Chervenak, Frank A., author. | Coverdale, John H., author.
Title: Professional ethics in obstetrics and gynecology / Laurence B. McCullough, Frank A. Chervenak, John H. Coverdale.
Description: Cambridge, United Kingdom; New York, NY: Cambridge University Press, 2020. | Includes bibliographical references and index.
Identifiers: LCCN 2019019466 | ISBN 9781316631492 (paperback)
Subjects: | MESH: Obstetrics – ethics | Gynecology – ethics | Decision Making – ethics | Problem Solving – ethics
Classification: LCC RG103 | NLM WQ 21 | DDC 174.2/98–dc23
LC record available at https://lccn.loc.gov/2019019466

ISBN 978-1-316-63149-2 Paperback

....

Cambridge University Press has no responsibility for the persistence or accuracy of URLs for external or third-party internet websites referred to in this publication and does not guarantee that any content on such websites is, or will remain, accurate or appropriate.

Every effort has been made in preparing this book to provide accurate and up-to-date information which is in accord with accepted standards and practice at the time of publication. Although case histories are drawn from actual cases, every effort has been made to disguise the identities of the individuals involved. Nevertheless, the authors, editors and publishers can make no warranties that the information contained herein is totally free from error, not least because clinical standards are constantly changing through research and regulation. The authors, editors, and publishers therefore disclaim all liability for direct or consequential damages resulting from the use of material contained in this book. Readers are strongly advised to pay careful attention to information provided by the manufacturer of any drugs or equipment that they plan to use.

For our patients, medical students, residents, fellows, and clinical colleagues
And for our mentors

Contents

Preface xxi
Acknowledgments xxiii

Section 1 Professional Ethics in Obstetrics and Gynecology

1 **Professional Ethics in Medicine** 1
  Goal 1
  Objectives 1
  Topics 1
  Key Concepts 2
  1.1 Professional Ethics in Medicine and Professional Ethics in Obstetrics and Gynecology 3
  1.2 Ethics and Ethical Reasoning 3
    1.2.1 Ethics 3
    1.2.2 Ethical Reasoning 4
      1.2.2.1 Clinical Judgment 4
      1.2.2.2 Ethical Judgment 4
      1.2.2.3 Two Components of Ethical Reasoning 4
      1.2.2.4 Preventing Common Errors in Ethical Reasoning 5
    1.2.3 The Discipline of Ethical Reasoning 6
    1.2.4 Critical Appraisal of Argument-Based Ethical Reasoning 6
    1.2.5 Two Approaches to Ethical Reasoning: The Quest for Certainty and the Quest for Reliability 6
      1.2.5.1 The Quest for Certainty 7
      1.2.5.2 The Quest for Reliability 7
      1.2.5.3 Professional Ethics in Medicine Is the Quest for Reliability 7
  1.3 Medical Ethics and Bioethics 7
    1.3.1 Medical Ethics 7
      1.3.1.1 Philosophical Medical Ethics 7
      1.3.1.2 Limitations of Medical Ethics 8
    1.3.2 Bioethics 8
      1.3.2.1 Limitations of Bioethics 9
  1.4 Ethical Principles and Virtues in Medical Ethics and Bioethics 9
    1.4.1 The Four Ethical Principles in Medical Ethics and Bioethics 9
      1.4.1.1 The Ethical Principle of Beneficence in Medical Ethics and Bioethics 9
      1.4.1.2 The Ethical Principle of Nonmaleficence in Medical Ethics and Bioethics 10
      1.4.1.3 Beneficence and Nonmaleficence in the History of Medical Ethics 10
      1.4.1.4 The Ethical Principle of Respect for Autonomy in Medical Ethics and Bioethics 10
      1.4.1.5 The Ethical Principle of Justice in Medical Ethics and Bioethics 10
      1.4.1.6 Putting Ethical Principles into Practice 11
  1.5 Professional Ethics in Medicine 11
    1.5.1 The Invention of Professional Ethics in Medicine 11
      1.5.1.1 Hippocratic Medical Ethics 11
      1.5.1.2 Friedrich Hoffmann on the Politic Physician 12
      1.5.1.3 John Gregory and Thomas Percival on Professional Ethics in Medicine 13
      1.5.1.4 Gregory's Professional Ethics in Medicine 13
      1.5.1.5 Percival's Professional Ethics in Medicine 14
      1.5.1.6 The Ethical Concept of Medicine as a Profession 14
  1.6 Professional Virtues and Ethical Principles in Professional Ethics in Medicine 15
    1.6.1 The Five Professional Virtues 15
      1.6.1.1 The Professional Virtue of Integrity 15

vii

Contents

- 1.6.1.2 The Professional Virtue of Humility 16
- 1.6.1.3 The Professional Virtue of Compassion 16
- 1.6.1.4 The Professional Virtue of Self-Effacement 16
- 1.6.1.5 The Professional Virtue of Self-Sacrifice 17
- 1.6.2 The Four Ethical Principles in Professional Ethics in Medicine 17
  - 1.6.2.1 The Ethical Principle of Beneficence in Professional Ethics in Medicine 17
  - 1.6.2.2 The Concept of a Medically Reasonable Alternative 17
  - 1.6.2.3 The Ethical Principle of Nonmaleficence in Professional Ethics in Medicine 18
  - 1.6.2.4 The Ethical Principle of Respect for Autonomy in Professional Ethics in Medicine 18
  - 1.6.2.5 The Ethical Principle of Healthcare Justice in Professional Ethics in Medicine 18
- 1.7 Advantages of Professional Ethics in Medicine 19
- 1.8 Why Should Physicians Commit to the Ethical Concept of Medicine as a Profession? 19
- References 22

2 Professional Ethics in Obstetrics and Gynecology 24
- Goal 24
- Objectives 24
- Topics 24
- Key Concepts 25
- 2.1 Professional Ethics in Obstetrics and Gynecology 26
- 2.2 Professional Virtues and Ethical Principles in Professional Ethics in Gynecology 26
  - 2.2.1 The Female Patient 26
    - 2.2.1.1 Gregory on Ethical Obligations to the Female Patient 27
  - 2.2.2 The Five Professional Virtues in Professional Ethics in Gynecology 27
    - 2.2.2.1 The Professional Virtue of Integrity in Professional Ethics in Gynecology 27
    - 2.2.2.2 The Professional Virtue of Humility in Professional Ethics in Gynecology 27
    - 2.2.2.3 The Professional Virtue of Compassion in Professional Ethics in Gynecology 27
    - 2.2.2.4 The Professional Virtue of Self-Effacement in Professional Ethics in Gynecology 28
    - 2.2.2.5 The Professional Virtue of Self-Sacrifice in Professional Ethics in Gynecology 28
  - 2.2.3 Ethical Principles in Professional Ethics in Gynecology 29
    - 2.2.3.1 The Ethical Principle of Beneficence in Professional Ethics in Gynecology 29
    - 2.2.3.2 The Concept of a Medically Reasonable Alternative 29
    - 2.2.3.3 The Ethical Principle of Nonmaleficence in Professional Ethics in Gynecology 29
    - 2.2.3.4 The Ethical Principle of Respect for Autonomy in Professional Ethics in Gynecology 29
    - 2.2.3.5 The Ethical Principle of Healthcare Justice in Professional Ethics in Gynecology 29
- 2.3 Professional Virtues and Ethical Principles in Professional Ethics in Obstetrics 30
  - 2.3.1 The Five Professional Virtues in Professional Ethics in Obstetrics 30
    - 2.3.1.1 The Professional Virtue of Integrity in Professional Ethics in Obstetrics 30
    - 2.3.1.2 The Professional Virtue of Humility in Professional Ethics in Obstetrics 30
    - 2.3.1.3 The Professional Virtue of Compassion in Professional Ethics in Obstetrics 30
    - 2.3.1.4 The Professional Virtue of Self-Effacement in Professional Ethics in Obstetrics 31
    - 2.3.1.5 The Professional Virtue of Self-Sacrifice in Professional Ethics in Obstetrics 31
  - 2.3.2 Ethical Principles in Professional Ethics in Obstetrics 32

- 2.3.2.1 The Ethical Principle of Beneficence in Professional Ethics in Obstetrics 32
- 2.3.2.2 The Concept of a Medically Reasonable Alternative 32
- 2.3.2.3 The Ethical Principle of Nonmaleficence in Professional Ethics in Obstetrics 32
- 2.3.2.4 The Ethical Principle of Respect for Autonomy in Professional Ethics in Obstetrics 32
- 2.3.2.5 The Ethical Principle of Healthcare Justice in Professional Ethics in Obstetrics 32

2.4 The Ethical Concept of the Fetus as a Patient 33
- 2.4.1 Five Decades of the Discourse of the Fetus as a Patient 33
- 2.4.2 A Preliminary: The Ethical Concept of Moral Status 34
  - 2.4.2.1 Dominance of Independent Moral Status in Medical Ethics and Bioethics 34
  - 2.4.2.2 Problems with the Concept of Independent Moral Status 35
- 2.4.3 The Ethical Concept of the Fetus as a Patient 35
  - 2.4.3.1 The Viable Fetus as a Patient 36
  - 2.4.3.2 The Periviable Fetus as a Patient 36
  - 2.4.3.3 The Previable Fetus as a Patient 36
  - 2.4.3.4 The Obstetrician's Prima Facie Beneficence-Based Obligations to the Fetal Patient 36
  - 2.4.3.5 Limits on Prima Facie Beneficence-Based Obligations to the Pregnant Patient 37
  - 2.4.3.6 Enforcement of Prima Facie Beneficence-Based Ethical Obligations to the Fetal Patient 37

2.5 Advantages of the Ethical Concept of the Fetus as a Patient 38
- 2.5.1 The Ethical Concept of the Fetus as a Patient Avoids the Philosophical and Clinical Paralysis of "Right to Life" 38
- 2.5.2 The Ethical Concept of the Fetus as a Patient Avoids Reducing Moral Status to Independent Moral Status 38
- 2.5.3 The Ethical Concept of the Fetus as a Patient Avoids Rights-Based Absolutism 39
- 2.5.4 The Fetus Is a Separate Patient: A Failed Critique of the Ethical Concept of the Fetus as a Patient 40

2.6 Delivery Makes a Difference: Professional Ethics in Perinatal Medicine 41

References 42

3 **Decision Making By, With, and For Patients** 45
Goal 45
Objectives 45
Topics 45
Key Concepts 47

3.1 Decision Making By, With, and For Patients 47
3.2 A Decision Made *By* and *With* the Patient: Simple and Informed Consent 47
- 3.2.1 The Presumption of Decision-Making Capacity in Adult Patients 47
- 3.2.2 The Presumption of Decision-Making Capacity in Minors with Legal Authority over Themselves 47
- 3.2.3 "Competence" and "Capacity": Two Names for the Same Clinical Phenomenon 48
- 3.2.4 Seven Components of Decision-Making Capacity 48
- 3.2.5 Consent: Simple and Informed 49
  - 3.2.5.1 Simple Consent 49
  - 3.2.5.2 Informed Consent Process 51

3.3 Informed Refusal: A Strict Legal Obligation with a Preventive Ethics Component 55
- 3.3.1 The Strict Legal Obligation 55
- 3.3.2 The Preventive Ethics Component 56

3.4 How Attitudes Can Distort Clinical Judgment 56
3.5 Who Should Obtain Simple Consent? 57
3.6 Who Should Lead the Informed Consent Process? 57
3.7 Projecting Decision Making into the Future: Advance Directives 57

Contents

3.8 A Decision *By* the Patient *With* the Obstetrician-Gynecologist and Others Who Assist in the Decision-Making Process: Assisted Decision Making 58
   3.8.1 Assessment of Decision-Making Capacity 58
   3.8.2 Risk-Adjusted Assessment of Decision-Making Capacity: Proceed with Great Caution 58
   3.8.3 Decision-Making Capacity Is Task Specific and Time Specific 58
      3.8.3.1 Task-Specific Decision-Making Capacity 58
      3.8.3.2 Time-Specific Decision-Making Capacity 59
      3.8.3.3 Ulysses Contract 59
   3.8.4 When One or More Components of Decision-Making Capacity Are Diminished 59
3.9 A Decision *By* Others but *With* the Patient: Pediatric and Geriatric Assent 59
3.10 A Decision *By* Others *For* the Patient but *Not With* the Patient: Surrogate Decision Making 61
   3.10.1 Two Standards for Surrogate Decision Making 61
      3.10.1.1 Substituted Judgment Standard 61
      3.10.1.2 The Best Interests Standard 62
3.11 Clinical Ethical Topics in Decision Making for Patients 62
   3.11.1 Variants of Impaired Autonomy 62
      3.11.1.1 Chronic and Variable Impairment of Autonomy 62
      3.11.1.2 Chronic and Invariable Impairment of Autonomy 63
      3.11.1.3 Chronic and Progressive Impairment of Autonomy 63
      3.11.1.4 Chronic and Decreasing Impairment of Autonomy 63

3.12 Surrogate Decision Making about Termination of Pregnancy 64
3.13 Surrogate Decision Making about Prevention of Pregnancy 64
3.14 Managing Doubts about the Reliability of a Surrogate Decision Maker 65
3.15 Managing Refusal of a Family Member to Accept the Legally Designated Surrogate 65
3.16 Medical Emergencies 66
References 66

4 **Confidentiality** 68
Goal 68
Objectives 68
Topics 68
Key Concepts 69
4.1 Confidentiality in Professional Ethics in Obstetrics and Gynecology 69
   4.1.2 History of the Obligation 69
      4.1.2.1 The Hippocratic Oath 69
      4.1.2.2 Friedrich Hoffmann on the Politic Physician as Taciturn 69
      4.1.2.3 John Gregory on Keeping Patients' Secrets 70
      4.1.2.4 Thomas Percival on Keeping Patients' Secrets 71
      4.1.2.5 The Shift from an Absolute to Prima Facie Ethical Obligation 71
      4.1.2.6 Confidentiality: A Prima Facie Ethical Obligation 72
4.2 Setting Ethically Justified Limits on the Prima Facie Ethical Obligation of Confidentiality in Obstetrics and Gynecology 72
4.3 Ethical Challenges to Fulfilling the Prima Facie Ethical Obligation of Confidentiality 73
   4.3.1 Emergency Medical Care 73
   4.3.2 Disclosure to Family Members during and after Procedures Requiring Sedation or Anesthesia 73
   4.3.3 Inquiries by the Patient's Employer 74
   4.3.4 Insurance Claims 74
   4.3.5 Electronic Medical Record 75

4.3.6 Implications of Genetic and Genomic Information for Individuals Other than the Patient 75
4.3.7 Patients with Sexually Transmitted Disease Engaging in Behavior Known to Transmit Disease 76
4.3.8 Health Insurance Portability and Accountability Act 76
4.3.9 Electronic Communication with Patients 77
4.3.10 Use of Social Media 77
References 77

5 Conflicts of Interest and Conflicts of Commitment 79
Goal 79
Objectives 79
Topics 79
Key Concepts 80
5.1 Conflicts of Interest and Conflicts of Commitment in Historical Perspective 80
5.2 Conflicts of Interest 80
  5.2.1 Entrepreneurial versus Professional Relationships 80
  5.2.2 Conflict of Interest Defined 81
  5.2.3 John Gregory on Conflicts of Interest 81
  5.2.4 Thomas Percival on Conflicts of Interest 82
  5.2.5 Conceptual Confusion about Conflicts of Interest 83
  5.2.6 Professionally Responsible Management of Conflicts of Interest 83
    5.2.6.1 Use of Imaging 83
    5.2.6.2 Payment for Clinical Practice 83
    5.2.6.3 Cosmetic Procedures 84
    5.2.6.4 Research 84
5.3 Conflicts of Commitment 85
  5.3.1 Conflict of Commitment Defined 85
  5.3.2 Percival on Conflicts of Commitment 85
  5.3.3 Professionally Responsible Management of Conflicts of Commitment 85
  5.3.4 Preventing Conflation of Conflicts of Interest with Conflicts of Commitment 86
5.4 The Ethics of Romantic and Sexual Relationships with Patients 86
  5.4.1 An Historical Perspective 86
  5.4.2 Contemporary Perspective 88
5.5 Conscientious Objection: A Conflict of Commitment 89
  5.5.1 Conscientious Objection Defined 89
  5.5.2 A Useful Historical Analogy 89
  5.5.3 Conscientious Objection in Residency Training 89
  5.5.4 Conscientious Objection to Contraception 89
  5.5.5 Conscientious Objection to Referral for Induced Abortion and Feticide 90
    5.5.5.1 Invoking Individual Conscience Bears the Burden of Proof 90
    5.5.5.2 Beneficence-Based and Autonomy-Based Indications 90
    5.5.5.3 Beneficence-Based Direct Referral 90
    5.5.5.4 Autonomy-Based Indirect Referral 91
    5.5.5.5 Polarized Positions Are Unnecessary 91
References 92

Section 2 Pedagogy of Professional Ethics in Obstetrics and Gynecology

6 Teaching Professional Ethics in Obstetrics and Gynecology 93
Goal 93
Objectives 93
Topics 93
Key Concepts 94
6.1 Teaching the Basics of Professional Ethics in Obstetrics and Gynecology 94
6.2 Teaching the Discipline of Ethical Reasoning 95
  6.2.1 Precision of Thought and Speech 95

- 6.2.2 Going Where Arguments Take One and Nowhere Else 95
- 6.3 Pedagogical Tools 96
  - 6.3.1 Formal Assessment Tool for the Normative Ethics Literature 96
    - 6.3.1.1 Does the Article Address a Focused Ethics Question? 96
    - 6.3.1.2 Are the Results of the Article Valid? 97
    - 6.3.1.3 What Are the Results? 98
    - 6.3.1.4 Will the Results Help Me in Clinical Practice? In Innovation and Research? In Organizational Culture? In Health Policy and Advocacy? 98
  - 6.3.2 Structured Reviews of the Normative Ethics Literature 98
- 6.4 Pedagogical Methods 98
  - 6.4.1 Case-Based Teaching Using an Ethics Workup 98
  - 6.4.2 "Fast Ethics": Teaching Ethics on Rounds 99
  - 6.4.3 Preparing a Grand Rounds Presentation on Professional Ethics in Obstetrics and Gynecology 99
  - 6.4.4 What Makes a Great Teacher of Professional Ethics in Obstetrics and Gynecology? 100
- 6.5 A Distinctive Challenge in Graduate Medical Education: Preventing Drift Away from Professionalism 101
  - 6.5.1 The Commitment to the Ethical Concept of Medicine as a Profession 101
  - 6.5.2 Drift Away from an Organizational Culture of Professionalism 102
    - 6.5.2.1 Restricted Duty Hours 102
    - 6.5.2.2 Supervision by Attending Physicians 103
    - 6.5.2.3 Compounding Factors 103
- 6.6 A Preventive Ethics Response to Reduced Accountability 103
  - 6.6.1 Performing a Critical Appraisal of the Organizational Culture of the Residency 104
  - 6.6.2 Defining Components of Professional Accountability in Milestones 104
  - 6.6.3 Mastering the Skillset of Patient Safety and Quality 104
  - 6.6.4 Enhancing the Role of ACGME 105
- References 105

Section 3 Professionally Responsible Clinical Practice

7 Prevention of Pregnancy 107
- Goal 107
- Objectives 107
- Topics 107
- Key Concepts 108
- 7.1 The Biopsychosocial Concept of Fertility 108
  - 7.1.1 The Role of the Biologic Concept of Sex in the Biopsychosocial Concept of Fertility 108
  - 7.1.2 The Biologic Concept of Fertility: A Clinical Condition with Two Meanings 108
  - 7.1.3 The Biopsychosocial Concept of Fertility 108
- 7.2 Medically Reasonable Alternatives for the Prevention of Pregnancy 109
  - 7.2.1 Four Groups of Methods to Prevent Pregnancy 109
- 7.3 Decision Making about the Management of Fertility 109
  - 7.3.1 Beneficence-Based Deliberative Clinical Judgment 109
  - 7.3.2 Autonomy-Based Clinical Judgment 109
  - 7.3.3 The Role of Directive Counseling 109
  - 7.3.4 The Role of Shared Decision Making 110
  - 7.3.5 Impermissible Scope of Beneficence-Based Deliberative Clinical Judgment 110
- 7.4 Assisted Decision Making 111
  - 7.4.1 Assisted Decision Making with Patients with Major Mental Disorders 111
- 7.5 Pediatric Assent 112
- 7.6 Surrogate Decision Making 112
- 7.7 Organizational Policy 113
- 7.8 Healthcare-Justice–Based Deliberative Clinical Judgment and Advocacy 113

7.8.1 Access to Clinical Management of Fertility   113
7.8.2 Court-Ordered Clinical Management of Fertility   113
References   114

8 Initiation of Pregnancy   115
Goal   115
Objectives   115
Topics   115
Key Concepts   116
8.1 Two Roles of the Obstetrician-Gynecologist in the Initiation of Pregnancy   116
  8.1.1 Assisted Reproduction   116
  8.1.2 Preconception Counseling   116
8.2 Precision of Thought and Speech   117
  8.2.1 The In Vitro Meaning of "Embryo" in Reproductive Medicine   117
  8.2.2 The In Vivo Meaning of "Embryo" in Reproductive Medicine   117
8.3 In Vitro Assisted Reproduction   117
  8.3.1 The Ethical Concept of Moral Status   117
    8.3.1.1 Does an Embryo Have Independent Moral Status?   117
    8.3.1.2 Does an Embryo Have Dependent Moral Status?   118
    8.3.1.3 How Many Embryos Should Be Transferred?   118
    8.3.1.4 Preimplantation Analysis of the In Vitro Embryo   119
    8.3.1.5 Responding to Requests for a High Number of Embryos to Be Transferred   120
    8.3.1.6 Seamless Patient Care   120
8.4 Manipulation of the In Vitro Embryo: Clinical Innovation and Research   120
8.5 Preconception Counseling   120
  8.5.1 Anticipating Moral Risk   121
  8.5.2 Counseling about Obstetric Management   121
References   121

9 Induced Abortion and Feticide   123
Goal   123
Objectives   123
Topics   123
Key Concepts   124
9.1 Ethical Challenges of Counseling Pregnant Women about Induced Abortion and Feticide   124
9.2 Precision of Thought and Speech   124
9.3 Induced Abortion and Feticide before Viability in Professional Ethics of Obstetrics   125
9.4 Offering Induced Abortion and Feticide   125
  9.4.1 After Viability   125
  9.4.2 Before Viability: Beneficence-Based Justifications   126
    9.4.2.1 When Pregnancy Poses a Threat to the Health or Life of the Pregnant Patient   126
    9.4.2.2 When Pregnancy Poses a Threat to the Life or Health of the Coexistent Fetus(es)   126
  9.4.3 Before Viability: Autonomy-Based Justifications   126
9.5 Recommending Induced Abortion or Feticide   127
  9.5.1 Risk to the Health or Life of the Pregnant Woman   127
  9.5.2 Increased Risk to the Health or Life of the Fetus(es)   127
  9.5.3 Diagnosis of a Serious Fetal Anomaly   128
  9.5.4 Complications that Threaten the Health or Life of the Pregnant Woman and Fetal Salvage Is Hopeless   128
  9.5.5 Ethical Justifications   128
9.6 Decision Making With, By, and For Patients with Depression and Psychoses   128
9.7 Conscientious Objection to Offering or Recommending Induced Abortion or Feticide   129
9.8 Performing Induced Abortion and Feticide   129
9.9 Invoking Conscientious Objection to Performing Induced Abortion or Feticide   130
9.10 Confidentiality   131
9.11 Referring for Induced Abortion and Feticide   131
  9.11.1 Direct Referral   131
  9.11.2 Indirect Referral   131
References   131

Contents

10 **Fetal Analysis** 133
  Goal 133
  Objectives 133
  Topics 133
  Key Concepts 134
  10.1 Fetal Analysis and Decision Making about Obstetric Management 134
  10.2 Providing Clinical Information about Options for Fetal Analysis Using Precise Nomenclature 134
    10.2.1 Deceptively Imprecise Current Nomenclature 134
    10.2.2 Replacement Nomenclature: Noninvasive Fetal Analysis or Invasive Fetal Analysis 135
      10.2.2.1 Fetal Analysis 135
      10.2.2.2 Noninvasive or Invasive Method 135
      10.2.2.3 New Nomenclature 135
    10.2.3 Communication among Obstetricians 135
    10.2.4 Communication with Patients 135
  10.3 Nondirective Counseling or Shared Decision Making 136
  10.4 How Pregnant Women Will Respond to an Offer of Fetal Analysis 136
    10.4.1 Refusal of All Forms of Fetal Analysis 137
    10.4.2 Election of Invasive Fetal Analysis 137
    10.4.3 Election of Noninvasive Fetal Analysis 137
      10.4.3.1 Free Fetal DNA Analysis 137
    10.4.4 Uncertainty about What to Do 138
  10.5 Use of Results from Fetal Analysis 138
  References 138

11 **Periviability** 139
  Goal 139
  Objectives 139
  Topics 139
  Key Concepts 140
  11.1 Viability 140
  11.2 Periviable Birth 140
  11.3 Professional Ethics in Perinatal Medicine 140
    11.3.1 The Obstetric Component of Professional Ethics in Perinatal Medicine 141
    11.3.2 The Pediatric Component of Professional Ethics in Perinatal Medicine 141
  11.4 The Continuum of Deliberative Clinical Judgment about the Clinical Management of Periviability 142
    11.4.1 Intrapartum Management 142
      11.4.1.1 Consensus Statement from the American College of Obstetricians and Gynecologists and the Society for Maternal–Fetal Medicine 142
      11.4.1.2 Limits of Deliberative Clinical Obstetric Judgment 143
    11.4.2 Evaluation of the Neonatal Patient for Clinical Application of Specified Concepts of Futility 143
    11.4.3 Resuscitation as a Trial of Intervention 143
    11.4.4 Neonatal Critical Care as a Trial of Intervention 143
  11.5 A Multidisciplinary Team Approach to Counseling before Delivery 143
    11.5.1 Clarifying Who Is the Decision Maker with the Perinatal Team 143
    11.5.2 A Multidisciplinary Approach 144
  11.6 Responding to Requests to "Do Everything" 144
    11.6.1 A Preventive Ethics Approach 144
    11.6.2 Addressing Incomplete or Inaccurate Information 144
    11.6.3 Moral Theological Considerations 145
    11.6.4 Hope and Coping with Loss 145
  References 145

12 **Intrapartum Management** 147
  Goal 147
  Objectives 147
  Topics 147
  Key Concepts 148

12.1 The Continuum of Vaginal Delivery and Cesarean Delivery 149
12.2 Preventive Ethics for Cesarean Delivery 149
   12.2.1 Preventive Ethics 149
   12.2.2 The Goal of Preventive Ethics 149
   12.2.3 The Informed Consent Process as Preventive Ethics 150
   12.2.4 The Role of Recommendations 150
   12.2.5 When Both Vaginal and Cesarean Delivery Are Medically Reasonable 150
12.3 Cephalocentesis 151
   12.3.1 Isolated Fetal Hydrocephalus 151
   12.3.2 Hydrocephalus with Severe Associated Abnormalities 151
   12.3.3 Hydrocephalus with Other Associated Anomalies 152
12.4 Refusal of Cesarean Delivery 152
   12.4.1 Refusal of Cesarean Delivery and Termination of Relationship with the Obstetrician 152
   12.4.2 Refusal of Cesarean Delivery and Election of the Medically Reasonable Alternative of Vaginal Delivery 152
   12.4.3 Refusal of Cesarean Delivery When It Is the Only Medically Reasonable Alternative: A Negative Right Coupled to a Positive Right 152
      12.4.3.1 The Role of the Professional Virtue of Integrity in Professional Ethics in Obstetrics and Gynecology 152
   12.4.4 Antepartum Refusal 153
   12.4.5 Intrapartum Refusal 153
      12.4.5.1 Refusal of Cesarean Delivery for Well-Documented, Intrapartum, Complete Placenta Previa and for Severe Placental Abruption 153
      12.4.5.2 Refusal of Cesarean Delivery for Severe Fetal Distress and Prolapsed Umbilical Cord 154
   12.4.6 Court Orders for Forced Cesarean Delivery 154
12.5 Decision Making With, By, and For Pregnant Patients with Mental Disorders and Illnesses 154
   12.5.1 Managing Powerful Responses 154
   12.5.2 Informed Consent, Assisted Consent, and Surrogate Decision Making 155
      12.5.2.1 Assessment of Decision-Making Capacity 155
      12.5.2.2 The Informed Consent Process 155
      12.5.2.3 Assisted Decision Making 155
      12.5.2.4 Surrogate Decision Making 155
   12.5.3 Treatment Is Accepted by the Patient 155
   12.5.4 Treatment Is Not Accepted by the Patient 157
      12.5.4.1 Attempt Assent 157
      12.5.4.2 When Beneficence-Based Ethical Obligations Should Guide Clinical Management 157
12.6 Continuing a Pregnancy in a Patient in a Permanent Vegetative State and in a Cadaver 157
   12.6.1 Continuing Pregnancy Is an Experiment 157
12.7 Responding to Requests for Cesarean Delivery 158
   12.7.1 Preventing Involuntary Requests 158
12.8 Planned Home Birth 158
   12.8.1 Planned Home Birth Is Inconsistent with Patient Safety 158
   12.8.2 Implications for Counseling Women Who Express an Interest in a Planned Home Birth 159
      12.8.2.1 The Role of Recommendations 159
      12.8.2.2 Making Recommendations Supports, Not Impairs, Patient Autonomy 160
References 160

13 The Perfect Baby 163
Goal 163
Objectives 163
Topics 163
Key Concepts 164
13.1 The Perilous Logic of the Belief that Medicine Can Control Human Biology 164
   13.1.1 The Quest for Control over Human Biology 164
   13.1.2 A Perilous Logic 164
13.2 Creative Literature in Ethical Reasoning 164
13.3 The Perils of Belief in Control and Expectation of Perfection: A Cautionary Tale from American Literature 164
   13.3.1 Nathaniel Hawthorne's "The Birth-Mark" 165
13.4 The Perils of the Logic of Belief in Control and Pursuit of Perfection 165
   13.4.1 An Antidote: Preventive Ethics 165
   13.4.2 The Interaction of Clinical and Social Conditions that Promote the Concept of the Perfect Baby 165
      13.4.2.1 Fetal Imaging 165
      13.4.2.2 Baby Pictures 165
      13.4.2.3 Belief in Control over Human Biology 165
      13.4.2.4 Consumer Rights Movement 166
13.5 Fashioning the Informed Consent Process to Defuse the Expectation That Medicine Can Control Human Reproductive Biology 166
   13.5.1 No Guarantee of a Perfect Baby 167
   13.5.2 What Obstetricians Should Know 167
   13.5.3 What Patients Need to Know 167
   13.5.4 Limits of Fetal Diagnosis 168
   13.5.5 Experimental Maternal–Fetal Intervention 169
13.6 Perfection in Pregnancy Is Not Attainable 169
References 170

14 Cancer and Pregnancy 171
Goal 171
Objectives 171
Topics 171
Key Concepts 172
14.1 Ethical Challenges of Cancer and Pregnancy 172
14.2 Congruent and Noncongruent Beneficence-Based Ethical Obligations of the Obstetrician 172
   14.2.1 Congruent Beneficence-Based Ethical Obligations to the Pregnant and the Fetal Patient 172
   14.2.2 Noncongruent Beneficence-Based Ethical Obligations to the Pregnant and the Fetal Patient 172
14.3 The Informed Consent Process 173
   14.3.1 The Informed Consent Process When the Fetus Is Previable 173
   14.3.2 The Informed Consent Process When the Fetus Is Viable 173
      14.3.2.1 Congruent Beneficence-Based Obligations to the Pregnant and the Fetal Patient 174
      14.3.2.2 Noncongruent Beneficence-Based Obligations to the Pregnant Patient 174
      14.3.2.3 Noncongruent Beneficence-Based Obligations to the Pregnant Patient and the Fetal Patient 174
14.4 Advance Directives 176
References 176

15 Setting Ethically Justified Limits on Life-Sustaining Treatment 177
Goal 177
Objectives 177
Topics 177
Key Concepts 178
15.1 Two Goals of Life-Sustaining Treatment 178
15.2 Beneficence-Based and Autonomy-Based Limits of Life-Sustaining Treatment 178
15.3 Historical Perspective 179
   15.3.1 The Hippocratic Tradition of Declaring Gravely Ill Patients Incurable and Abandoning Them 179
   15.3.2 John Gregory's Reversal of the Hippocratic Tradition of Abandoning Dying Patients 179

- 15.3.3 The Influence of Enthusiasm in American Critical Care   180
- 15.3.4 The Influence of American Common Law   180
- 15.3.5 An Emerging Consensus   180
- 15.3.6 The Influence of a Landmark Article   180
- 15.4 An Algorithm for the Role of the Obstetrician-Gynecologist in Decision Making about Setting Ethically Justified Limits on Life-Sustaining Treatment   181
  - 15.4.1 Steps of the Algorithm   182
  - 15.4.2 Preventing Unacceptable Opportunity Costs to Other Patients   183
- 15.5 Why the Groningen Protocol Should Be Rejected in Professional Ethics in Perinatal Medicine   184
- 15.6 A Preventive Ethics Approach to Setting Ethically Justified Limits on Life-Sustaining Treatment   184
- 15.7 Responding to Inappropriate Requests for Life-Sustaining Treatment   185
  - 15.7.1 The Role of the Professional Virtue of Integrity in Professional Ethics in Obstetrics and Gynecology and in Perinatal Medicine   185
  - 15.7.2 Why Requests to "Do Everything" Are Made: A Hypothesis from Qualitative Research on End-of-Life Surrogate Decision Making   185
  - 15.7.3 Responding to Requests to "Do Everything"   185
  - 15.7.4 The Essential Role of Hospital Policy and Commitment to It by Hospital Leadership   186
- References   186

Section 4 Professionally Responsible Leadership

16 **Leadership**   189
  - Goal   189
  - Objectives   189
  - Topics   189
  - Key Concepts   190
  - 16.1 Ethical Challenges in Organizational Leadership   190
  - 16.2 Leadership as a Philosophy   190
    - 16.2.1 Plato on Leadership   191
    - 16.2.2 Peter Drucker on Leadership   191
    - 16.2.3 John Gregory and Thomas Percival on Professional Virtues in Leadership   191
      - 16.2.3.1 The Professional Virtue of Self-Effacement   191
      - 16.2.3.2 The Professional Virtue of Self-Sacrifice   192
      - 16.2.3.3 The Professional Virtue of Compassion   192
      - 16.2.3.4 The Professional Virtue of Integrity   192
      - 16.2.3.5 The Professional Virtue of Humility   192
  - 16.3 Gregory and Percival on Organizational Culture   192
    - 16.3.1 Professional Treatment of Colleagues   192
    - 16.3.2 Professional Resource Management   193
      - 16.3.2.1 The Perils of a Utilitarian Organizational Culture   193
      - 16.3.2.2 The Perils of a Libertarian Organizational Culture   193
    - 16.3.3 Professional Use of Power   193
      - 16.3.3.1 Thomas Hobbes on Power   193
      - 16.3.3.2 Monopoly Power and Monopsony Power   193
    - 16.3.4 Organizational Dysfunction: A Progressive Disorder   194
      - 16.3.4.1 Machiavellian Organizational Culture   194
      - 16.3.4.2 A Cynical Organizational Culture   194
      - 16.3.4.3 A Wonderland Organizational Culture   194
      - 16.3.4.4 A Kafkaesque Organizational Culture   194

16.3.4.5 A Postmodern Organizational Culture 194
16.3.4.6 Common Signs of Progressive Organizational Dysfunction 195
16.4 Managing Guild Interests 195
16.4.1 Guild Interests: An Insidious Threat to a Professional Organizational Culture 195
16.4.2 Two Potentially Insidious Incentives 196
16.4.2.1 Productivity Incentives 196
16.4.2.2 Regulatory and Compliance Demands 196
16.4.3 A Powerful Antidote: An Organizational Culture that Subordinates Guild Interests to Professionalism 196
16.4.3.1 Setting Reasonable Limits on Self-Sacrifice 197
16.4.3.2 Preventing Incremental Subordination of Professionalism to Guild Self-Interest 197
16.5 Navigating the Perilous Waters of Scylla and Charybdis 197
References 198

Section 5 Professionally Responsible Innovation and Research

17 **Clinical Innovation and Research in Obstetrics and Gynecology** 201
Goal 201
Objectives 201
Topics 201
Key Concepts 202
17.1 Clinical Innovation and Research 202
17.2 Maternal–Fetal Intervention 202
17.2.1 The Role of Animal Models 203
17.2.2 Prospective Oversight of Maternal–Fetal Innovation: The Perinatal Innovation Review Committee 203
17.2.3 Prospective Oversight of Maternal–Fetal Research by the Institutional Review Board 203
17.2.4 Professionally Responsible Transition to Clinical Practice 205
17.3 The MOMS Clinical Trial: A Model for Maternal–Fetal Research 205
17.4 Minimizing Risk to the Fetal Patient of Maternal–Fetal Research for Fetal Benefit 205
17.5 The Transition into Clinical Practice 206
17.6 Ethically Justified Criteria for Maternal–Fetal Innovation and Research and for the Transition to Clinical Practice 206
17.6.1 Ethically Justified Criteria for Maternal–Fetal Innovation and Early-Phase Maternal–Fetal Clinical Research for Efficacy and Safety for Fetal Benefit 206
17.6.2 Ethically Justified Criteria for Randomized Controlled Trials for Fetal Benefit 206
17.6.3 Ethically Justified Criteria for the Professionally Responsible Transition to Clinical Practice 207
17.6.4 The Informed Consent Process 207
17.7 Research with Pregnant Patients with Mental Illnesses and Disorders 207
17.7.1 Guidance from the Council for International Organizations of Medical Societies 208
17.7.1.1 Balance of Benefits and Risks to the Pregnant Patient 208
17.7.1.2 Balance of Benefits and Risks to the Fetal Patient 208
17.7.1.3 Balance of Benefits and Risks to the Neonatal and the Pediatric Patient 209
17.7.1.4 Overall Ethical Evaluation 209
17.7.2 Ethically Justified Study Design 210
17.7.2.1 Phase of Study 210
17.7.2.2 The Informed Consent Process 210
References 212

Section 6 Professionally Responsible Health Policy and Advocacy

18 **Health Policy and Advocacy** 215
   Goal 215
   Objectives 215
   Topics 215
   Key Concepts 216
   18.1 Healthcare Justice, Health Policy, and Advocacy 216
   18.2 Advocacy: Women and Children First 217
      18.2.1 Healthcare-Justice–Based Ethical Framework 217
      18.2.2 Challenges to Justice in the Allocation of Healthcare Resources to Women and Children 218
         18.2.2.1 Challenges to Substantive Justice 218
         18.2.2.2 Challenges to Procedural Justice 220
   18.3 Antidote to Cynicism about the Ethical Principle of Healthcare Justice 221
      18.3.1 Identifying and Addressing Social Conditions that Impede Healthcare Justice 221
      18.3.2 The Impact of Climate Change on the Life and Health of Female, Pregnant, and Neonatal Patients 222
   18.4 "Women and Children First – or Last?" The New York Declaration of the International Academy of Perinatal Medicine 222
   References 223

Glossary of Key Concepts 225
Index 235

Preface

This is the first book on professional ethics in obstetrics and gynecology. Its origins, however, are in eighteenth-century Britain, where professional ethics in medicine was invented by two extraordinary physician-ethicists, John Gregory (1724–1773) of Scotland and Thomas Percival (1740–1804) of England. They invented the ethical concept of medicine as a profession, which they intended to be transcultural, transnational, and transreligious. Their goal has been realized in professional ethics in obstetrics and gynecology, as this book attests.

Chapter 1 shows that professional ethics in medicine is based on Gregory and Percival's ethical concept of medicine as a profession, marking a strong and distinctive contrast between professional ethics in medicine, on the one hand, and contemporary medical ethics and bioethics, on the other hand. Chapter 2 shows that professional ethics in obstetrics and gynecology, in turn, is based on professional ethics in medicine and the ethical concepts of the female patient, pregnant patient, fetal patient, and (in perinatal medicine) neonatal patient. These ethical concepts play an essential role in professional ethics in obstetrics and gynecology, marking another important contrast with contemporary medical ethics and bioethics.

After this historical, philosophical, and clinical introduction to professional ethics in obstetrics and gynecology, Section 1 goes on to examine three dimensions of professional ethics in obstetrics and gynecology that permeate clinical practice, organizational cultures and their leadership, clinical innovation and research, and healthcare advocacy and policy for female, pregnant, fetal, and neonatal patients: decision making by, with, and for patients; confidentiality; and management of conflicts of interest and conflicts of commitment. A unique feature of this book is its sustained exploration of professional ethics in the intersection of obstetrics and gynecology, on the one hand, and psychiatry, on the other. Chapter 3 initiates this exploration with its emphasis on a continuum of decision making by, with, and for patients – simple consent, informed consent, assisted decision making, assent, and surrogate decision making. This exploration continues in subsequent chapters.

Undergraduate medical education introduces medical students to obstetrics and gynecology as an essential component of the general education of a professional physician and also to set the stage for specialty training for medical students who elect this professional pathway. As every experienced medical educator knows, much of clinical teaching comprises teaching the basics again and again to each successive generation of learners. We have therefore included a chapter, in Section 2, on teaching the basics of professional ethics in obstetrics and gynecology. Professionalism is a core competency in graduate medical education. Chapter 6 addresses the ethical obligation of faculty to prevent drift by residents away from professionalism.

To support teaching the material in the other chapters of this book, each chapter starts with a goal and objectives, a topics list, and a list of key concepts that shape the ethical reasoning in each chapter. A comprehensive Glossary of Key Concepts, with definitions, appears at the end of the book.

The clinical practice of obstetrics and gynecology affects the entire human life cycle – from conception, pregnancy, and birth, through adolescence to adulthood, to chronic conditions and end-of-life care. Professional ethics in the clinical practice of obstetrics and gynecology is addressed in Section 3. These chapters describe ethical frameworks, based on professional ethics in obstetrics and gynecology, that provide ethically justified, clinically grounded, and practical guidance on prevention of pregnancy, initiation of pregnancy, induced abortion and feticide, fetal analysis (a new phrase used in a proposed new nomenclature), periviability, intrapartum management, the perfect baby, cancer and pregnancy, and setting ethically justified limits on clinical management of patients' conditions and diagnosis, especially at the end of the their lives.

Gregory and Percival added to their history-of-medicine-changing creation of the ethical concept of medicine as a profession the profound insight that the commitment to this ethical concept by obstetrician-gynecologists and other physicians does not succeed in isolation. Organizational cultures have become essential for obstetrician-gynecologists to make and sustain their commitment to the ethical concept of medicine over a lifetime of clinical practice. Professionally responsible leadership by obstetrician-gynecologists in healthcare organizations has therefore become an essential dimension of professional ethics in obstetrics and gynecology and is addressed in Section 4.

Section 5 addresses professionally responsible clinical innovation and research, which play an indispensable role in improving the quality and safety of patient care in maternal–fetal intervention for maternal or fetal benefit. Professional ethics in obstetrics provides the basis for an ethical framework to guide clinical innovation and research on maternal–fetal interventions for fetal or maternal benefit. The ethical concept of the fetus as a patient constitutes a unique component of this ethical framework, adding to it a set of ethical and clinical considerations not found in US federal human subjects research regulations or elsewhere. This ethical framework is deployed to address the ethical challenges of clinical innovation and research for fetal and maternal benefit in the case of pregnant women with mental illnesses and disorders.

The ethical principle of healthcare justice expands the scope of professional ethics in obstetrics and gynecology to include the clinical needs of populations of female, pregnant, fetal, and neonatal patients. This ethical principle requires that allocation of resources be guided by the ethical obligation created by the ethical principle of healthcare justice in professional ethics in obstetrics and gynecology: to see to it that all female, pregnant, fetal, and neonatal patients have access to and receive medically reasonable clinical management of their conditions and diagnoses. Health policy and advocacy for "Women and Children First" is addressed in Section 6.

To aid readers – and teachers – of this book, we have provided multiple points of access to its content. The topics lists in the Contents and at the beginning of each chapter guide the reader to text that he or she might need to responsibly manage, or teach, a specific topic in professional ethics in obstetrics and gynecology. To ensure that each topic and subtopic is self-sufficient for the reader's or teacher's purposes, there is deliberate repetition within and across chapters. Our goal in taking this approach has been to minimize the need for the reader, teacher, or learner to flip back and forth among topics and subtopics. The Glossary of Key Concepts at the end of the book contains all key concepts from the chapters and succinct definitions, creating a unique resource for progressing to mastery of the conceptual vocabulary of professional ethics in obstetrics and gynecology. The content of the book can also be accessed from the the comprehensive Index that appears after the Glossary of Key Concepts at the end of the book.

Two of us (LBM and FAC) have collaborated on professional ethics in obstetrics and gynecology for 36 years. Dr. Coverdale joined this collaboration 30 years ago, bringing a sustained focus on the intersection of obstetrics, gynecology, and psychiatry. We collaboratively developed the ethical reasoning that we then presented in our scholarship (portions of which have been included or adapted in 11 of the chapters that follow and as documented in the Acknowledgments section). This scholarship became the basis for our clinical teaching of medical students, residents, fellows, and clinical colleagues, and the results of this teaching were fed back into our scholarship. We set our results before readers, teachers, and learners in the chapters that follow.

Without the commitment of our learners to professional ethics in obstetrics and gynecology, we could not have created and benefited from this wonderful synergy of clinical teaching and scholarship. Without the commitment of our learners to professional ethics in obstetrics and gynecology, this book would not exist. In response to their intellectual generosity, we dedicate this book to our patients and learners who, in the ancient tradition of medical education, became our teachers. We are also indebted – beyond what words can express – to our mentors, *sine quibus non*.

Acknowledgments

Parts of the following chapters include or adapt portions of the listed articles with permission:

Chapter 5: Conflicts of Interest and Conflicts of Commitment
Chervenak FA, McCullough LB. The ethics of direct and indirect referral for termination of pregnancy. Am J Obstet Gynecol 2008; 199: 232.e1–3.

Chervenak FA, McCullough LB, Coverdale JH. Ethically justified guidelines for defining sexual boundaries between obstetrician-gynecologists and their patients. Am J Obstet Gynecol 1996; 175: 496–500.

Chapter 6: Teaching Professional Ethics in Obstetrics and Gynecology
Chervenak FA, McCullough LB, Grünebaum A. Preventing incremental drift away from professionalism in graduate medical education. Am J Obstet Gynecol 2018; 219: 589.e1–589.e3.

McCullough LB, Coverdale JH, Chervenak FA. Argument-based ethics: a formal tool for critically appraising the normative medical ethics literature. Am J Obstet Gynecol 2004; 191: 1097–1102.

Chapter 9: Induced Abortion and Feticide
Chervenak FA, McCullough LB. An ethically justified practical approach to offering, recommending, performing, and referring for induced abortion and feticide. Am J Obstet Gynecol. 2009; 201: 560.e1–6.

Coverdale J, Chervenak FA, McCullough LB, Bayer T. Ethically justified clinically comprehensive guidelines for the management of the depressed pregnant patient. Am J Obstet Gynecol 1996; 174: 169–173.

McCullough LB, Coverdale J, Chervenak FA. Ethical challenges of decision making with pregnant patients who have schizophrenia. Am J Obstet Gynecol 2002; 187: 696–702.

Chapter 10: Fetal Analysis
Chervenak FA, McCullough LB, Dudenhausen J. Fetal analysis with invasive method (FA-I) and fetal analysis with non-invasive method (FA-NI): replacing current, deceptively imprecise clinical nomenclature. J Perinat Med 2017; 45: 985–987.

Chervenak FA, McCullough LB, Sharma G, Davis J, Gross G. Enhancing patient autonomy with risk assessment and invasive diagnosis: an ethical solution to a clinical challenge. Am J Obstet Gynecol 2008; 199: 19.e1–19.e4.

Chapter 12: Intrapartum Management
Babbitt KE, Bailey KJ, Coverdale JH, Chervenak FA, McCullough LB. Professionally responsible intrapartum management of patients with major mental disorders. Am J Obstet Gynecol 2014; 210: 27–31.

Chervenak FA, McCullough LB. Ethical dimensions of fetal neurology. Semin Fetal Neonatal Med 2012; 17: 252–255.

Chervenak FA, McCullough LB. Preventive ethics for cesarean delivery: the time has come. Am J Obstet Gynecol 2013; 209: 166–167.

Coverdale J, Chervenak FA, McCullough LB, Bayer T. Ethically justified clinically comprehensive guidelines for the management of the depressed pregnant patient. Am J Obstet Gynecol 1996; 174: 169–173.

Grünebaum A, McCullough LB, Arabin B, Chervenak FA. Critical appraisal of defenses of planned home birth. Am J Obstet Gynecol 2019; 22: 30–34.

McCullough LB, Coverdale J, Chervenak FA. Ethical challenges of decision making with pregnant patients who have schizophrenia. Am J Obstet Gynecol 2002; 187: 696–702.

Acknowledgments

Chapter 13: The Perfect Baby
Chervenak FA, McCullough LB, Brent RL. The perils of the imperfect expectation of the perfect baby. Am J Obstet Gynecol 2010; 203: 101.e1–101.e5.

Chapter 14: Cancer and Pregnancy
Chervenak FA, McCullough LB, Knapp RC, Caputo TA, Barber HRK. A clinically comprehensive ethical framework for offering and recommending cancer treatment before and during pregnancy. Cancer 2004: 100; 215–222.

Chapter 15: Setting Ethically Justified Limits on Life-Sustaining Treatment
Chervenak FA, McCullough LB, Arabin B. Why the Groningen Protocol should be rejected. Hastings Cent Rep 2006; 36: 30–33.

Chapter 16: Leadership
Chervenak FA, McCullough LB. Responsibly managing the medical school – teaching hospital relationship. Acad Med 2005; 80: 690–693.

Chervenak FA, McCullough LB. The diagnosis and management of progressive dysfunction of healthcare organizations. Obstet Gynecol 2005; 105: 882–887.

Chervenak FA, McCullough LB, Brent RL. The professional responsibility model of physician leadership. Am J Obstet Gynecol 2013; 208: 97–101.

Chervenak FA, McCullough LB, Hale RW. Guild interests: an insidious threat to professionalism in obstetrics and gynecology. Am J Obstet Gynecol 2018; 219: 581–584.

Chapter 17: Clinical Innovation and Research in Obstetrics and Gynecology
Chervenak FA, McCullough LB. An ethically justified framework for clinical investigation to benefit pregnant and fetal patients. Am J Bioeth 2011; 11: 39–49.

McCullough LB, Coverdale JH, Chervenak FA. Is pharmacologic research on pregnant women with psychoses ethically permissible? J Perinat Med 2015; 43: 439–444.

Chapter 18: Health Policy and Advocacy
Chervenak FA, McCullough LB. "Women and Children First:" Transforming an historic defining moment into a contemporary ethical imperative. Am J Obstet Gynecol 2009; 201: 351.e1–5.

The text of "Women and Children First or Last?" of the International Academy of Perinatal Medicine is included in its entirety in Chapter 18 and is used with permission

Chervenak FA, McCullough LB, and the International Academy of Perinatal Medicine. Women and children first or last? The New York Declaration. Am J Obstet Gynecol 2009; 201: 335. Available at www.ajog.org/article/S0002-9378(09)00772-8/pdf (accessed March 1, 2019).

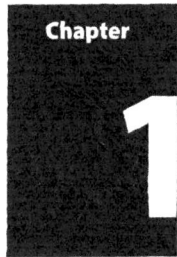

Section 1 Professional Ethics in Obstetrics and Gynecology

Chapter 1

Professional Ethics in Medicine

GOAL
This chapter provides a historical and philosophical introduction to professional ethics in medicine, based on the ethical concept of medicine as a profession.

OBJECTIVES
On completing study of this chapter, the reader will:

Define ethics, medical ethics, bioethics

Define professional ethics in medicine

Describe the two components of ethical reasoning

Identify the discipline of ethical reasoning

Describe the ethical concept of medicine as a profession

Describe the five professional virtues of professional ethics in medicine

Describe the four ethical principles of professional ethics in medicine

Describe the advantages of professional ethics in medicine

Answer the question: Why should physicians commit to the ethical concept of medicine as a profession?

TOPICS

1.1	Professional Ethics in Medicine and Professional Ethics in Obstetrics and Gynecology	3
1.2	Ethics and Ethical Reasoning	3
	1.2.1 Ethics	3
	1.2.2 Ethical Reasoning	4
	1.2.2.1 Clinical Judgment	4
	1.2.2.2 Ethical Judgment	4
	1.2.2.3 Two Components of Ethical Reasoning	4
	1.2.2.4 Preventing Common Errors in Ethical Reasoning	5
	1.2.3 The Discipline of Ethical Reasoning	6
	1.2.4 Critical Appraisal of Argument-Based Ethical Reasoning	6
	1.2.5 Two Approaches to Ethical Reasoning: The Quest for Certainty and the Quest for Reliability	6
	1.2.5.1 The Quest for Certainty	7
	1.2.5.2 The Quest for Reliability	7
	1.2.5.3 Professional Ethics in Medicine Is the Quest for Reliability	7
1.3	Medical Ethics and Bioethics	7
	1.3.1 Medical Ethics	7
	1.3.1.1 Philosophical Medical Ethics	7

Section 1: Professional Ethics in Obstetrics and Gynecology

        1.3.1.2 Limitations of Medical Ethics   8
    1.3.2 Bioethics   8
        1.3.2.1 Limitations of Bioethics   9
1.4 Ethical Principles and Virtues in Medical Ethics and Bioethics   9
    1.4.1 The Four Ethical Principles in Medical Ethics and Bioethics   9
        1.4.1.1 The Ethical Principle of Beneficence in Medical Ethics and Bioethics   9
        1.4.1.2 The Ethical Principle of Nonmaleficence in Medical Ethics and Bioethics   10
        1.4.1.3 Beneficence and Nonmaleficence in the History of Medical Ethics   10
        1.4.1.4 The Ethical Principle of Respect for Autonomy in Medical Ethics and Bioethics   10
        1.4.1.5 The Ethical Principle of Justice in Medical Ethics and Bioethics   10
        1.4.1.6 Putting Ethical Principles into Practice   11
1.5 Professional Ethics in Medicine   11
    1.5.1 The Invention of Professional Ethics in Medicine   11
        1.5.1.1 Hippocratic Medical Ethics   11
        1.5.1.2 Friedrich Hoffmann on the Politic Physician   12
        1.5.1.3 John Gregory and Thomas Percival on Professional Ethics in Medicine   13
        1.5.1.4 Gregory's Professional Ethics in Medicine   13
        1.5.1.5 Percival's Professional Ethics in Medicine   14
        1.5.1.6 The Ethical Concept of Medicine as a Profession   14
1.6 Professional Virtues and Ethical Principles in Professional Ethics in Medicine   15
    1.6.1 The Five Professional Virtues   15
        1.6.1.1 The Professional Virtue of Integrity   15
        1.6.1.2 The Professional Virtue of Humility   16
        1.6.1.3 The Professional Virtue of Compassion   16
        1.6.1.4 The Professional Virtue of Self-Effacement   16
        1.6.1.5 The Professional Virtue of Self-Sacrifice   17
    1.6.2 The Four Ethical Principles in Professional Ethics in Medicine   17
        1.6.2.1 The Ethical Principle of Beneficence in Professional Ethics in Medicine   17
        1.6.2.2 The Concept of a Medically Reasonable Alternative   17
        1.6.2.3 The Ethical Principle of Nonmaleficence in Professional Ethics in Medicine   18
        1.6.2.4 The Ethical Principle of Respect for Autonomy in Professional Ethics in Medicine   18
        1.6.2.5 The Ethical Principle of Healthcare Justice in Professional Ethics in Medicine   18
1.7 Advantages of Professional Ethics in Medicine   19
1.8 Why Should Physicians Commit to the Ethical Concept of Medicine as a Profession?   19

Key Concepts

Absolute ethical obligation
Absolute ethical principle
Argument-based ethical reasoning
Beneficence-based clinical judgment
Bioethics
Biopsychosocial concept of health and disease
Common morality
Conflict of commitment
Conflict of interest
Consequentialism
Deliberative clinical judgment
Discipline of ethical reasoning
Distress
Enthusiasm
Ethical analysis
Ethical argument
Ethical concept of medicine as a profession
Ethical judgment

Ethical obligation
Ethical principle
Ethical principle of beneficence in medical ethics and bioethics
Ethical principle of beneficence in professional ethics in medicine
Ethical principle of healthcare justice in professional ethics in medicine
Ethical principle of justice in medical ethics and bioethics
Ethical principle of nonmaleficence in medical ethics and bioethics
Ethical principle of nonmaleficence in professional ethics in medicine
Ethical principle of respect for autonomy in medical ethics and bioethics
Ethical principle of respect for autonomy in professional ethics in medicine
Ethical reasoning
Ethically impermissible
Ethically ideal
Ethically obligatory
Ethically permissible
Ethics
"First do no harm"
Harm principle
Judgment
Medical ethics
Medically reasonable alternative
Moral science
Moral philosophy
Moral theology
Morality
Morally ideal
Morally impermissible
Morally obligatory
Morally permissible
Organizational culture
Pain
Patient
Prima facie ethical obligation
Prima facie ethical principle
Professional ethics in medicine
Professional virtue of compassion
Professional virtue of humility
Professional virtue of integrity
Professional virtue of self-effacement
Professional virtue of self-sacrifice
Public trust
Quest for certainty
Quest for reliability
Secular ethical reasoning
Specification
Speculation
Suffering
Virtues
Voluntary

1.1 Professional Ethics in Medicine and Professional Ethics in Obstetrics and Gynecology

In this book we provide an historical, philosophical, clinically comprehensive, and practical account of professional ethics in obstetrics and gynecology. The goal of professional ethics in obstetrics and gynecology is to identify what is ethically permissible, ethically obligatory, ethically impermissible, and ethically ideal in patient care, clinical innovation and research, organizational culture, and health policy and advocacy concerning female, pregnant, and fetal patients.

In this book we understand professional ethics in obstetrics and gynecology to be a subfield of professional ethics in medicine. We therefore begin with an account of professional ethics in medicine in this chapter and then adapt this account to obstetrics and gynecology in Chapter 2. In this chapter we distinguish professional ethics in medicine from medical ethics and from bioethics and then set out the commitment to the ethical concept of medicine as a profession, which serves as the basis of professional ethics in medicine. To set the stage for these two explanatory tasks, we begin by introducing the reader to ethics and ethical reasoning.

1.2 Ethics and Ethical Reasoning

Diagnostic and prognostic reasoning both require precision of thought and speech so that each team member's thinking can be reliably communicated to other team members. The safety and quality of patient care depend on precision of thought and speech, because errors in communication pose preventable threats to patient safety and quality. For example, the patient's feet are inferior to the patient's pelvis, even when the patient in the operating room is in the Trendelenburg position. The patient's sternum is anterior to the patient's heart, even when the patient is face down on an examination table.

1.2.1 Ethics

Ethics is an essential component of patient care, clinical innovation and research, organizational culture, and health policy advocacy. Ethics deploys concepts – ethical principles and virtues – that have a precise meaning, making effective identification and professionally responsible management of ethical challenges possible. Indeed, "ethics" itself has a precise meaning and so we begin with an account of ethics and ethical reasoning.

Ethics is the disciplined study of morality with the goal of incrementally improving it, based on reasoned ethical judgments. *Morality* comprises our actual beliefs about behavior and character that are morally impermissible, morally permissible, morally obligatory, and morally ideal. *Morally impermissible* means that a form of behavior or character should not occur, e.g., sexual abuse of patients. *Morally permissible* means that a form of behavior may occur in circumstances in which there are multiple forms of behavior or character supported by ethical reasoning, e.g., waiving professional fees when volunteering in an international medical mission. *Morally obligatory* means that a form of behavior or character should occur, e.g., leading a professionally responsible informed consent process for hysterectomy with an adult patient with intact decision-making capacity. *Morally ideal* behavior invokes perfectionism: always striving for a perfect and therefore highly valued outcome even while knowing that one may fall short, e.g., providing adequate emergency management in the field in response to a mass-casualty event.[1,2] Morally ideal also means that it is morally obligatory to make incremental progress toward the highly valued outcome.

Morality is formed from multiple sources, including family, geography, group, history, law, personal opinion, philosophy, religion, and tribe. Morality is thus pluralistic, which can become a source of conflict about what is morally impermissible, morally permissible, morally obligatory, and morally ideal.

1.2.2 Ethical Reasoning

1.2.2.1 Clinical Judgment

Judgment is the process of reliably classifying an entity by applying clear and justified criteria. When these criteria are idiosyncratic, a judgment has value only for the individual who has formed it. When these criteria are authoritative – drawn from a source that others should acknowledge as important and applicable – a judgment has value both for the individual who formed it and for others.

Consider clinical judgment, which begins with the facts of the matter: signs; symptoms; and the results of history and physical examination, laboratory analysis, and imaging. Evidence-based causal explanations are then formed to explain these results in terms of pathology: abnormal anatomy, or pathophysiology. These explanations are then arrayed by probability in a differential diagnosis based on biopsychosocial criteria for normal and pathological anatomy and physiology. This process results in clinical diagnosis, prognosis, and plan of care, all of which vary directly in reliability by strength of evidence for them. The reliability of clinical judgment is a function of being deliberative: evidence-based (an appeal to the best available, critically appraised evidence), rigorous (especially in the effort to identify and reduce the influence of bias), transparent (the physician can explain his or her judgment to other clinicians, especially team members, and the patient), and accountable (to meet accepted standards of patient safety and quality). Even when evidence is lacking, the other components of deliberative clinical judgment can and therefore should be satisfied. The common response that "there isn't evidence for everything" does not apply to deliberative clinical judgment.

Deliberative clinical judgment is intellectually authoritative for physicians and other clinicians and therefore for patients. Patients should take seriously deliberative clinical judgment about their condition and its clinical management in their subsequent decision-making process with their physicians. The intellectual authority of deliberative clinical judgment has the potential to influence the patient's decision-making process. It is a mistake, however, to conclude that this intellectual authority controls her decision making.

1.2.2.2 Ethical Judgment

Ethical judgments about what is ethically permissible, obligatory, impermissible, and ideal are analogous. Authoritative ethical judgments are reasoned judgments. Reasoned ethical judgments result from an intellectually rigorous process that always starts with the facts of the matter, to avoid *enthusiasm* (beliefs that lack an evidence base) and *speculation* (beliefs that do not pass muster even as plausible hypotheses). Reasoned ethical judgments apply clear criteria to classify character, behavior, organizational culture, and health policy and advocacy as ethically permissible, ethically obligatory, ethically impermissible, and ethically ideal.

1.2.2.3 Two Components of Ethical Reasoning

Criteria must be relevant to the facts of the matter and must also be justified, i.e., supported by reasons that appeal clearly expressed ethical concepts: principles and virtues. This is known as *ethical analysis*. The implications of these clearly expressed concepts must then be precisely identified and shown to follow from the clearly expressed concepts. This is known as *ethical argument*. The result of this intellectually rigorous, practical process is reliable classification of behavior, character traits, organizational culture, or health policy and advocacy as ethically permissible, obligatory, impermissible, or ideal. This classification varies in reliability directly by the strength of the basis of the criteria in ethical principles and virtues and the rigor of the application of such criteria to the facts of the matter.

Ethically impermissible means that a form of behavior, character, organizational culture, or health policy and advocacy should not occur. *Ethically permissible* means that a form of behavior, character, organizational culture, or health policy and advocacy may occur in circumstances in which there are multiple forms of behavior, character, organizational culture, or health policy and advocacy supported by ethical reasoning. *Ethically obligatory* means that a form of behavior, character, organizational culture, or health policy and advocacy should occur. *Ethically ideal* behavior invokes perfectionism: always striving for a perfect outcome even while knowing that one may fall short. Health policy is sometimes expressed as an ideal, e.g., the goal of providing every patient with a source of payment, such as universal health insurance.

1.2.2.4 Preventing Common Errors in Ethical Reasoning

Clinical judgment aims to improve patient care by preventing common errors in clinical reasoning and its communication. So too, ethical judgments aim to improve morality, by preventing errors in ethical reasoning and its communication. (See Table 1.1.) Common errors in ethical reasoning include (1) starting with conclusions about what is ethically permissible, obligatory, impermissible, or ideal and then searching for friendly reasons, i.e., ethical concepts and their implications (or, more technically, premises), which gets ethical reasoning backwards; (2) mere opinion, which is the assertion of a conclusion without any effort to identify relevant premises; (3) appeal to majority opinion, which is always at high and unmanageable risk of biases of various kinds, including biases of which those in the majority may be unaware; (4) appeal to one's position of power in an organizational hierarchy, which establishes only that one has and may exercise such power but does not establish how one *ought* to do so; (5) equating legal judgment about what is impermissible, permissible, obligatory in the law with what is impermissible, permissible, obligatory in the professional ethics of medicine and of obstetrics and gynecology; (6) intuitions or initial, untested judgments that must be examined critically before they become eligible for being authoritative;[3,4] (7) making the most noise or otherwise being good at gaining the attention of others, which is not a form of reasoning at all; (8) speculation, i.e., making up hypothetical clinical situations (also known as "thought experiments") that have little or no bearing on clinical reality, e.g., exploring the ethics of genetic manipulation in patients on the assumption that such intervention is clinically safe;[5] and (9) not situating argument in context of other arguments, i.e., failing to identify and respond to already existing ethical reasoning on a topic, especially those that differ from one's own ethical reasoning.

Table 1.1 Errors in ethical reasoning.

Name of error	Error made
Starting with conclusions and searching for friendly reasons	Gets ethical reasoning backward, because ethical reasoning starts with reasons to reach conclusions
Mere opinion	Asserts a conclusion with no supporting reasons
Appeals to majority opinion	No prevention of bias in reasons and conclusion
Appeal to power	Replaces authority of reasoning with organizational authority
Equating legal judgment with ethical reasoning	Accepts legal reasoning with no critical appraisal from the perspective of professional ethics in medicine
Appeal to intuitions	Accepts initial judgment without critical appraisal from the perspective of professional ethics in medicine
Making the most noise	Gaining attention of others without the support of ethical reasoning
Speculation	Making up examples that lack clinical application
Not situating argument in context of other arguments	Failing to identify and respond to already ethical reasoning on a topic, especially those that differ from one's own ethical reasoning.

1.2.3 The Discipline of Ethical Reasoning

One achieves the discipline of ethical reasoning by always and only making judgments that result from ethical analysis and argument. More colloquially, one achieves the discipline of ethical reasoning by going where ethical analysis and argument take one and nowhere else. This is also known as argument-based reasoning.[6] (See Chapter 6.) If the ethical judgment that results from ethical reasoning is considered unacceptable, one must (1) critically appraise the ethical reasoning by identifying and correcting errors of ethical analysis and argument and (2) produce an alternative, well-reasoned ethical judgment. If critical appraisal does not result in an alternative ethical judgment, one must consider oneself intellectually prohibited from dismissing the initial ethical judgment as unacceptable. One must therefore change one's mind by adopting the initial judgment.

If one does not submit to the intellectual discipline of ethical reasoning, one should not expect to be taken seriously by those committed to professional ethics in medicine and therefore to professional ethics in obstetrics and gynecology. Instead, one should expect to be challenged and then supported by those committed to the discipline of ethical reasoning to achieve well-reasoned ethical judgments. One should not take such a response personally, but professionally, by recommitting to the discipline of ethical reasoning.

1.2.4 Critical Appraisal of Argument-Based Ethical Reasoning

Argument-based ethical reasoning can be critically appraised for its clinical utility in managing ethically challenging cases, just as evidence-based clinical judgment and practice can be appraised. The critical appraisal of evidence-based clinical reasoning is systematic and disciplined; so too for argument-based ethical reasoning. Critical appraisal is an essential component of the discipline of ethical reasoning and has four steps.

1. Does the article address a focused ethics question?
2. Are the arguments that support the results of the article valid?
3. What are the results?
4. Will the results help me in clinical practice?[6]

Like all clinically applicable literature, a paper in the professional ethics of obstetrics and gynecology should have a focused clinical ethical question, for example: How should a gynecologist respond when a premenopausal patient who has no symptoms or pathology requests a hysterectomy to prevent future pregnancies? The validity of ethical argument has three components. First, as explained in Section 1.2.2.3, ethical analysis should produce concepts that are clearly stated. Second, ethical argument is deployed to identify the implications of these clearly expressed concepts. Third, ethical analysis and argument should be grounded in a review of the pertinent literature, to catalog concepts that are clinically pertinent and how they have been clearly or unclearly expressed. Ideally, this should be a structured review with the search terms and databases specified. We should note, however, that many papers in normative ethics lag behind the standards of the evidence-based literature. The results should be expressed in a way that is clinically applicable. Results should be considered helpful when they provide clear guidance to clinical decision making and behavior based on it. Finally, articles that are identified in a structured review can be scored for their answers to these four questions.[7]

There is a continuum in professional ethics in obstetrics and gynecology literature from opinion without supporting argument to rigorous work based on rigorous ethical analysis and argument. Using the preceding four questions as a critical appraisal tool will equip the reader to distinguish the quality of ethical reasoning along this continuum. The lower the score assigned to a paper, the greater is the potential for bias and the need to take recommendations with a jaundiced eye. (See Chapter 6 for teaching critical appraisal of argument-based ethical reasoning.)

1.2.5 Two Approaches to Ethical Reasoning: The Quest for Certainty and the Quest for Reliability

In the history of Western philosophical ethics (also known as moral philosophy) there are two main approaches to ethical reasoning. Diego Gracia has characterized these as the *Quest for Certainty* and the *Quest for Reliability*.[8]

1.2.5.1 The Quest for Certainty

The quest for certainty assumes that the moral life requires certainty of ethical judgment deriving from foundations that are beyond doubt. This approach originates in the philosophy of Plato (ca. 427–ca. 347 BCE), with its appeal to unchanging, eternal "forms" as the basis of all knowledge. The quest for certainty is also known as foundationalism, typified by the appeal to Reason in the moral philosophy of Immanuel Kant (1724–1804) and its famous categorical imperative to treat all persons as ends in themselves and never as merely means. This categorical imperative can be denied only by embracing irrationality.[8]

1.2.5.2 The Quest for Reliability

The quest for reliability, in strong contrast, aims for ethical judgments that we can act on with confidence that we have good reasons, which always remain open to revision and improvement. The quest for reliability requires a commitment to the virtue of humility, which is a corollary of the professional virtue of integrity. The quest for reliability originates in the moral philosophy of Aristotle (384–322 BCE), who, it should be noted, was also a physician and scientist and thus already comfortable with judgments characterized by reliability and not certainty.

This approach continued in the work of the eighteenth-century Scottish moral sense theorists, such as David Hume (1711–1776)[9] and the American pragmatist William James (1842–1910)[10]. Hume took himself to be doing moral science and reporting his primary discovery, the principle of sympathy. Sympathy is a constitutive, causal process in human moral physiology (seated in the heart) that naturally inclines us, as a matter of habit, to enter into the lived experience of others and thereby become motivated to protect and promote their interests as our primary concern and motivation.[9] In the early twentieth century, a philosophy of reliability known as pragmatism emerged, pioneered by James,[10] which appeals to shared commitments to what ought to be valued as the basis of ethical judgment.[8] These commitments create their truth in our lives and the lives of others. For example, it is true that the United States is a secular, democratic republic provided that enough people in the United States commit to the rule of law grounded in the United States Constitution.

1.2.5.3 Professional Ethics in Medicine Is the Quest for Reliability

Clinical judgment is a quest, not for certainty, but for reliability of clinical judgments about the condition of the patient and its professionally responsible clinical management. Ethical reasoning should reflect the context in which it is deployed, as Aristotle teaches in his *Nicomachean Ethics*.[11] We will therefore understand professional ethics in medicine and in obstetrics and gynecology as the quest for reliability, not the quest for certainty.

1.3 Medical Ethics and Bioethics

The discourse of professional ethics in medicine is often equated with the discourse of medical ethics or the discourse of bioethics. In this book we emphasize the differences between professional ethics in medicine and medical ethics and bioethics. (See Table 1.2.)

1.3.1 Medical Ethics

Medical ethics is the disciplined study of the morality of physicians and patients, clinical innovation and research, and health policy and advocacy, with the aim of improving medical morality. A major source for medical ethics, in its millennia-long history, is moral theology, because religions give meaning to the life cycle, for the stages of which physicians are often present. Other sources include family, geography, group, history, law, personal opinion, philosophy, religion, and tribe. Medical ethics is a global tradition of inquiry found in all cultures and regions, dating from Before the Common Era (BCE), based on the sacred texts of Judaism, Buddhism, and Hinduism and philosophical texts such as those of Confucius (551–479 BCE) and Plato.[12]

From its ancient origins medical ethics has been pluralistic, drawing on diverse and potentially incompatible sources to guide physicians, patients, and communities in matters of clinical practice and, starting as early as the eighteenth century, research. In the long history of medical ethics no single approach has arisen with the intellectual authority to transcend this pluralism. As a result, medical ethics is neither transreligious, nor transcultural, nor transnational.

1.3.1.1 Philosophical Medical Ethics

A potential exception should be noted: Philosophical medical ethics claims to be transreligious, transcultural, and transnational. This claim has initial plausibility,

Table 1.2 Medical ethics, philosophical medical ethics, bioethics, and professional ethics in medicine.

	Medical ethics	Philosophical medical ethics	Bioethics	Professional ethics in medicine
Transreligious	No	Yes	No	Yes
Transcultural	No	No	No	Yes
Transnational	No	No	No	Yes

because philosophical discourse is secular in that it makes no appeal to sources of divine or transcendent, cultural, or political origin. Philosophical medical ethics thus reliably claims to be transreligious. However, the claim of philosophical medical ethics to be transcultural and transnational is suspect, because there are profound and irresolvable methodological differences in world philosophy.

Consider a distinct contrast. Western moral philosophy endorses the "moral point of view" in which each individual counts for one and no more than one in ethical reasoning, which is a way of expressing the concept of equality. The moral point of view is highly abstract and is therefore not based on human relationships. Confucianism rejects this approach, making the relationship between the obedient child and his parents central, in which family counts for more than one. This is known as "filial piety." One has ethical obligations to everyone to benefit them but one's obligations to one's family always take precedence. This relationship-based approach rejects an appeal to the moral point of view and its highly abstract concept of equality.

There are also major differences within contemporary Western medical ethics. For example, the concept of solidarity (we are all in this together and should come to each other's aid) plays a central role in European medical ethics. Solidarity can be understood as a powerful response to the physical, natural, moral, and human catastrophe of World War II: solidarity can prevent recurrence of such catastrophe. Solidarity, at best, plays but a peripheral role in American medical ethics. The United States had a very different experience of World War II, from which it emerged with comparatively very limited physical, natural, and human cost. American individualism, many believed, had triumphed. It should come as no surprise that respect for individual autonomy is *a* central ethical concept (for those who quest for reliability) or *the* central ethical concept (for those who quest for certainty) in American bioethics.

No single approach has emerged in the long history of global philosophical ethics that successfully transcends these profound philosophical differences. Thus, while the claim that philosophical medical ethics is transreligious holds up well, the claim to be both transcultural and transnational does not withstand close scrutiny.

1.3.1.2 Limitations of Medical Ethics

The discourses of medical ethics are thus limited. This limitation has implications for the successful deployment of medical ethics, which should occur in four steps: (1) specifying the disciplinary source(s) invoked, followed by ethical analysis and ethical argument as used in that discipline; (2) identifying whether the quest is for certainty or reliability; (3) identifying the implications for what is ethically permissible, obligatory, impermissible, and ideal for physicians and patients in clinical practice, clinical innovation and research, organizational culture, and health policy and advocacy; and (4) acknowledging the religious, cultural, and national limits of resulting ethical judgments in a pluralistic society and pluralistic world.

1.3.2 Bioethics

Bioethics is the disciplined study of the morality of healthcare professionals, patients, healthcare organizations, innovation, biomedical and clinical research, healthcare policy, and advocacy with the aim of improving bioethical morality. Since its origins in the later 1960s and early 1970s (some claim the United States as the country of origin,[13] others the United Kingdom[14]), bioethics has become a global field of inquiry.[15] The result is a multidisciplinary field of inquiry, the sources of which include allied health professions, law, literature, medicine, moral theology, narrative studies, nursing, philosophy, policy studies, qualitative and quantitative social sciences, and religious studies (a secular discipline).[16]

In the United States the field of bioethics was first created by physicians (who were sophisticated students of moral theology and moral philosophy), moral theologians, religious studies scholars, legal scholars, and moral philosophers. With a handful of exceptions, the humanities and legal scholars specialized in traditional areas of their disciplines; specialization in bioethics came later.[13] Bioethics is now robustly multidisciplinary.

1.3.2.1 Limitations of Bioethics

The distinctive strength of bioethics is that it is a remarkably pluralistic field. This strength is also a limitation. Like medical ethics – and for the very reasons described in Section 1.3.1 – bioethics is neither transreligious, nor transcultural, nor transnational. This limitation has implications for the successful deployment of bioethics, which should occur in four steps: (1) specifying the disciplinary source(s) invoked, followed by ethical analysis and ethical argument as used in that discipline; (2) identifying whether the quest is for certainty or reliability; (3) identifying the implications for healthcare professionals and patients, healthcare organizations, and health policy and advocacy for what is ethically permissible, obligatory, impermissible, and ideal in clinical practice, clinical innovation and, organizational culture, and healthcare policy; and (4) acknowledging the religious, cultural, and national limits of resulting ethical judgments in a pluralistic society and pluralistic world.

1.4 Ethical Principles and Virtues in Medical Ethics and Bioethics

The ethical concepts deployed in both medical ethics and bioethics are known as ethical principles, sometimes deployed alone and sometimes in conjunction with virtues. Ethical principles function as guides to ethical judgment and behavior based on it. Ethical principles can be absolute, i.e., not subject to justified limits. A pacifist, for example, may adopt an exceptionless respect for human life and therefore judge all forms of killing human beings to be ethically impermissible, even in self-defense. Ethical principles can also be limited: they guide ethical judgment and behavior unless in ethical reasoning they are shown to be overridden by another ethical principle or virtue. Limited ethical principles are known as prima facie ethical principles.[17] For example, in Roman Catholic moral theology there is an ethical obligation not to kill human beings as prima facie: induced abortion and capital punishment are ethically impermissible but killing in self-defense and in war that meets the criteria for being a just war are ethically permissible.

In the quest for certainty in ethical reasoning, ethical principles are typically classified as absolute. In the quest for reliability in ethical reasoning, ethical principles are always classified as prima facie. In this book, ethical reasoning in professional ethics of medicine and of obstetrics and gynecology appeals to prima facie ethical principles, as explained in the text that follows and in Chapter 2.

Virtues are traits of character that are judged to be worth cultivating because they also guide ethical judgment and behavior based on it. The pluralism of methods in medical ethics and bioethics is especially evident in the wide range of virtues to which various forms of medical ethics and bioethics appeal, including caring, compassion, discernment, trustworthiness, integrity, and conscientiousness.[17, pp. 34–44] There is, however, no agreement in medical ethics or bioethics on the relevant virtues. In the professional ethics of medicine and of obstetrics and gynecology, as explained in Section 1.5, the core *professional virtues* comprise integrity, humility, compassion, self-effacement, and self-sacrifice, as we will explain later in this chapter. Virtues play little or no role in the quest for certainty in ethical reasoning. In striking contrast, virtues are essential in the quest for reliability in ethical reasoning and therefore for professional ethics in medicine generally and professional ethics in obstetrics and gynecology specifically.

1.4.1 The Four Ethical Principles in Medical Ethics and Bioethics

1.4.1.1 The Ethical Principle of Beneficence in Medical Ethics and Bioethics

In moral philosophy, ethical principles tend to be expressed in general, often highly abstract terms. The ethical principle of beneficence in medical ethics and bioethics generates the prima facie ethical obligation to act in a way that results in a net balance of good over harmful consequences for those affected by one's behavior. In the technical discourse of moral philosophy, beneficence is a consequentialist principle.[17] Beauchamp and Childress, coauthors of one of the most important and influential books on bioethics, put it concisely: "The principle of beneficence refers to a statement of moral obligation to act for the benefit of others."[17, p. 203] "Good" and "harmful" are explicated in diverse ways, depending on the variant of philosophical consequentialism from which these concepts are drawn.

1.4.1.2 The Ethical Principle of Nonmaleficence in Medical Ethics and Bioethics

The ethical principle of nonmaleficence in medical ethics and bioethics generates the prima facie ethical obligation to act in a way that prevents or does not cause a net balance of harmful over good consequences for those affected by one's behavior. Beauchamp and Childress again put it concisely: "One ought not to inflict evil or harm."[17, p. 151] "Harm" is explicated in diverse ways, depending on the variant of philosophical consequentialism from which these concepts are drawn. Some texts use instead the word "nonmalfeasance." This is a mistake, inasmuch as malfeasance refers to misconduct of elected and other government officials who violate their oath of office or the criminal or civil law.

1.4.1.3 Beneficence and Nonmaleficence in the History of Medical Ethics

The ethical principles of beneficence and nonmaleficence have deep roots in the history of medical ethics. Thomas Percival (1740–1804), who wrote the first text in the global history of medical ethics entitled *Medical Ethics*, may have been the first to use the word "beneficence."[18] A version of nonmaleficence can be found in the Hippocratic text *Epidemics*, the unknown author of which enjoins physicians "to help, or at least to do no harm."[19] Another version of nonmaleficence is the very common injunction, "first do no harm." The Latinized variant, "primum non nocere," is attributed to the American physician and medical ethicist Worthington Hooker (1806–1867).[20] Note that "first do no harm" is not the discourse of *Epidemics*, which makes beneficence the primary principle, with nonmaleficence secondary. Thus understood, "to help, or at least to do no harm" can be read as nonmaleficence functioning as a limiting principle on beneficence: when the physician has a weak evidence base for clinical judgment and a proposed course of clinical management based on such weak clinical judgment, the physician should proceed with great caution, to prevent net clinical harm to the patient.

1.4.1.4 The Ethical Principle of Respect for Autonomy in Medical Ethics and Bioethics

The discourse of rights appears in the global history of medical ethics as early as 1772, in the first text on professional medical ethics, John Gregory's (1724–1773) *Lectures on the Duties and Qualifications of a Physician*[21]: "Every man has a right to speak where his own life is concerned, or that of a friend."[21, p. 33] This right derives from the physician's sympathy-based obligation (taken from David Hume (1711–1776)) to identify and respond to the lived experience of illness of the patient. The concept of rights based on the capacity for autonomous decision making and action comes much later, with the invention of the field of bioethics in the late 1960s and early 1970s.

We rely, again, on the concise formulation of the ethical principle of respect for autonomy in medical ethics and bioethics provided by Beauchamp and Childress: "To respect autonomous agents is to acknowledge their right to hold views, to make choices, and to take actions based on their values and beliefs."[17, p. 106] Autonomous agents "act (1) intentionally, (2) with understanding, and (3) without controlling influences that determine their action."[17, p. 104] The ethical principle of respect for autonomy creates the prima facie ethical obligation to acknowledge and implement the informed and voluntary decisions of others and not interfere with behavior based on such decisions, except when behavior creates a significant potential to result in harm to others, especially serious, far-reaching, and irreversible harm. This is known as the harm principle in bioethics, a variant of the ethical principle of nonmaleficence.

1.4.1.5 The Ethical Principle of Justice in Medical Ethics and Bioethics

The fourth ethical principle in medical ethics and bioethics is the ethical principle of *justice*. The general formulation of this ethical principle is "attributed to Aristotle: Equals must be treated equally and unequals must be treated unequally."[17, p. 250] The ethical principle of justice in medical ethics and bioethics creates the prima facie ethical obligation to treat groups of individuals equally or with fairness. There is profound disagreement in the histories of Western and global philosophical ethics and moral theology about how the "justice," "equality," and "fairness" should be understood. The reader should be suspicious of any claim that an author is presenting *the* theory of justice in medical ethics or bioethics.

1.4.1.6 Putting Ethical Principles into Practice

To be put into practice, as effective guides to ethical judgment and behavior based on it, these abstract ethical principles must be *specified*: "Specification is a process of reducing the indeterminacy of abstract norms [such as principles and virtues] and generating rules with action-guiding content,"[17, p. 17] which Beauchamp and Childress base on the pioneering work of Henry Richardson.[22] For all four ethical principles, the first step in specification is to clarify whether the principle is absolute or prima facie. For beneficence or nonmaleficence to function as an effective action guide, one must also specify an account of the goods and harms that are relevant in a specific context and how they should be balanced and establish the authority for providing such an account. For respect for autonomy to function as an effective action guide, the scope of autonomous agents also must be specified, especially by providing justified criteria for who should be considered an autonomous agent. For justice, the respect in which individuals are equal or unequal must be clarified and justified criteria presented for making this crucial distinction.

Specifications of ethical principles should explain why the perspective from which such an account is articulated should have intellectual and therefore moral authority for others. In medical ethics and bioethics, even when agreement exists on how to specify these ethical principles, there remain competing accounts for the authority of such specifications, further reflecting the pluralism of medical ethics and bioethics. In professional ethics in medicine and professional ethics in obstetrics and gynecology the requisite intellectual and moral authority for specifying these and other ethical principles derives from the ethical concept of medicine as a profession. This approach differentiates professional ethics in medicine and in obstetrics and gynecology from medical ethics and bioethics.

1.5 Professional Ethics in Medicine

Professional ethics in medicine is the disciplined study of the morality of physicians and patients in clinical practice, clinical innovation and research, organizational culture, and health policy and advocacy with the aim of improving them, based on the ethical concept of medicine as a profession. Professional ethics in medicine is *not* pluralistic, because it is based on a single philosophical concept, the ethical concept of medicine as a profession. This concept was invented to be, and remains, transreligious, transnational, and transcultural.[9]

1.5.1 The Invention of Professional Ethics in Medicine

1.5.1.1 Hippocratic Medical Ethics

It is commonly assumed that professional ethics in medicine originated in the Hippocratic oath[23] and the ethical texts of the *Hippocratic Corpus*, the body of works written over more than a century and therefore by multiple authors. Jacques Jouanna points out in his masterful biography of Hippocrates[24] that the physicians of the Hippocratic or Coan school of medicine ran short of sons and needed to recruit other young men. Until this time, the Coan school functioned as a family-based guild, protecting market share in an unforgivingly competitive world of medical practice and adding sons of members whose loyalty to the guild could be safely assumed.

Once a guild recruits nonfamily members, loyalty cannot be assumed but must be made explicit. Oaths have played the role of solemnizing a promise of loyalty for millennia. The Hippocratic oath is no exception. Indeed, the oath in its opening section characterizes itself as a "written covenant"[23] between initiates to the Coan school and its master physicians. A covenant is among the most solemn of promises. The initiate promises to protect *techné*, the unchanging and unchangeable doctrine of the four humors, interactions among which explain disease. The initiate also promises to protect "reputation" or the positive estimations of potential customers of Coan school physicians, which are essential for gaining and retaining market share. Only men were permitted to become initiates.

The oath is not based on science, which is changing and changeable by its very nature. It is not based on a constitutive trait of character such as professional integrity. The oath could not be taken by women. It is therefore completely inadequate as the origin of professional ethics in medicine. The oath and the ethical texts of the *Hippocratic Corpus* are best understood as texts in medical ethics and a flawed medical ethics at that. These texts should not be understood to be texts about professional ethics in medicine.

Even if this were not the case, there is no millennia-long tradition of swearing to the Hippocratic oath by physicians or trainees.[25] The practice died out in the early centuries of the Common Era. Administration of the oath was revived in the early decades of the twentieth century in the United States, during a period in which medicine was a socially and economically fragile social institution. Vivian Nutton points out that the purpose of doing so was to invoke the revered historical figure of Hippocrates to shore up this weak social standing,[25] even though the Hippocratic authors would reject the emergence of scientific medicine, which we now – and correctly – celebrate as one of the great achievements of the profession of medicine. The revered figure of Hippocrates has frequently been invoked to give value to ideas and practices with which the Hippocratic physicians would be unfamiliar.[26]

1.5.1.2 Friedrich Hoffmann on the Politic Physician

Hippocratic medical ethics is the medical ethics of market exchanges, in which two parties of similar power enter into contracts to provide services in exchange for payment. By the early eighteenth century municipalities and principalities were hiring physicians. Physicians became subordinate to the power of government or royalty, resulting in a relationship of unequals. Friedrich Hoffmann (1660–1742) was a professor of medicine at the University of Halle, in southern modern-day Germany and also a physician at a number of royal courts. He therefore had direct experience with these new forms of medical practice that were becoming available to his medical students.

Hoffmann's response was the concept of *medicus politicus*, or the "politic physician."[27] By this phrase Hoffmann did not mean the "political" physician but rather the physician who knew how to comport himself when subject to unaccountable power. Princes could hire and fire court physicians at will. Economic security, to which physicians are now accustomed, did not exist. The task was to survive. Survival is grounded in the virtue of prudence, which schools one in the discipline of identifying and then acting to protect one's legitimate interest.

Hoffmann based his medical ethics on the virtue of prudence but prudence based on enlightened self-interest. This is Hoffmann's distinctive contribution to the history of medical ethics and marks a significant differentiation from Hippocratic, entrepreneurial medical ethics. Enlightened self-interest takes into account the interests of those who have power over one. Melding one's self-interests with the interests of those with power over one results in prudence based on enlightened self-interest. For example, the principalities and royal courts of the time derived their authority from Christianity. Hoffmann therefore begins his *Medicus Politicus* with the injunction that the "physician should be a Christian."[27] That is, the politic physician publicly embraces the religion of the royal courts. Privately, the physician may believe otherwise. This was the strategy of the Marranos in medieval Spain, Jews who publicly converted to Christianity and submitted publicly to Christian morality and law but kept their Jewish faith alive in the privacy of their homes. The Marrano Jews were politic.

Hoffmann prescribes a set of rules, designed with the goal of surviving court power in mind. For example, the physician should comport himself as a man worthy of a good reputation:

> Based on the virtues from moral philosophy, the physician ought to accomplish his work with diligence. And so he should be merciful, mild, and humane. Just as from the plague, he should flee from a dissolute life, evil words, drunkenness, and all illicit games and everything else that would lose the trust of the sick.[27]

Hoffmann's account of prudence based on enlightened self-interest has contemporary relevance. Prudence as enlightened self-interest becomes the basis for the concept of the physician's legitimate self-interests: self-interest melded with the health-related interests of patients as understood in beneficence-based clinical ethical judgment. The legitimate self-interests of a physician align with the health-related interests of the patient. For example, Hoffmann enjoins physicians to be "chaste" when treating female patients.[27] Chastity is a virtue that blunts sexual attraction. The result is to protect the female patient from sexual predation and, at the same time, the reputation of the physician as trustworthy by the female patient and – crucially – her husband. (See Chapter 4 and 5.) Improving one's fund of knowledge and clinical skills benefits patients clinically, making the time and expense of doing so a legitimate self-interest of every physician. Aligning oneself with the interests of insurance companies in providing evidence-based clinical management of one's patients protects and promotes the health of one's patients and also protects the business model of one's clinical practice.

1.5.1.3 John Gregory and Thomas Percival on Professional Ethics in Medicine

Hoffmann's politic physician addressed circumstances in which the patient and payers had power over the physician. The invention of professional ethics in medicine responded to a different problem: the power that physicians came to have over patients.

Two eighteenth-century British physician-ethicists, John Gregory (1724–1773) of Scotland and Thomas Percival (1740–1804) of England, invented professional medical ethics.[9,28] Gregory trained in Scotland and the Netherlands and experienced first-hand the transreligious, transnational, and transcultural method of science based in Francis Bacon's (1561–1626) philosophy of science in Edinburgh and then in Leiden, where Herman Boerhaave's (1668–1738) legacy in experienced-based (for Bacon's usage of "experience" as roughly equivalent of "evidence,"[9] see Section 1.5.1.5.). At the University of Edinburgh, where Gregory was professor of medicine (1766–1773), he taught multireligious, multicultural, multinational students. Some of these students came from persecuted, "dissenting" faith communities in England who would not accept the teachings and therefore the theological authority of the Church of England. Percival also trained in Scotland and the Netherlands and came from the dissenting faith community of Unitarians in Warrington, near Manchester. In their works on professional ethics in medicine, both of these remarkable physician-ethicists self-consciously wanted medicine to become a profession that would be transreligious, transnational, and transcultural.

1.5.1.4 Gregory's Professional Ethics in Medicine

Gregory wrote his professional ethics in medicine in response to a crisis of lost trust in physicians, surgeons, apothecaries, and other practitioners. Keep in mind the context. This was more than a century before the enactment of pure drug statutes and the creation of the Food and Drug Administration in the United States in the early twentieth century and its considerable regulatory powers over both prescription and over-the-counter medications. In response to illness, the sick first self-diagnosed and self-treated, which was known as "self-physicking." Guides to self-physicking for the layperson became popular, for example, William Buchan's *Domestic Medicine*.[9]

Seeking help from a medical practitioner was undertaken with trepidation born of rampant distrust. Dorothy and Roy Porter have documented this epidemic of distrust among the sick.[29] The sick did not believe that medical practitioners knew what they were doing. For example, there were almost as many theories of disease and remedies as there were physicians. Physicians offered "nostrums" to their patients, compound medications the contents of which practitioners who made and sold these remedies kept secret and which practitioners did not produce under conditions of quality control. These nostrums often contained opium, which induced euphoria and increased sales. In addition to this intellectual distrust, the sick experienced moral distrust. The sick could not be confident that the recommendations of medical practitioners were motivated more by their self-interest in income and reputation than by a sustained commitment to the well-being of the sick. Hoffmann's concept of prudence as enlightened self-interest, it would appear, did not take hold in Britain.

Physicians and surgeons were often considered therefore to be "men of interest,"[9] i.e., men motivated primarily by individual self-interest and guild self-interest (e.g., physicians competing with surgeons, "man-midwives" – the forerunners of modern obstetricians – with female midwives) and not an obligation to protect and promote the health and life of the sick. It is therefore telling that the first topic that Gregory addresses in *Lectures* is the distinction between medicine undertaken by these men of interest and medicine undertaken as a profession for the benefit of the sick. (See Chapter 5.)

Gregory was also concerned that in the new secular charitable hospitals, known as royal infirmaries, physicians, surgeons, and apothecaries gained power over the sick. This stood in sharp contrast to the private practice of medicine, a small market of services provided to the well-to-do in their homes. In this setting, physicians were subordinate to the power of the wealthy, because he who pays the piper calls the tune. Today, physicians are still subordinate to the power of payers, especially as the insurance market consolidates into ever-larger companies with growing monopsony power. Medicare exerts growing influence over hospital practice.

The infirmaries were established by the aristocracy and owners of factories, coal fields, shipyards, and other industries of the nascent industrial revolution, to provide free medical and surgical care to their employees, the working sick poor. In infirmaries physicians and surgeons for the first time gained power over the sick that derived from an organization that the sick poor depended on for care paid for by their employers, who valued a healthy workforce, and by the aristocracy as an act of charity.[9]

Gregory wanted to create a professional ethics of medicine to guide that power so that it was used primarily for the benefit of patients and not primarily for individual self-interest or group self-interest as the competition among physicians, surgeons, and apothecaries that was already intense in the private sphere became even more intense in the institutional setting. Finally, Gregory was teaching clinical medicine and ethics to students of remarkable diversity. Because they would not subscribe to the articles of faith of the Church of England, English dissenters came north, attracted by the culture of *Lehrenfreiheit* or freedom to teach (perhaps the first expression of academic freedom) for which the University of Edinburgh was increasingly well known. Students of different faiths also came from the North American British colonies. Some of them were revolutionaries, notably Benjamin Rush (1746–1813), a signer of the Declaration of Independence for Pennsylvania in 1776 and later Surgeon General of the ultimately victorious Continental Army.[9] Medical ethics would not do; a professional ethics of medicine was required that would transcend potential divisive differences of religion, culture, and nationality.

1.5.1.5 Percival's Professional Ethics in Medicine

Percival was equally concerned to create a transreligious professional ethics for medicine. As a dissenter, he had experienced oppression first hand: he would not in conscience submit to the Articles of Faith of the Church of England and thus could not attend medical school at Oxford or Cambridge. He attended medical school at the University of Edinburgh, leaving for Leiden for continued study the year before Gregory took up his professorship at Edinburgh in 1766. Percival also experienced religiously based violence when the dissenter meeting house he attended in Warrington was set afire by an angry mob.

Percival was determined to take on the politics of the Royal Infirmary of Manchester, which was controlled by two powerful medical families, resulting in bitter feuds between those families and physicians and surgeons in the community who wanted appointments to the "faculty" of the infirmary. Many of the latter were scientifically and clinically superior to the former. These feuds threatened to paralyze the infirmary, the trustees of which asked Percival to write an ethics text to guide physicians, surgeons, and apothecaries on a basis that transcended individual and group self-interest. Percival had an earned reputation as a moralist, based on his many writings.[30]

Percival's solution was to create an ethics of cooperation to guide the growing, organizationally derived power of physicians and surgeons over patients.[9] Percival characterized his text as "Professional Ethics."[18] *Medical Ethics* was the first book in the global history of medical ethics with this title. By its very nature, an ethics of cooperation must be transreligious, transnational, and transcultural. So, too, for professional ethics in medicine.

Both Gregory and Percival, reflecting the enduring scientific influence of Boerhaave's Leiden, as it was known after his death, first adopted the philosophy of science and of medicine of Bacon. Bacon insisted that science be based on "experience," carefully conducted natural experiments (observational studies of the course of disease and its responses to medical or surgical management, i.e., morbidity and mortality) and controlled experiments (designed studies, e.g., of the separate components of compound drugs to identify which components, alone or in combination, produced the results attributed to the compound). Bacon should be credited with inventing a nascent form of what is now known as evidence-based medicine.[9]

Both Gregory and Percival turned to the best moral philosophy of their time, the moral science, respectively, of Hume and Richard Price (1723–1791).[9] As explained in Section 1.4.1.4, the core discovery of this moral science was sympathy (also called "humanity"), a natural process of entering into the lived experience of others that then motivates one to protect and promote their interests as one's primary concern and motivation and to keep individual and group self-interest systematically secondary.

1.5.1.6 The Ethical Concept of Medicine as a Profession

Drawing on these powerful intellectual resources, Gregory and Percival invented the ethical concept of medicine as a profession, which can be read as requiring three commitments of professional physicians and surgeons (see Table 1.3):

> To become and remain scientifically and clinically competent, by adopting Baconian "experience"-based scientific method or, as we would now say, by

Table 1.3 The ethical concept of medicine as a profession.

To become and remain scientifically and clinically competent, by submitting to the discipline of deliberative clinical judgment and clinical practice and research based on it

To make protection and promotion of the patient's health-related interests one's primary concern and motivation, keeping individual self-interest systematically secondary

To make protection and promotion of the patient's health-related interests one's primary concern and motivation, keeping group or guild self-interest systematically secondary

---

submitting to the discipline of deliberative clinical judgment and clinical practice and research based on it;

To make protection and promotion of the patient's health-related interests one's primary concern and motivation, keeping *individual* self-interest systematically secondary; and

To make protection and promotion of the patient's health-related interests one's primary concern and motivation, keeping *group* self-interest systematically secondary. Percival called for medicine to become a "public trust," rather than the creature of the group self-interests of families or the various medical and surgical guilds, then (and still) known as the Royal Colleges.[31,32]

For Gregory and Percival, making these commitments transforms the physician as medical practitioner acting primarily from self-interest, i.e., as a "man of interest," into the physician as medical professional. The contractual relationship between a sick person and a self-interested medical practitioner breeds distrust, the belief that the physician does not know what he is doing and is not primarily committed to protecting and promoting the health-related interests of the sick person on the basis of experienced-based, i.e., deliberative, clinical judgment. The professional relationship stands in sharp contrast: the sick individual is now under the competent, dedicated protection of a medical professional. The sick person thus becomes a patient: a living human being who is presented to a professional physician and there exist forms of clinical management that are reliably predicted to result in net clinical benefit for that human being. This conceptual shift appears in the language of Gregory's *Lectures*, in that he uses both "the sick" and "patient" with similar frequency. Percival uses "patient" far more often. The use of "patient" subsequently became increasingly common and taken for granted, masking the conceptual accomplishment of Gregory and Percival in inventing professional ethics in medicine.

1.6 Professional Virtues and Ethical Principles in Professional Ethics in Medicine

The professional relationship of physicians to patients, the physician–patient relationship, depends for its authority on professional virtues and the ethical principles of beneficence, nonmaleficence, respect for autonomy, and justice. The professional virtues ground the physician–patient relationship in a sustained concern for the health and life of each patient. Ethical principles provide guidance to physicians in how to implement this concern in clinical practice and research. This order of virtues and principles differentiates professional ethics in medicine and in obstetrics and gynecology from the primacy of ethical principles in medical ethics and, especially, in bioethics. This crucial difference cannot be overemphasized.

1.6.1 The Five Professional Virtues

There are five professional virtues in professional ethics in medicine. (See Table 1.4.)

1.6.1.1 The Professional Virtue of Integrity

The bedrock professional virtue is the professional virtue of integrity. Integrity in ethics generally is a virtue that integrates one's intellectual and moral life into a coherent whole and thus makes one's life worth living. Specifying this virtue requires that one identify the basis for this integration and then why this integration is worth pursuing.

The ancient Greek philosophers, Plato especially, understood that the pursuit and experience of intellectual and moral excellence alone integrates one's intellectual and moral life.[33] The ethical concept of medicine as a profession provides the basis for both intellectual integrity and moral integrity and their integration. Intellectual integrity is achieved by making the life-long commitment to becoming and remaining scientifically and clinical competent. Moral

Table 1.4 Professional virtues.

Integrity	The habit of living by and not compromising the commitment to the ethical concept of medicine as a profession
Humility	The habit of recognizing the limits of one's ethical judgments and working persistently to improve them
Compassion	The habit of recognizing when one's patient experiences pain, distress, or suffering or is at risk for doing so and acting to prevent and effectively manage and prevent pain, distress, or suffering
Self-effacement	The habit of identifying and then minimizing the influences on one's clinical judgment and clinical management of features of the patient that are irrelevant in clinical judgment and put clinical judgment at preventable risk of bias
Self-sacrifice	The habit of taking reasonable risks of harm to one's legitimate self-interest in patient care, research, and advocacy

integrity is achieved by making the life-long commitment to the priority of protecting and promoting the health-related interests of the patient and to the systematically secondary status of individual self-interest and group or guild self-interest. Living out these three commitments of the ethical concept of medicine as a profession makes the pursuit of excellence in service to biomedical science and patients central in the professional life of a physician. Only the experience of excellence in medicine possesses the capacity to sustain physicians throughout their practice lives, especially when their patients do not do well.

The professional virtue of integrity creates the strong, prima facie ethical obligation to live by and not to compromise the physician's commitment to the ethical concept of medicine as a profession. The burden of proof for defeating this ethical obligation is very steep, perhaps insurmountable, because without professional integrity there is no profession of medicine.

1.6.1.2 The Professional Virtue of Humility

An important corollary of the professional virtue of integrity, related especially to intellectual integrity, is the professional virtue of humility: the habit of recognizing the limits of one's ethical judgments and working persistently to improve them. Gregory identified a key component of humility, which he called "candor" or being "open" to new evidence from whatever source it may come, including patients or competitors, and changing one's mind, as required by the strength of the evidence.[9,21] Without candor, it is impossible to develop the professional virtue of humility.

1.6.1.3 The Professional Virtue of Compassion

The professional virtue of compassion creates a two-step prima facie ethical obligation. The first step is to recognize when one's patient experiences pain, distress, or suffering or is at risk of doing so. The second step is to act promptly and effectively to clinically manage or prevent pain, distress, or suffering. Pain is the report in the central nervous system of tissue damage (some add threat of tissue damage) accompanied by awareness. Distress is the experience of disruption of one's behavioral repertoire. Suffering is the experience of one's aims and intentions for current or future well-being becoming blocked or impeded to some degree. One can be in pain without being in distress or suffering, although pain can cause either or both. One can be in distress without being in pain or suffering, although distress can cause suffering. One can be suffering without being in pain or distress. The phrase "mental pain" is used imprecisely to mean either suffering or being in pain and suffering. Loss of precision of thought and speech can be prevented by not using the phrase "mental pain."

1.6.1.4 The Professional Virtue of Self-Effacement

The professional virtue of self-effacement creates the prima facie ethical obligation to identify and then minimize the influences on one's clinical judgment and clinical management of features of the patient that are irrelevant in clinical judgment and put clinical judgment at preventable risk of bias if these features are, mistakenly, considered clinically relevant. The financial status or social standing of a patient is clinically irrelevant. Gregory was concerned that physicians, like many human beings, can be dazzled by great wealth or higher social standing and therefore should ignore them, because bedazzlement with wealth or power can lead to overtreatment, especially in response to what may be experienced as undeniable requests.

Gregory provided the antidote. The clinical conditions of both the wealthy and the economically disadvantaged, the powerful and the powerless, should be managed alike.[9,21] The ethics of triage in military medicine invokes self-effacement with its commitment to set priority for clinical management based on the patient's condition and the likelihood of success of treatment. Triage ethics therefore considers the uniform worn by a state combatant to be irrelevant to the fact that that human being is a patient: he or she has been presented to the physician and there exist forms of clinical management that are reliably predicted to produce net clinical benefit. There is ethical controversy about whether triage ethics should apply to wounded nonstate combatants, i.e., terrorists.

1.6.1.5 The Professional Virtue of Self-Sacrifice

The professional virtue of self-sacrifice creates the prima facie ethical obligation to take reasonable risks of harm to one's legitimate self-interest in patient care, research, and advocacy. Implementing this virtue requires the physician to distinguish between legitimate self-interest and mere self-interest. (See Chapter 5.) Risking mere self-interest should become routine. Risking legitimate self-interest without limit, however, can become the vice of recklessness. For example, if a 250-pound, muscularly well-developed man who has ingested phencyclidine (PCP) is brought to the emergency department by the police and becomes violent, a 110-pound (nonanorectic) female medical student may unnecessarily risk her life or health in trying to control the patient, when police officers and emergency department security personnel have been trained in effectively and safely (for the patient and for themselves) bringing such a patient under physical control. The professional virtue of self-sacrifice becomes essential for the professionally responsible management of conflicts of interest, i.e., conflicts between ethical obligations to patients or research subjects, on the one hand, and legitimate self-interests, on the other hand. Where to set justified limits on self-sacrifice, e.g., of the business model of a group practice, requires very well-reasoned ethical analysis and argument.

Conflicts of interest differ from – but are often conflated with – conflicts of commitment. (See Chapter 5.) Conflicts of commitment exist when the physician's ethical obligations to patients or research subjects become incompatible with the physician's ethical obligations to other people in his or her life, especially family members. Self-sacrifice can justifiably require abandoning self-interest, sometimes to a considerable degree. Self-sacrifice of commitments to people other than patients or research subjects requires strong justification, because these others may not agree to release the physician from ethical obligations to them. The "work–life balance" should be understood not just in terms of conflicts of interest but also conflicts of commitment, which is why judgments and organizational policies about work–life balance become so challenging.

1.6.2 The Four Ethical Principles in Professional Ethics in Medicine

Professional ethics in medicine specifies the ethical principles of beneficence, nonmaleficence, respect for autonomy, and justice in ways that differ from their specification in medical ethics and bioethics. (See Table 1.5.) The results are distinctive practical clinical guides to patient care, clinical innovation and research, organizational culture and its leadership, and health policy and advocacy. These specifications differ from the specifications of ethical principles in medical ethics and bioethics.

1.6.2.1 The Ethical Principle of Beneficence in Professional Ethics in Medicine

The ethical principle of beneficence in professional ethics in medicine creates the prima facie ethical obligation of the physician to provide clinical management that in deliberative clinical judgment is predicted to result in net clinical benefit for the patient and therefore protect and promote the patient's health-related interests. The strength of the obligation varies directly with the strength of the evidence for predicted net clinical benefit.

1.6.2.2 The Concept of a Medically Reasonable Alternative

When a form of clinical management is both technically feasible and supported in beneficence-based clinical judgment, it is known as "medically reasonable." We cannot overemphasize that it is an egregious error to consider a form of clinical management to be medically reasonable solely because it is technically feasible.

17

Section 1: Professional Ethics in Obstetrics and Gynecology

Table 1.5 Ethical principles in the professional ethics of medicine.

Beneficence	An ethical principle creates the prima facie ethical obligation of the physician to provide clinical management that in deliberative clinical judgment is predicted to result in net clinical benefit for the patient and therefore protect and promote the patient's health-related interests.
Nonmaleficence	An ethical principle that sets the limiting condition on the ethical principle of beneficence: when in deliberative clinical judgment the evidence for a medically reasonable alternative becomes weak, the physician must become alert to the increasing strength of the prediction that net clinical harm could be the outcome for the patient. There is a nonmaleficence-based prima facie ethical obligation to prevent such an outcome.
Respect for Autonomy	An ethical principle that creates the prima facie ethical obligation to empower the patient to make informed and voluntary decisions about the management of her clinical condition by providing her with information about the medically reasonable alternatives for its clinical management.
Healthcare Justice	An ethical principle that applies to populations of patients and creates the prima facie ethical obligation of the physician to see to it that each patient is treated equally or fairly as "equally" and "fairly" are understood clinically: each patient is to be provided medically reasonable clinical management of her condition or diagnosis.

Failure to keep this is mind creates preventable ethical challenges in critical care obstetrics and gynecology. (See Chapter 15.)

1.6.2.3 The Ethical Principle of Nonmaleficence in Professional Ethics in Medicine

The ethical principle of nonmaleficence in professional ethics in medicine sets the limiting condition on the ethical principle of beneficence. When in deliberative clinical judgment the evidence for a medically reasonable alternative becomes weak, the physician should become alert to the increasing strength of the prediction that net clinical harm could be the outcome. There is a strong nonmaleficence-based prima facie ethical obligation to prevent such an outcome, which is fulfilled by identifying other medically reasonable alternatives with a stronger evidence base. When these are not available, the physician should proceed with great caution. In some cases, especially for end-stage disease, the only medically reasonable alternative will become palliative and hospice care. (See Chapter 15.)

1.6.2.4 The Ethical Principle of Respect for Autonomy in Professional Ethics in Medicine

Beneficence creates the prima facie ethical obligation to identify all of the medically reasonable alternatives for the clinical management of the patient's condition. The ethical principle of respect for autonomy in professional ethics in medicine creates the prima facie ethical obligation to empower the patient to make informed and voluntary decisions about the management of her clinical condition by providing her with information about her condition and the medically reasonable alternatives for its clinical management. A patient's decision is informed if she has an adequate understanding of the nature of her condition, the medically reasonable alternatives for its clinical management, the strength of evidence supporting the clinical judgment of medical reasonableness, and the nature and probability of the clinical benefits and risks of each medically reasonable alternative. When patients indicate the need for support in processing this information or seem to be challenged by this task, e.g., because of complex cognitive demands, the ethical principle of respect for autonomy creates the ethical obligation to offer the patient psychosocial support. A patient's decision making is voluntary when it is not controlled by internal or external controlling influences.[17] The physician should be alert to such influences and act to blunt them.

1.6.2.5 The Ethical Principle of Healthcare Justice in Professional Ethics in Medicine

The ethical principle of healthcare justice applies to populations of patients and specifies the general ethical principle of justice. Healthcare justice creates the prima facie ethical obligation of the physician to see to it that each patient is treated equally as "equality" is understood clinically: each patient is to be provided medically reasonable clinical management of her condition.[34] Patients are equal with respect to a shared condition or diagnosis and are unequal when their conditions differ. For example, the time required for an antenatal office visit for a patient whose pregnancy has been and remains uncomplicated will be less than that required for a patient who has experienced significant risks to her health or life, e.g., newly recurrent cancer. This unequal difference in time allocated does not violate healthcare justice. Healthcare justice prohibits rationing, where "rationing" in its precise use means that some patients are denied access to any medically reasonable alternative.

1.7 Advantages of Professional Ethics in Medicine

Professional ethics in medicine enjoys several advantages over medical ethics and bioethics. The latter are pluralistic, drawing on both theological and nontheological resources. Professional ethics in medicine appeals to a single clinically oriented, philosophical concept, the ethical concept of medicine as a profession. This concept is not the product of a specific philosophical method and is thus immune to methodological disputes in moral philosophy. Professional ethics in medicine is secular. Its three defining commitments make no reference to deity, transcendent reality, sacred texts, or religious tradition for their authority. Nor is secular reasoning necessarily hostile to religion and faith communities, as secular, professional ethics in medicine is transreligious.

For Beauchamp and Childress ethical principles and virtues originate in a "common morality," or "norms about right and wrong conduct that are so widely shared that they form a stable social compact."[17, pp. 2–3] This claim is doubtful on both empirical grounds, as the earlier example of solidarity shows, and on philosophical grounds, the absence of a single authoritative method in moral philosophy. Professional ethics in medicine does not invoke – and need not invoke – common morality with all of its potentially disabling problems.

The concept of being a patient in professional ethics in medicine does not originate in the patient but in the professional relationship created by making the three commitments of the ethical concept of medicine as a profession. As a result, to be a patient does not require that one is a person,[35] a rational, self-conscious entity that is capable of giving itself value and thus possessing autonomy. To say the least, the concept of being a person invokes complex metaphysics, which is not always acknowledged in the literature of medical ethics and bioethics that invokes the concept of being a person as the basis for the ethical principle of respect for autonomy. The ethical concept of being a patient in professional ethics in medicine is emphatically not a metaphysical concept nor is it required to be. Professional ethics in medicine, and therefore professional ethics in obstetrics and gynecology, is thus completely free of the metaphysical challenges that plague medical ethics and bioethics and are frequently ignored.

The most common way to express the ethical concept of being a patient in the literature of medical ethics and bioethics is to invoke the concept of a right, the claim of an individual against others to be treated in a specified way. The discourse of rights comes with another metaphysical problem: what kind of entity has rights that originate in it? There is no agreement on the authoritative method for addressing the question. There is therefore no convincing answer to the question. This is not a problem for professional ethics in medicine, and therefore for professional ethics in obstetrics and gynecology, because the ethical concept of being a patient is beneficence based. Beneficence-based reasoning does not require invocation of the concept of a right. Indeed, doing so conflates the ethical principles of beneficence and respect for autonomy, a major methodological error in ethical reasoning from which professional ethics in medicine is immune.

1.8 Why Should Physicians Commit to the Ethical Concept of Medicine as a Profession?

Gregory and Percival answered this question by appealing to Hume's discovery of sympathy: a constitutive, causal process in individuals that incentivizes them naturally to enter into the lives of others and respond to their vulnerability to disease, injury, and death.[9] Percival also invokes intuition or the capacity to recognize moral qualities in others. This concept comes from the moral science of Richard Price, with whose student, John Taylor (1694–1761), Percival studied at the Warrington Academy.[9]

Two centuries later both appeals are problematic. Hume, Gregory, and Percival did their work before Charles Darwin (1809–1882) did his work on evolution. A core concept of evolutionary biology is the variation of traits. Not all members of a species exhibit all of the traits thought to be typical of that species. This means that some human beings lack sympathy and are therefore heartless. In the professional discourse of psychiatry such individuals are classified as sociopathic, a personality disorder for which there is no effective treatment.

The concept of an intuition is not exact, as Robert Audi has shown.[36] The idea that we have the capacity to directly apprehend moral qualities in others and to do so without risk of bias does not withstand close scrutiny from the perspective of behavioral psychology. This scientific discipline has, unwittingly, recaptured a scientific finding that Bacon reported four centuries ago: human judgment, including immediate, nondiscursive judgments labeled intuitions, is intrinsically at risk of being biased.[3,4] Biases must therefore always be identified and their distorting influence responsibly managed to a minimum. These are precisely the tasks of deliberative clinical judgment in clinical practice and research.

These two major scientific differences between our time and that of Gregory and Percival mean that we cannot appeal to sympathy or intuition, cognitive or affective capacities that are constitutive of the nature of all human beings and that are free from bias. Instead, we have to appeal to what the experience of clinical practice would be like for physicians and their patients and what the experience of clinical innovation and research would be like for clinical investigators and their research subjects if so many physicians failed to commit to the ethical concept of medicine as a profession that the profession of medicine ceased to exist.

The history of medicine tells us what these experiences would be like, because the best guide to the future is the past. As noted in Section 1.5.1.4, before Gregory and Percival invented the ethical concept of medicine as a profession, there was epidemic distrust of the sick toward medical practitioners of all kinds, and especially toward physicians and surgeons.[9,29] The sick stayed away from medical practitioners because the sick did not trust physicians or surgeons to know what they were doing and did not trust that physicians and surgeons were doing what they did primarily for the benefit of the sick individual. This distrust was corrosive for the sick and also, crucially, for physicians who found themselves the object of distrust. The practice of medicine, as every physician and trainee knows, is very cognitively and affectively demanding, especially when risk of morbidity and disability increase, when a patient suffers functional decline, and when a patient dies. The demands of clinical innovation and research are equally high, especially when unexpected adverse events occur or when clinical investigation does not yield the definitive results hoped for from it. These demands would become impossible to manage in an atmosphere of epidemic distrust. Epidemic distrust would doom advocacy and health policy to failure. Making and sustaining the commitment to the ethical concept of medicine becomes an essential and powerful antidote to distrust and therefore vital to the successful management of the demands of clinical practice and research, which, in turn, is essential for patient safety and quality. This is crucial in clinical practice and research with patients with experience-based distrust of physicians, especially patients of color. Put simply, the sustained commitment to the ethical concept of medicine as a profession creates the intellectual and moral excellence of medicine. The experience of this intellectual and moral excellence makes being a physician a way of life with value for physicians, their patients, their families, and society.

Clinical practice now must conform to and support the requirements of an organizational culture of patient safety and quality. Team care is not a slogan; team care is the indispensable means by which an organizational culture of safety and quality is created and sustained. Team care requires an ethics of cooperation based on the shared commitment to the ethical concept of medicine as a profession.

Gregory wrote professional ethics in medicine to unify medicine and surgery, the boundaries of which were then hotly contested, for which patients paid dearly.[9] The desired unification of medicine and surgery required an ethics of cooperation, which commitment to the ethical concept of medicine as a profession creates. Gregory paints a compelling portrait of the clinical consequences of physicians spurning cooperation and accountability:

> An obstinate adherence to an unsuccessful method of treating a disease, must be owing to a high degree of self-conceit, and a belief of the infallibility of a system. This error is the more difficult to cure, as it generally proceeds from ignorance. True knowledge

and clear discernment may lead one into the extreme of diffidence and humility; but are inconsistent with self-conceit. It sometimes happens too, that this obstinacy proceeds from a defect in the heart. Such physicians see that they are wrong; but are too proud to acknowledge their error, especially if it be pointed out to them by one of the profession. To this species of pride, a pride incompatible with true dignity and elevation of mind, have the lives of thousands been sacrificed.[21, pp. 28-29]

Percival was explicit about creating an ethics of cooperation among physicians, surgeons, and apothecaries in the Royal Infirmary of Manchester. In the first chapter of *Medical Ethics* Percival goes into considerable detail about the creation of registries (what we now call databases about the processes and outcomes of clinical care and research), the creation of regular clinical conferences to review challenging cases (thus anticipating tumor boards and morbidity and mortality conferences by a century), and a committee to oversee clinical research (thus anticipating Institutional Review Boards by a century-and-a-half).[7] These forms of cooperation are required, Percival maintained, by the commitment to the ethical concept of medicine as a profession.

Finally, the transnational, transcultural, and transreligious nature of the ethical concept of medicine as a profession makes possible the creation of international societies of physicians in the various specialties, such as the International Federation of Gynecology and Obstetrics (FIGO),[37] World Association of Perinatal Medicine,[38] the International Academy of Perinatal Medicine,[39] as well as transnational nongovernmental organizations such as the World Medical Association[40] and the World Health Organization.[41] These international and transnational organizations issue statements on a wide range of ethical challenges in clinical practice, clinical innovation and research, and health policy and advocacy. The global intellectual and moral authority of such statements for physicians everywhere originates in the ethical concept of medicine as a profession. FIGO, for example, has made its commitment to the ethical concept of medicine as a profession explicit.[42]

These justifications for committing to the ethical concept of medicine as a profession do not comprise what in ethical reasoning is known as a "principled argument" or an appeal to concepts that originate in the "moral point of view" that, as explained in Section 1.3.1.1, is taken to apply in all circumstances because it invokes timeless philosophical concepts such as the common morality. A principled argument is in the tradition of the quest for certainty and requires physicians to consider the ethical concept of medicine as a profession to be timeless and adherence to it required by unassailable argument.

Principled ethical reasoning differs from the ethical reasoning of Gregory and Percival, because these two physician-ethicists made their cases for professional ethics in medicine in the tradition of the quest for reliability, in two ways. The first is the style of persuasion of Gregory and Percival. In an argument of persuasion one offers, as we have here, a set of considerations, none of which is "principled" and therefore decisive. Instead, their ethical reasoning aims to persuade because the destructive consequences for physicians, their patients, and clinical innovators and investigators and their subjects, organizational culture, and health policy and advocacy of not having a profession of medicine are unacceptable.

The second is the pragmatic nature of professional medical ethics. James' pragmatism is distinctive for its emphasis on truth as something that is made, especially the truth of social practices and institutions such as the profession of medicine.[10] When physicians make and sustain their commitment to the ethical concept of medicine as a profession, they validate that there is a profession of medicine. Put another way, the profession of medicine is not some timeless idea that, because it is timeless, sustains itself and is thus immune from intellectual and moral damage that results when enough physicians abandon the ethical concept of medicine as a profession. Philosophers engaged in the quest for certainty must be committed to timeless ideas but the history of ideas and concepts, including the histories of medical ethics and of professional ethics in medicine, makes such a commitment implausible. The profession of medicine is the invention, not of the authors of the Hippocratic texts or of Hoffmann, but of two remarkable physician-ethicists of the eighteenth century, John Gregory and Thomas Percival. Their invention will not sustain itself but it is very much worth sustaining when we consider medical practice and research that is not professional or, worse, unprofessional.

References

1. McCullough LB. Taking seriously the "what then?" question: an ethical framework for the responsible management of medical disasters. J Clin Ethics 2011; 21: 321–327.
2. Chervenak FA, McCullough LB. An ethical framework for the responsible management of pregnant patients in a medical disaster. J Clin Ethics 2011; 22: 20–24.
3. Brody BA. Life and Death Decision Making. New York: Oxford University Press, 1988.
4. Brody BA. Taking Issue: Pluralism and Casuistry in Bioethics. Washington, DC: Georgetown University Press, 2003.
5. Buchanan A, Brock DW, Daniels D, Wikler D. From Chance to Choice: Genetics and Justice. New York: Cambridge University Press, 2000.
6. McCullough LB, Coverdale JH, Chervenak FA. Argument-based ethics: a formal tool for critically appraising the normative medical ethics literature. Am J Obstet Gynecol 2004; 191: 1097–1102.
7. McCullough LB, Coverdale JH, Chervenak FA. Constructing a systematic review for argument-based clinical ethics literature: the example of concealed medications. J Med Philos 2007; 32: 65–76.
8. Gracia D. Philosophy: ancient and contemporary approaches. In Sugarman J, Sulmasy DP, eds. Methods in Medical Ethics, 2nd ed. Washington, DC: Georgetown University Press, 2010: 55–72.
9. McCullough LB. John Gregory and the Invention of Professional Medical Ethics and the Profession of Medicine. Dordrecht, the Netherlands: Springer, 1998.
10. James W. The Will to Believe and Other Essays in Popular Philosophy. The Floating Press, 2010. www.thefloatingpress.com. Originally published 1896.
11. Aristotle. Nicomachean Ethics. Crisp R, trans. and ed. New York: Cambridge University Press, 2000.
12. Baker RB, McCullough LB, eds. The Cambridge World History of Medical Ethics. New York: Cambridge University Press, 2009.
13. Jonsen AR. The discourses of bioethics in the United States. In Baker RB, McCullough LB, eds. The Cambridge World History of Medical Ethics. New York: Cambridge University Press, 2009: 477–485.
14. Boyd K. The discourses of bioethics in the United Kingdom. In Baker RB, McCullough LB, eds. The Cambridge World History of Medical Ethics. New York: Cambridge University Press, 2009: 486–489.
15. Baker RB, McCullough LB. What is the history of medical ethics? In Baker RB, McCullough LB, eds. The Cambridge World History of Medical Ethics. New York: Cambridge University Press, 2009: 3–15.
16. Jonsen AR. The Birth of Bioethics. New York: Oxford University Press, 1998.
17. Beauchamp TL, Childress JF. Principles of Biomedical Ethics, 7th ed. New York: Oxford University Press, 2013.
18. Percival T. Medical Ethics; or, A Code of Institutes and Precepts, adapted to the Professional Conduct of Physicians and Surgeons. London: Johnson & Bickerstaff, 1803.
19. Hippocrates. Epidemics. In Jones WHS, trans., Hippocrates, vol. 1. Cambridge, MA: Harvard University Press, 1923: 165.
20. Baker RB, Burns CR. Worthington Hooker. In Baker RB, McCullough LB, eds. The Cambridge World History of Medical Ethics. New York: Cambridge University Press, 2009: 709.
21. Gregory J. Lectures on the Duties and Qualifications of a Physician. London: W. Strahan and T. Cadell, 1772. Reprinted in McCullough LB, ed. John Gregory's Writings on Medical Ethics and the Philosophy of Medicine. Dordrecht, the Netherlands: Kluwer Academic, 1998: 161–248.
22. Richardson HS. Specifying norms as a way to resolve concrete ethical problems. Philos Public Aff 1990; 19: 270–310.
23. von Staden H. "In a pure and holy way:" personal and professional conduct in the Hippocratic Oath. J Hist Med Allied Sci 1996; 51: 404–437.
24. Jouanna J. Hippocrates, trans. DeBevoise MB. Baltimore, MD: Johns Hopkins University Press, 2001.
25. Nutton V. The discourses of European practitioners in the tradition of the Hippocratic texts. In Baker RB, McCullough LB, eds. The Cambridge World History of Medical Ethics. New York: Cambridge University Press, 2009: 359–362.
26. Gálvao-Sobrinho CR. Hippocratic ideals, medical ethics, and the practice of medicine in the early middle ages: the legacy of the Hippocratic Oath. J Hist Med Allied Sci 1996; 51: 438–455.
27. Hoffmann F. Medicus politicus; sive, regulae prudentiae secundum quas medicus juvenis studia sua & vitae rationem dirigere debet. Leiden, Philip Bonk, 1738. (The Politic Doctor, or Rules of Prudence according to which a Young Physician Should Direct his Studies and Reason of Life).
28. Baker RB, McCullough LB. The discourses of philosophical medical ethics. In Baker RB, McCullough LB, eds. The Cambridge World History of Medical Ethics. New York: Cambridge University Press, 2009: 281–311.
29. Porter D, Porter R. Patient's Progress: Doctors and Doctoring in Eighteenth Century England. Cambridge: Cambridge University Press, 1989.
30. Percival T. The Works, Literary, Moral, and Medical of Thomas Percival, M.D. 4 vols. New York: Cambridge University Press, 2014. Originally published by J. Johnson, St. Paul's Church-Yard, London, 1807.
31. Chervenak FA, McCullough LB, Brent RL. The professional responsibility model of obstetric ethics: avoiding the perils of clashing rights. Am J Obstet Gynecol 2011; 205: 315.e1–5.
32. McCullough LB. The ethical concept of medicine as a profession: its origins in modern medical ethics and implications for physicians. In Kenny N, Shelton W, eds. Lost Virtue: Professional Character Development in Medical Education. New York: Elsevier, 2006: 17–27.
33. Plato. Republic. In Cooper JM, Hutchinson DS, eds. Plato Complete Works. Indianapolis, IN: Hackett, 1997: 971–1223.
34. Chervenak FA, McCullough LB. Healthcare justice and human rights in perinatal medicine. Semin Perinatol 2016; 40: 234–236.
35. Ruddick W, Wilcox W. Operating on the fetus. Hastings Cent Rep 1982; 12: 10–14.

36. Audi R. Intuition and its place in ethics. J Am Philos Assoc 2015; 1: 57–77.
37. International Federation of Gynecology and Obstetrics. Available at www.figo.org/ (accessed March 1, 2019).
38. World Association of Perinatal Medicine. Available at www.wapm.info/ (accessed March 1, 2019).
39. International Academy of Perinatal Medicine. Available at https://iaperinatalmedicine.org/ (accessed March 1, 2019).
40. World Medical Association. Available at www.wma.net/ (accessed March 1, 2019).
41. World Health Organization. Available at www.who.int/ (accessed March 1, 2019).
42. FIGO Committee for the Ethical Aspects of Human Reproduction and Women's Health. Professionalism in obstetric and gynecologic practice. Int J Gynaecol Obstet 2017; 36: 249–251.

Chapter 2: Professional Ethics in Obstetrics and Gynecology

GOAL
This chapter provides an introduction to professional ethics in obstetrics and gynecology based on the ethical concept of medicine as a profession and the ethical concepts of the female patient, pregnant patient, and fetal patient. There is also an introduction to professional ethics in perinatal medicine.

OBJECTIVES
On completing study of this chapter, the reader will:

Identify five professional virtues in professional ethics in obstetrics and gynecology

Identify four ethical principles in professional ethics in obstetrics and gynecology

Describe the ethical concept of the fetus as a patient

Describe professional ethics in perinatal medicine

Describe the best interests of the child standard

Describe implications of the ethical concept of the fetus as a patient for clinical practice

Prepare for the clinical application of professional ethics in obstetrics and gynecology and professional ethics in perinatal medicine, as detailed in subsequent chapters

TOPICS

2.1 Professional Ethics in Obstetrics and Gynecology	26
2.2 Professional Virtues and Ethical Principles in Professional Ethics in Gynecology	26
2.2.1 The Female Patient	26
2.2.1.1 Gregory on Ethical Obligations to the Female Patient	27
2.2.2 The Five Professional Virtues in Professional Ethics in Gynecology	27
2.2.2.1 The Professional Virtue of Integrity in Professional Ethics in Gynecology	27
2.2.2.2 The Professional Virtue of Humility in Professional Ethics in Gynecology	27
2.2.2.3 The Professional Virtue of Compassion in Professional Ethics in Gynecology	27
2.2.2.4 The Professional Virtue of Self-Effacement in Professional Ethics in Gynecology	28
2.2.2.5 The Professional Virtue of Self-Sacrifice in Professional Ethics in Gynecology	28
2.2.3 Ethical Principles in Professional Ethics in Gynecology	29
2.2.3.1 The Ethical Principle of Beneficence in Professional Ethics in Gynecology	29
2.2.3.2 The Concept of a Medically Reasonable Alternative	29
2.2.3.3 The Ethical Principle of Nonmaleficence in Professional Ethics in Gynecology	29
2.2.3.4 The Ethical Principle of Respect for Autonomy in Professional Ethics in Gynecology	29
2.2.3.5 The Ethical Principle of Healthcare Justice in Professional Ethics in Gynecology	29
2.3 Professional Virtues and Ethical Principles in Professional Ethics in Obstetrics	30

2.3.1 The Five Professional Virtues in Professional Ethics in Obstetrics ... 30
    2.3.1.1 The Professional Virtue of Integrity in Professional Ethics in Obstetrics ... 30
    2.3.1.2 The Professional Virtue of Humility in Professional Ethics in Obstetrics ... 30
    2.3.1.3 The Professional Virtue of Compassion in Professional Ethics in Obstetrics ... 30
    2.3.1.4 The Professional Virtue of Self-Effacement in Professional Ethics in Obstetrics ... 31
    2.3.1.5 The Professional Virtue of Self-Sacrifice in Professional Ethics in Obstetrics ... 31
2.3.2 Ethical Principles in Professional Ethics in Obstetrics ... 32
    2.3.2.1 The Ethical Principle of Beneficence in Professional Ethics in Obstetrics ... 32
    2.3.2.2 The Concept of a Medically Reasonable Alternative ... 32
    2.3.2.3 The Ethical Principle of Nonmaleficence in Professional Ethics in Obstetrics ... 32
    2.3.2.4 The Ethical Principle of Respect for Autonomy in Professional Ethics in Obstetrics ... 32
    2.3.2.5 The Ethical Principle of Healthcare Justice in Professional Ethics in Obstetrics ... 32
2.4 The Ethical Concept of the Fetus as a Patient ... 33
  2.4.1 Five Decades of the Discourse of the Fetus as a Patient ... 33
  2.4.2 A Preliminary: The Ethical Concept of Moral Status ... 34
    2.4.2.1 Dominance of Independent Moral Status in Medical Ethics and Bioethics ... 34
    2.4.2.2 Problems with the Concept of Independent Moral Status ... 35
  2.4.3 The Ethical Concept of the Fetus as a Patient ... 35
    2.4.3.1 The Viable Fetus as a Patient ... 36
    2.4.3.2 The Periviable Fetus as a Patient ... 36
    2.4.3.3 The Previable Fetus as a Patient ... 36
    2.4.3.4 The Obstetrician's Prima Facie Beneficence-Based Obligations to the Fetal Patient ... 36
    2.4.3.5 Limits on Prima Facie Beneficence-Based Obligations to the Pregnant Patient ... 37
    2.4.3.6 Enforcement of Prima Facie Beneficence-Based Ethical Obligations to the Fetal Patient ... 37
2.5 Advantages of the Ethical Concept of the Fetus as a Patient ... 38
  2.5.1 The Ethical Concept of the Fetus as a Patient Avoids the Philosophical and Clinical Paralysis of "Right to Life" ... 38
  2.5.2 The Ethical Concept of the Fetus as a Patient Avoids Reducing Moral Status to Independent Moral Status ... 38
  2.5.3 The Ethical Concept of the Fetus as a Patient Avoids Rights-Based Absolutism ... 39
  2.5.4 The Fetus Is a Separate Patient: A Failed Critique of the Ethical Concept of the Fetus as a Patient ... 40
2.6 Delivery Makes a Difference: Professional Ethics in Perinatal Medicine ... 41

Key Concepts

Best interests of the child standard
Biopsychosocial concept of health and disease
Conflict of commitment
Conflict of interest
Deliberative clinical judgment
Dependent moral status
Ethical concept of the fetus as a patient
Ethical concept of medicine as a profession
Ethical principle of beneficence in professional ethics in gynecology
Ethical principle of beneficence in professional ethics in obstetrics
Ethical principle of healthcare justice in professional ethics in gynecology
Ethical principle of healthcare justice in obstetrics
Ethical principle of nonmaleficence in professional ethics in obstetrics and gynecology

Ethical principle of respect for autonomy in professional ethics in gynecology
Ethical principle of respect for autonomy in professional ethics in obstetrics
Female patient
Fetus as a patient
Independent moral status
Medically reasonable alternative
Moral status
Pregnant patient
Professional ethics in gynecology
Professional ethics in obstetrics
Professional ethics in obstetrics and gynecology
Professional ethics in pediatrics
Professional ethics in perinatal medicine
Professional virtue of compassion
Professional virtue of humility
Professional virtue of integrity
Professional virtue of self-effacement
Professional virtue of self-sacrifice

2.1 Professional Ethics in Obstetrics and Gynecology

Professional ethics in obstetrics and gynecology is the disciplined study of the morality of physicians in the care of female patients, pregnant patients, and fetal patients in clinical practice; clinical innovation and research; organizational culture; and health policy and advocacy, based on the ethical concept of medicine as a profession and the ethical concept of the fetus as a patient. Professional ethics in perinatal medicine is the disciplined study of the morality of obstetrics and the morality with pediatrics in the care of peripartum fetal patients and neonatal patients, based on the ethical concept of medicine as a profession. Professional ethics in obstetrics and gynecology and in perinatal medicine are *not* pluralistic, because each is based on a single philosophical concept, the ethical concept of medicine as a profession, which was invented to be, and remains, transreligious, transnational, and transcultural, as we saw in Chapter 1. Professional ethics in gynecology addresses clinical practice, clinical innovation and research, organizational culture, and health policy and advocacy with regard to the female patient. Professional ethics in obstetrics addresses clinical practice, clinical innovation and research, organizational culture, and health policy and advocacy with regard to pregnant and fetal patients. One outcome of pregnancy is livebirth, resulting in a neonatal patient. The professional ethics of perinatal medicine addresses clinical practice, clinical innovation and research, organizational culture, and health policy and advocacy with regard to peripartum fetal and neonatal patients. Female patients and pregnant patients can be adults or minors. Decision making with regard to adults comes under the professional ethics of informed consent, while decision making with regard to minors comes under the professional ethics of pediatric assent and surrogate decision making, both of which are addressed in Chapter 3.

This chapter identifies the key concepts of professional ethics in gynecology, obstetrics, and perinatal medicine with a focus on specifying professional virtues and ethical principles for gynecology, obstetrics, and perinatal medicine. Because the fetus is sometimes a patient, specification of the ethical principle of beneficence includes beneficence-based obligations to the fetal patient, a key concept of professional ethics in obstetrics that is explicated as part of the specification of the ethical principle of beneficence in obstetrics.

2.2 Professional Virtues and Ethical Principles in Professional Ethics in Gynecology

Professional ethics in gynecology is the disciplined study of the morality of physicians caring for female patients in clinical practice, innovation and research, organizational culture, and health policy and advocacy, based on the ethical concept of medicine as a profession.

2.2.1 The Female Patient

A living human being becomes a female patient when she is presented to a gynecologist (or other healthcare professional) and there exist forms of clinical management that are reliably predicted to result in net clinical benefit for her. A woman can present herself to a gynecologist or she can be presented by others, e.g., by emergency medical personnel who have been summoned to bring her to the emergency department because she collapsed at work from vaginal hemorrhaging. In short, becoming a female patient is a beneficence-based concept that does not include consent as an essential component. Being a female patient does not originate in autonomy but adult female patients have autonomy, which originates autonomy-based ethical obligations to them.

2.2.1.1 Gregory on Ethical Obligations to the Female Patient

John Gregory (1724–1773) devotes a considerable portion of his landmark *Lectures on the Duties and Qualifications of a Physician* to the distinctive ethical obligations to the female patient. For example, he addresses the clinical care of patients with what were then known as "nervous ailments," patients who are now known as the "worried well," including – but not by any means limited to – female patients.[1]

> There is a numerous class of patients who put a physician's good-nature and patience to a severe trial; those I mean who suffer under nervous ailments. Although the fears of these patients are generally groundless, yet their sufferings are real; and the disease is as much seated in the constitution as a rheumatism or a dropsy. To treat their complaints with ridicule or neglect, from supposing them the effect of a crazy imagination, is equally cruel and absurd.[1, pp. 23–24]

Put in more contemporary terms, the worried well can suffer – sometimes so severely that they are disabled in social settings – from real psychological disorders, including mental disorders such as anxiety to various degrees. The professional virtue of compassion creates the prima facie ethical obligation not to say to such a patient that "this is all in your head." Doing so only demeans and dismisses the patient's experience and increases her distress and suffering with no offsetting clinical benefit.

2.2.2 The Five Professional Virtues in Professional Ethics in Gynecology

2.2.2.1 The Professional Virtue of Integrity in Professional Ethics in Gynecology

The bedrock professional virtue is professional integrity. As explained in Chapter 1, the ethical concept of medicine as a profession provides the basis for both intellectual integrity and moral integrity and their integration. Intellectual integrity is achieved by making the life-long commitment to becoming and remaining scientifically and clinically competent in the care of the female patient. Moral integrity is achieved by making the life-long commitment to the priority of protecting and promoting the health-related interests of the female patient and to the systematically secondary status of individual self-interest and group or guild self-interest. The commitment to the ethical concept of medicine as a profession makes the pursuit of excellence in service to biomedical science and female patients central in the professional life of the gynecologist. Only the experience of excellence possesses the capacity to sustain gynecologists throughout their practice lives, especially when their female patients experience serious disease with poor outcomes, for example, gynecologic cancer that has metastasized to other organs. The professional virtue of integrity creates the strong, prima facie ethical obligation to practice, live by, and not compromise the commitment to the ethical concept of medicine as a profession. The burden of proof for defeating this ethical obligation is very steep, perhaps insurmountable, because without professional integrity there is no profession of medicine.

2.2.2.2 The Professional Virtue of Humility in Professional Ethics in Gynecology

An important corollary of the professional virtue of integrity, related especially to intellectual integrity, is the professional virtue of humility: the habit of recognizing the limits of one's ethical judgments and working persistently to improve them. As explained in Chapter 1, a key component of humility is what Gregory called "candor" or being "open" to new evidence from whatever source it may come, including female patients, and changing one's mind depending on the strength of the evidence.[1,2] Without candor, it is impossible to develop the professional virtue of humility. As Jack Coulehan has pointed out, "humility requires toughness and emotional resilience," not "weakness of self-abnegation."[3, p. 201]

2.2.2.3 The Professional Virtue of Compassion in Professional Ethics in Gynecology

The professional virtue of compassion creates a two-step ethical obligation. The first step is to recognize when a female patient experiences pain, distress, or suffering or is at risk of doing so. The second step is to act promptly to effectively clinically manage or prevent pain, distress, or suffering. Pain is the report in the central nervous system of tissue damage or perhaps the threat of tissue damage accompanied by awareness. Distress is the experience of disruption of one's behavioral repertoire. Suffering is the experience of one's aims and intentions for current or future well-being becoming blocked or impeded to some degree. One can be in pain without being in distress or suffering, although pain can cause either or both. One can be in distress without being in pain or suffering, although distress can cause suffering. One can be suffering without being in pain or distress. The phrase "mental pain" is used imprecisely for either suffering or being in pain and suffering. Precision of thought and speech requires not using the phrase "mental pain."

2.2.2.4 The Professional Virtue of Self-Effacement in Professional Ethics in Gynecology

Self-effacement names the habit of identifying and then not being influenced in one's clinical judgment and clinical management by features of the female patient that are irrelevant in clinical judgment and put clinical judgment at preventable risk of bias if these features are, mistakenly, considered clinically relevant. The financial status or social prominence of a patient is clinically irrelevant. Gregory was concerned that physicians, like many human beings, can be dazzled by great wealth or social prominence and therefore should ignore them.[1,2] The wealthy and the economically disadvantaged female patient should be managed alike. This can be put more generally: the professional virtue of compassion creates the prima facie ethical obligation to prevent the source of payment for the female patient from biasing clinical judgment about the diagnosis of the female patient's condition and its clinical management. The same is true for race, nationality, language spoken, and other social factors when they are clinically irrelevant.

2.2.2.5 The Professional Virtue of Self-Sacrifice in Professional Ethics in Gynecology

The professional virtue of self-sacrifice creates the prima facie ethical obligation to take reasonable risks to one's legitimate self-interest in the care of the female patient. Implementing this virtue requires the physician to distinguish between legitimate self-interest and mere self-interest. (See Chapter 5.) Legitimate self-interests align with the health-related interests of the patient and include the necessary conditions for professionally responsible clinical practice and research, such as rest and time for continuing medical education, and the necessary conditions for life–work balance.

Risking mere self-interest should become routine. Risking legitimate self-interest without limit, however, can become the vice of recklessness. A woman who has experienced sexual assault in her past may react physically to a vaginal examination, as an effect of posttraumatic stress disorder. Her response may escalate, despite the gynecologist's best efforts to mitigate her reaction. This response may include striking out at the gynecologist, perhaps involuntarily, or other decompensation. Recognition of the legitimate limits of the professional virtue of self-sacrifice should trigger implementation of a protocol for the management of a decompensating patient, which should include training for the gynecologist and other team members to deescalate the situation and to seek psychiatric input when needed.

The professional virtue of self-sacrifice becomes essential for the professionally responsible management of conflicts of interest, i.e., conflicts between ethical obligations to patients or research subjects, on the one hand, and legitimate self-interests, on the other hand. Where to set justified limits on group or guild self-sacrifice, e.g., in the business model of a group practice, requires well-reasoned ethical analysis and argument. (See Chapter 5.)

Conflicts of interest differ from – but are often conflated with – conflicts of commitment. Conflicts of commitment exist when the physician's ethical obligations to patients or research subjects become incompatible with the physician's ethical obligations to other people in his or her life, especially family members. Self-sacrifice can justifiably require abandoning self-interest, sometimes to a considerable degree. Self-sacrifice of commitments to people other than patients or research subjects requires strong justification, because these others may not agree to release the physician from ethical obligations to them. The "work–life balance" should be understood not just in terms of conflicts of interest but also conflicts of commitment, which is why judgments and organizational policies about work–life balance become so challenging. (See Chapter 5.)

2.2.3 Ethical Principles in Professional Ethics in Gynecology

2.2.3.1 The Ethical Principle of Beneficence in Professional Ethics in Gynecology

The ethical principle of beneficence in professional ethics in gynecology creates the prima facie ethical obligation of the gynecologist to provide clinical management that in deliberative (evidence-based, rigorous, transparent, and accountable) clinical judgment is predicted to result in net clinical benefit for the female patient and therefore protect and promote her health-related interests. The strength of the obligation varies directly with the strength of the evidence.

2.2.3.2 The Concept of a Medically Reasonable Alternative

The concept of a medically reasonable alternative in professional ethics in gynecology is beneficence based. A form of clinical management is to be classified as medically reasonable when two conditions are met: a form of clinical management is technically possible and supported in deliberative, beneficence-based clinical judgment. We cannot emphasize enough that both conditions, and not just the first, must be satisfied.

2.2.3.3 The Ethical Principle of Nonmaleficence in Professional Ethics in Gynecology

The ethical principle of nonmaleficence in professional ethics in gynecology sets the limiting condition on the ethical principle of beneficence. When the evidence for a medically reasonable alternative becomes weak, the gynecologist must become alert to the increasing strength of the prediction that net clinical harm could be the outcome, e.g., another round of chemotherapy for a gynecologic cancer that stopped responding to previous rounds. There is a prima facie nonmaleficence-based ethical obligation to prevent the net harmful outcomes of overtreatment, i.e., treatment that does not result in net balance of clinical good over harms but a net balance of clinical harms over clinical goods. In such clinical circumstances, this ethical obligation is fulfilled by identifying other medically reasonable alternatives with a stronger evidence base. Sometimes the only medically reasonable alternative for the clinical management of end-stage disease is hospice and palliative care. (See Chapter 15.)

2.2.3.4 The Ethical Principle of Respect for Autonomy in Professional Ethics in Gynecology

Beneficence creates the prima facie ethical obligation to identify the medically reasonable alternatives for the clinical management of the patient's condition. The ethical principle of respect for autonomy in professional ethics in gynecology creates the prima facie ethical obligation to empower the female patient to make informed and voluntary decisions about the management of her clinical condition by providing her with information about the medically reasonable alternatives for its clinical management. A patient's decision is informed when she has an adequate understanding of the nature of her condition, the medically reasonable alternatives for its clinical management, the strength of evidence supporting the clinical judgment of medical reasonableness, and the nature and probability of the clinical benefits and risks of each medically reasonable alternative. When patients indicate the need for support in processing this information or seem to be challenged by this task, e.g., because of complex cognitive or affective demands, the ethical principle of respect for autonomy creates the ethical obligation to empower the female patient by offering psychosocial support. A patient's decision making is voluntary when it is not controlled by internal or external controlling influences.[4,5] The physician should be alert to such influences and act to blunt them.

2.2.3.5 The Ethical Principle of Healthcare Justice in Professional Ethics in Gynecology

The ethical principle of healthcare justice in professional ethics in gynecology applies to populations of female patients and creates the prima facie ethical obligation of the gynecologist to see to it that each female patient is provided medically reasonable clinical management of her condition. Patients are equal with respect to a shared condition and unequal when their conditions differ. For example, the time required to explain that the results of a Pap smear are normal will be less than the time required to explain the finding of atypical squamous cells of undetermined clinical significance. This unequal difference in time allocated does not violate healthcare justice; indeed this inequality is required by the ethical principle of healthcare justice.

2.3 Professional Virtues and Ethical Principles in Professional Ethics in Obstetrics

A pregnant woman becomes a pregnant patient when she is presented to an obstetrician (or other healthcare professional) and there exist forms of clinical management that are reliably predicted to result in net clinical benefit for her and for the fetal patient, when the fetus is a patient. A pregnant woman can present herself to an obstetrician or she can be presented by others, e.g., by emergency medical personnel who have been summoned to bring her to the emergency department because she collapsed at work and is in premature labor. In short, becoming a pregnant patient is a beneficence-based concept that does not include consent as an essential component. Being a pregnant patient does not originate in her autonomy. Adult pregnant patients have autonomy, which originates in autonomy-based ethical obligations to them.

Obstetrics is a unique medical specialty because the fetus can sometimes become a patient. The concept of the fetus as a patient is addressed in detail in Section 2.4. A live-born infant becomes a neonatal patient when the infant is born in the presence of an obstetrician or other healthcare professional. In the professional ethics of obstetrics, the obstetrician has ethical obligations not only to the pregnant patient and to the fetal patient (when the fetus is a patient) but also to the future neonatal patient, which will also be addressed in Section 2.6.

2.3.1 The Five Professional Virtues in Professional Ethics in Obstetrics

2.3.1.1 The Professional Virtue of Integrity in Professional Ethics in Obstetrics

The bedrock professional virtue is professional integrity. As explained in Chapter 1, the ethical concept of medicine as a profession provides the basis for both intellectual integrity and moral integrity and their integration. Intellectual integrity is achieved by making the life-long commitment to becoming and remaining scientifically and clinically competent in the care of the pregnant and the fetal patient. Moral integrity is achieved by making the life-long commitment to the priority of protecting and promoting the health-related interests of pregnant, fetal, and neonatal patients and to the systematically secondary status of individual self-interest and group or guild self-interest. Living out these three commitments of the ethical concept of medicine as a profession makes the pursuit of excellence in service to biomedical science and in the care of pregnant, fetal, and future neonatal patients central in the professional life of the obstetrician. Only the experience of excellence possesses the capacity to sustain obstetricians throughout their practice lives, especially when pregnancy has outcomes such as in utero fetal demise or stillbirth. The professional virtue of integrity creates the strong prima facie ethical obligation to practice and live by and not to compromise the commitment to the ethical concept of medicine as a profession. The burden of proof for defeating this ethical obligation is very steep, perhaps insurmountable, because without professional integrity there is no profession of medicine.

2.3.1.2 The Professional Virtue of Humility in Professional Ethics in Obstetrics

An important corollary of the professional virtue of integrity, related especially to intellectual integrity, is the professional virtue of humility: the habit of recognizing the limits of one's ethical judgments and working persistently to improve them. As explained in the previous chapter, a key component of humility is what Gregory called "candor" or being "open" to new evidence from whatever source it may come, including pregnant patients, and changing one's mind depending on the strength of the evidence.[1] Without candor, it is impossible to develop the professional virtue of humility. Coulehan has pointed out that "humility requires toughness and emotional resilience," not "weakness of self-abnegation."[3, p. 201]

2.3.1.3 The Professional Virtue of Compassion in Professional Ethics in Obstetrics

The professional virtue of compassion creates a two-step prima facie ethical obligation. The first step is to recognize when a pregnant patient experiences pain, distress, or suffering or is at risk of doing so, as required by the first commitment of the ethical concept of medicine as a profession. The second step is to act promptly to effectively clinically manage or prevent pain, distress, or suffering, as required by the second and third commitments of the ethical concept of medicine as a profession. Pain is the report in the central nervous system of tissue damage or perhaps threat of tissue damage accompanied by awareness. Distress is the experience of disruption of one's behavioral repertoire. Suffering is the experience of one's aims and intentions for current or future well-being becoming blocked or impeded to some degree. One can be in pain without being in distress or suffering, although pain can cause either or both. One can be in distress without being in pain or suffering, although distress can cause suffering. One can be suffering without being in pain or distress. The phrase "mental pain" is used imprecisely to mean suffering or being in pain and suffering. Precision of thought and speech requires not using the phrase "mental pain." A woman whose pregnancy has resulted from rape or incest should be considered to be at high risk for distress and suffering, which requires that the plan of care include management of this risk, e.g., by including a mental health professional on the care team.

2.3.1.4 The Professional Virtue of Self-Effacement in Professional Ethics in Obstetrics

Self-effacement designates the habit of identifying and then not being influenced in one's clinical judgment and clinical management by features of the pregnant patient that are irrelevant in clinical judgment and put clinical judgment at preventable risk of bias if these features are, mistakenly, considered clinically relevant. The financial status or social prominence of a patient is clinically irrelevant. Gregory was concerned that physicians, like many human beings, can be dazzled by great wealth or social prominence and therefore should ignore them. The wealthy and the economically disadvantaged pregnant patient should be managed alike. This can be put more generally: the source of payment for the pregnant patient should never influence and therefore bias clinical judgment about the diagnosis of the pregnant patient's condition and its clinical management. This is an especially important consideration as the percentage of pregnant patients covered by Medicaid (the federal–state program for the medically indigent) continues to increase.

2.3.1.5 The Professional Virtue of Self-Sacrifice in Professional Ethics in Obstetrics

The professional virtue of self-sacrifice creates the prima facie ethical obligation to take reasonable risks to one's legitimate self-interest in the care of the pregnant patient. Implementing this virtue requires the physician to distinguish between legitimate self-interest and mere self-interest. (See Chapter 5.) Legitimate self-interests should align with the health-related interests of pregnant, fetal, and neonatal patients and include the necessary conditions for professionally responsible clinical practice and research, such as rest and time for continuing medical education, and the necessary conditions for work–life balance.

Risking mere self-interest should become routine. Risking legitimate self-interest without limit, however, can become the vice of recklessness. Obstetrician-gynecologists who provide termination of pregnancy services have been publicly exposed, their homes have been picketed, and some have been violently – and in rare cases, lethally – assaulted. The professional virtue of self-sacrifice does not require unlimited exposure to personal risk to safety and life.

The professional virtue of self-sacrifice becomes essential for the professionally responsible management of conflicts of interest, i.e., conflicts between ethical obligations to patients or research subjects, on the one hand, and legitimate self-interests, on the other hand. Where to set justified limits on group self-sacrifice, e.g., in the business model of a group practice, requires very well-reasoned ethical analysis and argument. (See Chapter 5.)

Conflicts of interest differ from – but are often conflated with – conflicts of commitment. Conflicts of commitment exist when the physician's ethical obligations to patients or research subjects become incompatible with the physician's ethical obligations to other people in his or her life, especially family members. Self-sacrifice can justifiably require abandoning self-interest, sometimes to a considerable degree. Self-sacrifice of commitments to people other than patients or research subjects requires strong justification, because these others may not agree to release the physician from ethical obligations to them. The "work–life balance" should be understood not just in terms of conflicts of interest but also conflicts of commitment, which is why judgments and organizational policies about work–life balance become so challenging. (See Chapter 5.)

The concepts of conflicts of interest and conflicts of commitment should guide obstetrician-gynecologists in asserting conscientious objection. Because of the importance and complexity of this topic in the professional ethics of obstetrics and gynecology, we will address it separately in Chapter 5.

2.3.2 Ethical Principles in Professional Ethics in Obstetrics

2.3.2.1 The Ethical Principle of Beneficence in Professional Ethics in Obstetrics

The ethical principle of beneficence in professional ethics in obstetrics creates the prima facie ethical obligation of the obstetrician to provide clinical management that in deliberative clinical judgment is predicted to result in net clinical benefit for the pregnant patient and fetal patient (when the fetus is a patient) and to the future neonatal patient and therefore protect and promote their health-related interests. The strength of the obligation varies directly with the strength of the evidence.

2.3.2.2 The Concept of a Medically Reasonable Alternative

The concept of a medically reasonable alternative in professional ethics in obstetrics is beneficence based. A form of clinical management is to be classified as medically reasonable when each of two conditions is met: a form of clinical management is technically possible and supported in deliberative, beneficence-based clinical judgment. We cannot emphasize enough that both conditions, and not just the first, must be satisfied. Because the concept of a medically reasonable alternative is beneficence based in obstetrics it must take account of beneficence-based ethical obligations to both the pregnant patient and the fetal patient, when the fetus is a patient.

2.3.2.3 The Ethical Principle of Nonmaleficence in Professional Ethics in Obstetrics

The ethical principle of nonmaleficence in professional ethics in obstetrics sets the limiting condition on the ethical principle of beneficence. When the evidence for a medically reasonable alternative becomes weak, the obstetrician must become alert to the corresponding weakness of the prediction that net clinical benefit could be the outcome, e.g., not recommending cesarean delivery at the first indication of deceleration of fetal heart rate. There is a strong non-maleficence-based prima facie ethical obligation to prevent the net harmful outcomes for pregnant, fetal, and neonatal patients of unnecessary cesarean delivery for the current and future pregnancies. This obligation is fulfilled by recalling immediately to mind that the burden of proof is on recommending cesarean delivery, which burden is met by adhering to the discipline of intrapartum management based on deliberative clinical judgment. (See Chapter 12.)

2.3.2.4 The Ethical Principle of Respect for Autonomy in Professional Ethics in Obstetrics

Beneficence creates the prima facie ethical obligation to identify the medically reasonable alternatives for the clinical management of pregnancy and its maternal and fetal complications. The ethical principle of respect for autonomy in professional ethics in obstetrics creates the prima facie ethical obligation to empower the pregnant patient to make informed and voluntary decisions about the management of her pregnancy by providing her with information about the medically reasonable alternatives for its clinical management. A patient's decision is informed when she has an adequate understanding of the clinical condition of her pregnancy, the medically reasonable alternatives for its clinical management, the strength of evidence supporting the clinical judgment of medical reasonableness, and the nature and probability of the clinical benefits and risks of each medically reasonable alternative. When pregnant patients indicate the need for support in processing this information or seem to be challenged by this task, e.g., because of complex cognitive demands, the ethical principle of respect for autonomy creates the ethical obligation to offer the female patient psychosocial support. A patient's decision making is voluntary when it is not controlled by internal or external controlling influences.[4,5] The physician should be alert to such influences and act to blunt them. As explained in Chapter 3, sometimes the obstetrician has the autonomy-based ethical obligation to prevent family members, however well-meaning, from trying to usurp the voluntariness of the pregnant woman's decision-making processes.

2.3.2.5 The Ethical Principle of Healthcare Justice in Professional Ethics in Obstetrics

The ethical principle of healthcare justice applies to populations of pregnant, fetal, and neonatal patients and creates the prima facie ethical obligation of the physician to see to it that each pregnant patient and fetal patient is provided medically reasonable clinical management of their condition. Patients are equal with respect to a shared condition and are unequal when their conditions differ. For example, the time

Table 2.1 Ethical concept of the fetus as a patient.

Prima facie ethical obligations of the obstetrician-gynecologist	Patient	Nature of Obligation
Beneficence-based	Pregnant woman	Protect and promote health-related interests subject to the limit of her taking only reasonable risks to herself in current and future pregnancies
Autonomy-based	Pregnant woman	Empower her to make informed decisions about obstetric management
Beneficence-based	Fetus	Protect and promote health-related interests subject to the limit of the pregnant patient taking only reasonable risks to herself in current and future pregnancies
Prima facie ethical obligations of the pregnant woman		
Beneficence-based	Fetus	Protect and promote health-related interests subject to the limit of pregnant patient taking only reasonable risks to herself in current and future pregnancies

required to explain that a second-trimester ultrasound examination has detected no fetal anomalies will be less than the time required to explain a new diagnosis of clinically significant increased blood flow in the cerebral arteries of the fetus. This unequal difference in time allocated does not violate healthcare justice; indeed it is required by the ethical principle of healthcare justice.

2.4 The Ethical Concept of the Fetus as a Patient

2.4.1 Five Decades of the Discourse of the Fetus as a Patient

The discourse of the "fetal patient" and of the "fetus as a patient" (see Table 2.1) entered the medical literature as early as the early 1970s, when A. W. Liley referred to the fetus as a "personality."[6] A year earlier the editors of the 14th edition of *Williams Obstetrics* wrote: "Since World War II and especially in the last decade, knowledge of the fetus and his environment has increased remarkably. As an important consequence, the fetus has acquired the status as a patient to be cared for by the physician as he has long been accustomed to caring for the mother."[7, p. 199]

This emergence of the discourse of the fetus as a patient coincided with advances in fetal diagnosis, including ultrasound imaging and karyotyping, and the first efforts of direct fetal intervention in the form of experiments to treat the fetus by administering drugs to the pregnant woman, administering drugs to the fetus directly, and by direct intervention. These early efforts created the possibility that "prenatal diagnosis of a fetal malformation may now lead to treatment rather than abortion."[8, p. 777] Michael Harrison and colleagues extended this thinking directly into the realm of professional ethics in obstetrics when they wrote: "Our ability to diagnose fetal birth defects has achieved considerable sophistication. Treatment of several fetal diagnoses has proved feasible, and treatment of more complicated lesions will undoubtedly expand as techniques for fetal intervention improve. It seems likely that the fetus with a treatable birth defect is on the threshold of becoming a patient."[8, p. 777] Within a decade Harrison and N. Scott Adzick published a review entitled "The fetus as a patient."[9]

In the same issue of the *Journal of the American Medical Association* in which the paper by Harrison and colleagues appeared, John Fletcher (1931–2004), one of the founders of the field of bioethics, identified ethical issues that potential advances in maternal–fetal intervention create. These include how to balance the interests of the fetus with those of the pregnant woman, the potential conflict between treating the fetus with an anomaly and inducing abortion of the very same fetus, an ethical framework to guide clinical investigation, and setting priorities for federal and other funding of such investigation.[10] Michael Harrison, Mitchell Golbus, and Roy Filly's *The Unborn Patient* appeared shortly thereafter.[11]

This discourse of the fetal patient appears in the most current edition of *Williams Obstetrics* that makes it clear that the scope of obstetric practice includes "our second patient – the fetus."[12] This standard reference work for the specialty now includes a section entitled "The Fetal Patient," comprising eight chapters, ranging from prenatal diagnosis to fetal assessment and therapy.[13] The International Academy of Perinatal Medicine has an important affiliated society, The International Society of the Fetus as a Patient, which sponsors a scientific congress annually.[14]

Other publications in obstetrics and maternal–fetal medicine explicitly adopt the discourse of the fetal patient.[15–18] Other specialties have adopted the discourse of the fetus as a patient. The new subspecialties of fetal anesthesia and fetal imaging are illustrative. Regarding the former, consider: "Fetal surgery presents unique challenges in that there is the welfare of two patients to consider. Access to the fetal patient can be problematic, and consideration must be given to placental site, tocolysis, drug administration, and fetal monitoring."[19, p. 12] Regarding the latter, consider: "Knowledge of all fetal MRI possibilities and limitations by fetal medical specialists will allow its proper use and as a consequence can definitely optimize care of fetal patients."[20, p. 580] Leading outlets in the lay press have adopted this discourse.[21]

The five-decade discourse of the fetus as a patient, developing from fetus as a "personality" to the fetus as a "patient," to characterize the fetus has appealed to the notion that a change in status had occurred because of new interventions for fetal benefit had become clinical realities, e.g., intrauterine transfusion for the clinical management of Rh isoimmunization, or experiments to treat fetal malformations in utero. The discourse of the fetus as a patient has appealed implicitly to two ideas. The first was that invasive intervention for fetal benefit has become a clinical reality, e.g., intrauterine transfusion for the clinical management of Rh isoimmunization. The second was that surgical intervention for fetal benefit had begun to be investigated and promised to become an alternative to termination of pregnancy, as Harrison and colleagues noted.[8] In the mid-1980s two of us (FAC and LBM) presented the first explicit, practical, ethically reasoned account of the ethical concept of the fetus as a patient, based on prima facie beneficence-based ethical obligations to the pregnant and fetal patient and autonomy-based ethical obligations to the pregnant patient.[22]

2.4.2 A Preliminary: The Ethical Concept of Moral Status

The key to understanding this concept is the philosophical concept of moral status and its subconcepts of independent moral status and dependent moral status. As a preliminary to explicating the ethical concept of the fetus as a patient, we therefore need to explain the ethical concept of moral status. "Moral status" means that others have an ethical obligation to protect and promote the interests of an entity.[5] Moral status can originate in properties of an entity that it possesses independently of all other entities and that create the ethical obligation to protect and promote its interests. This is known as *independent moral status*. Moral status can also originate in a social role created by human beings, especially to protect human beings vulnerable to the power of others over them. This is known as *dependent moral status* because it depends on the creation and maintenance of social roles. There is no necessity to create such social roles, which are defined by the ethical obligations to entities reliably judged to occupy a specific social role. This stands in strong contrast to independent moral status, which necessarily creates ethical obligations to entities with such status.

2.4.2.1 Dominance of Independent Moral Status in Medical Ethics and Bioethics

In the medical ethics and bioethics literature, the concept of independent moral status dominates, reflecting the dominance of the concept in the literature of moral philosophy. This dominance can sometimes be taken for granted, especially in the quest for certainty about moral status.

The purpose of the concept of independent moral status becomes clear when we examine its history. This concept emerged during the various national enlightenments of the eighteenth century, especially the German and French national enlightenments.[23] The goal was to replace the concept that, as God's creation, each human being has moral status independent of the monarch or, more generally, the state. Such moral status is required to prevent the abuse of state power by those subject to it. Inasmuch as God transcends monarchs and modern states, being one of God's creatures creates the moral equality of individuals and those who claim state power over them. The dependent moral status of being one of God's creatures was very powerful indeed. The new concept of independent moral status had to be just as powerful. The version put forward by the German enlightenment philosopher, Immanuel Kant (1724–1804) fulfilled this goal. According to Kant, each person must be treated as a member of the "kingdom of ends" (which replaced the "kingdom of God"), which means that no person can be treated as a means merely, i.e., used for the purposes of others without consent. Kantian persons are no longer subjects of the monarch or the state but are independent and free.[24]

2.4.2.2 Problems with the Concept of Independent Moral Status

So powerful has the concept of independent moral status become, especially in the literature of bioethics, that its proponents fail to acknowledge persistent, considerable, and irresolvable disagreement about the properties that originate independent moral status. The austere Kantian account, that independent moral status originates in the capacity for rational self-consciousness, is not compatible with the view that independent moral status emerges from the capacity for consciousness or in the capacity to experience pain. No single philosophical method has emerged in the more than two centuries since Kant that resolved these differences in favor of *the* metaphysical account of independent moral status.

There is a further problem: each account of independent moral status fails to be clinically comprehensive because each leaves out many groups of patients. The Kantian account, for example, leaves out neonatal patients, patients with advanced dementias, patients with severe cognitive disabilities, and perhaps patients with severe mental disorders and diseases. These patients do not exhibit rational self-consciousness. There is no agreement in the bioethics literature about whether this outcome should be considered morally problematic and, if it is, how to manage it in a philosophically persuasive way. Professional ethics in obstetrics and gynecology and professional ethics in medicine both require a clinically comprehensive concept of moral status.

The invocation of independent moral status should not be taken for granted, because it has serious philosophical problems that its advocates have not been able to resolve. The quest for certainty, to which advocates of independent moral status are necessarily committed, has failed. The dominance of the concept of independent moral status in medical ethics and bioethics is therefore not philosophically or clinically justified. The alternative of dependent moral status therefore cannot be dismissed out-of-hand as philosophically unpersuasive.

2.4.3 The Ethical Concept of the Fetus as a Patient

The strongest point of differentiation of professional ethics in obstetrics from medical ethics and bioethics is the ethical concept of the fetus as a patient. As explained in Chapter 1, a living human being becomes a patient when that individual is presented to a physician or other healthcare professional and there exist forms of clinical management that in deliberative clinical judgment are predicted to result in net clinical benefit. A fetus becomes a patient when the fetus is presented to a physician or other healthcare professional and there exist forms of clinical management that in deliberative clinical judgment are predicted to result in net clinical benefit for the fetus. Understanding when the fetus should be considered "presented" to a physician or other healthcare professional is essential to understanding the ethical concept of the fetus as a patient. Whether the fetus is viable or not is the key, as explained in Section 2.4.3.1.

Being a patient is thus a function of the social role created by physicians committing themselves to the ethical concept of medicine as a profession and the existence of various forms of clinical management that have an evidence base of safety and effectiveness. Safety is oriented to the present: preventing unacceptable adverse events in the processes of patient care. The effectiveness of clinical management is understood in terms of the future, the predicted outcome of net balance of clinical goods over clinical harms. The general ethical concept of being a patient is thus beneficence based because this is the ethical principle that captures the ethical significance of clinical outcomes.

The ethical concept of the fetus as a patient is also future oriented: the outcomes for the child the fetus can become as a result of clinical management undertaken for fetal and therefore neonatal benefit. The fetus becomes a patient when there are reliable links between a fetus in the present and the neonatal patient it can later become.

When the fetus is a patient, the obstetrician has three prima facie ethical obligations, all of which in all clinical cases must be considered. The implications of the ethical principle of beneficence in professional ethics in

Table 2.2 When is the fetus a patient?

Previable	When the pregnant woman confers the moral status of being a patient and is presented for obstetric care
Viable	When the pregnant woman is presented for obstetric care

obstetrics and the ethical principle of respect for autonomy in professional ethics in obstetrics must be identified and balanced when not compatible. The obstetrician has prima facie beneficence-based and autonomy-based ethical obligations to the pregnant patient and prima facie beneficence-based obligations to the fetal patient. That all three ethical obligations are prima facie means that none automatically takes precedence over the other two. When these three obligations become incompatible, which, we emphasize, is rare, deliberative clinical judgment and ethical reasoning are required to reach an evidence-based and argument-based judgment about which obligation(s) should take precedence.

2.4.3.1 The Viable Fetus as a Patient

A fetus should be considered viable when its biological development permits survival ex utero with whatever level of technological support is required to prevent death, which supports a reliable prediction of live birth. It is a clinical and philosophical error to understand the concept of viability in solely biological terms; viability is a function of both a biological development and available technical capacity. When the fetus has become viable and when the pregnant woman is presented to a physician or other healthcare professional, there exist forms of clinical management that are reliably predicted to benefit the fetus and the child it can become because the fetus can survive to receive these benefits. (See Table 2.2.) Inasmuch as the technological capacity to prevent perinatal death differs among high-income, moderate-income, and low-income countries there is no single international gestational-age standard for viability, although the gestational-age range (23–24 weeks) applies in high-income countries.[25–28] This gestational age range may be considered ideal in healthcare-justice–based advocacy for increased healthcare funding for perinatal medicine. (See Chapter 18.) Viability at this gestational age range may be modified by such factors as multiple pregnancy, fetal sex, administration of steroids, and estimated fetal weight[29,30] given the limits of their application in obstetric clinical judgment.[31]

2.4.3.2 The Periviable Fetus as a Patient

The periviable fetus (see Chapter 11) may be considered a patient when deliberative clinical judgment supports a reliable prediction of live birth and survival with neonatal critical care.[25–28] Obstetricians and neonatologists should investigate whether such factors as birthweight, sex, singleton versus multiple pregnancy, and administration of steroids justify specification of previability into more precisely defined subpopulations.

2.4.3.3 The Previable Fetus as a Patient

The previable fetus (see Chapter 11) cannot survive ex utero even with the most advanced technological support.[25–28] This outcome results from biological immaturity for which current neonatal technology cannot compensate. The only link between a previable fetus and surviving to viability is the pregnant woman's decision to continue her pregnancy to viability, at which time her fetus becomes a patient, as explained in Section 2.4.3. (See Table 2.2.) The pregnant woman's right to make this decision is grounded in her autonomy. The pregnant woman may therefore take the view that the moral status of the fetus is so strong, e.g., as a matter of religious conviction, that she has an ethical obligation to continue her pregnancy. Other women may not share this view. The pluralism of claims in moral theology and in moral philosophy about the moral status of the fetus and the utter absence of a single authoritative method for identifying *the* correct account mean that no one – partner, spouse, family member, religious or spiritual advisor, or obstetrician – can decide for her what the moral status of her fetus is. She is therefore free to confer, withhold, or having once conferred withdraw, the moral status of being a patient on or from her fetus before viability.

2.4.3.4 The Obstetrician's Prima Facie Beneficence-Based Obligations to the Fetal Patient

The obstetrician has prima facie the beneficence-based ethical obligation to the fetal patient to identify and provide clinical management that is medically reasonable. In gynecology, this concept makes references only to the outcomes of clinical management of the female patient, as we saw in Section 2.2.1. In obstetrics, the concept becomes complicated by an implacable clinical reality: access to the fetus is available only through the pregnant patient's body. In making a clinical ethical judgment about the outcomes of clinical management for fetal benefit, the obstetrician must take account of the ethical implications of this implacable clinical ethical reality: prima facie beneficence-based and prime facie autonomy-based ethical obligations to the pregnant patient. All three ethical obligations must always be taken into account and balanced in ethically well-reasoned clinical ethical judgment. Because all three obligations are prima facie it is a clinical and philosophical error in ethical reasoning to treat any one of them as absolute, i.e., having automatic priority over the others or functioning as a default position that must be defeated by overwhelmingly convincing ethical reasoning. Clinical management for fetal benefit becomes medically reasonable if and only if there is an evidence base of (1) net clinical benefit for the fetal patient, (2) future child it can become, and (3) not-greater-than reasonable risk to the pregnant patient in her current and future pregnancies.

2.4.3.5 Limits on Prima Facie Beneficence-Based Obligations to the Pregnant Patient

The prima facie nature of the beneficence-based ethical obligation to the pregnant patient has an important implication: to protect and promote her own legitimate interests in her own life and health, her prima facie beneficence-based obligation to her fetus is to take only reasonable risks to her life and health. The judgment about what is "reasonable" is, in part, a clinical judgment concerning the probability of serious, far-reaching, and irreversible clinical harm to her in her current and future pregnancies and the probability for fetal benefit. In beneficence-based clinical judgment, there are three perspectives on such risk. When the probability of harm to the pregnant patient from intervention is high and the probability of harm from nonintervention to the fetal patient is low, the risks to her should be considered unreasonable by the obstetrician. When the probability of harm to the pregnant patient from intervention is low and the probability of harm to the fetal patient from nonintervention is high, these risks should be considered reasonable. When the probabilities are similar, a more nuanced clinical judgment is required and should be explained to the pregnant patient. The obstetrician has an autonomy-based ethical obligation to the pregnant patient to explain this crucial limitation on the risks she should be willing to take, especially as a preventive ethics response to women who think, mistakenly, that there are no justified limits on the risk that they should take to their own life and health for fetal benefit.

2.4.3.6 Enforcement of Prima Facie Beneficence-Based Ethical Obligations to the Fetal Patient

The prima facie beneficence-based ethical obligations of the obstetrician to the fetal patient do not differ from prima facie beneficence-based ethical obligations to any patient: to protect its life and health. It does *not* follow from the existence of prima facie ethical obligations to the fetal patient that the obstetrician, hospital, or legal authorities automatically have ethical justification to enforce these obligations. This is because the ethics of enforcing obligations to patients requires attention to additional, different ethical concepts and their implications that are independent of prima facie beneficence-based ethical obligation to a patient.

Such additional ethical concepts apply to the ethical justification of enforcement by a physician, e.g., threatening to contact hospital or even legal authorities. There is the prima facie nonmaleficence-based ethical obligation of every physician not to cause serious, far-reaching, and irreversible psychosocial harm to patients, including a pregnant woman's loss of trust in her own obstetrician and perhaps all healthcare professionals, which enforcement of ethical obligations risks. This nonmaleficence-based ethical obligation rises to the status of a prohibition when enforcement is in deliberative clinical judgment reliably predicted to be ineffective. In such circumstances it should be assumed that net psychosocial harm will ensue.

The use of state power to enforce prima facie beneficence-based ethical obligations also appeals to additional considerations. These include whether the legal enforcement is reliably predicted, based on past experience and expert judgment, to be effective. Even if effective, enforcement risks promoting disrespect for the law, an unacceptable outcome in a society that secures the security and freedom of its members by maintaining the rule of law. The possibility that civil courts might prohibit legal enforcement must also be considered.

This examination of the ethical justification of enforcing prima facie beneficence-based ethical obligations has a very important implication: Showing that there is no ethical justification for such enforcement does not show that the prima facie beneficence-based ethical obligation does not exist. This invalid line of reasoning often takes the following form: We would not force a patient do so X; therefore she has no ethical obligation to do X. This invalid reasoning has no place in professional ethics in obstetrics.

2.5 Advantages of the Ethical Concept of the Fetus as a Patient

2.5.1 The Ethical Concept of the Fetus as a Patient Avoids the Philosophical and Clinical Paralysis of "Right to Life"

In the professional ethics of obstetrics, the concept of a right, a justified claim to be treated in a specific fashion, does not apply to the fetal patient but only to the pregnant patient. In particular, the discourse of "right to life" of the fetus does not apply. The main reason is that beneficence-based ethical reasoning is not rights-based; it is based on the clinical ethical assessment of predictable outcomes and their evidence base. The discourse of rights fundamentally and impermissibly distorts the discourse of beneficence, twisting it into the discourse of independent moral status. Independent moral status, to be sure, provides the needed foundation for rights but is not relevant to the ethical concept of being a patient generally and the ethical concept of the fetus as a patient, specifically.

There is a further, unacceptable problem with the discourse of the right to life: failure to be clear at the stage of ethical analysis in ethical reasoning. To explain this problem, we need to distinguish four types of rights, based on the distinction between a negative right – the right to noninterference with one's decisions and behaviors – and a positive right – to the time, energy, and resources of others to advance one's interests. There can be prima facie negative right and absolute negative rights. There can be prima facie positive rights. Absolute positive rights are difficult to countenance because no one has the right to exhaust the resources of others and thus cause them serious, far-reaching, and irreversible harm with no offsetting benefit, which is ethically impermissible under the general ethical principle of nonmaleficence.

To use "right to life" with precision therefore requires the user to recognize that "right to life" invokes four distinct rights: the prima facie negative right not to be killed; the absolute negative right not to be killed; the prima facie positive right to the resources of others to advance one's own interest in continuing to live; and the absolute positive right to the resources of others to advance one's own interest in continuing to live. The latter is a theoretical right only, given the analysis just above of absolute positive rights. The discourse of "right to life" usually fails to provide ethical reasoning to explain the origin, i.e., independent moral status of the fetus, of the specific right invoked and its implications. The result is philosophical and clinical paralysis that makes the discourse of "right to life" irrelevant to professional ethics in obstetrics.

2.5.2 The Ethical Concept of the Fetus as a Patient Avoids Reducing Moral Status to Independent Moral Status

Contemporary moral philosophy is deeply shaped by the view that the only moral status that matters is independent moral status, as explained in Section 2.4.2.2. The philosopher Mary Ann Warren captures this point of view when she writes:

> Ascriptions of moral status serve to represent very general claims about the ways in which moral agents ought to conduct themselves toward entities of particular sorts. Thus, one important feature of the concept of moral status is its generality. Moral status is usually ascribed to members of a group, rather than merely to specific individuals. Moreover, it is usually ascribed on the basis of some property or properties that are thought to be possessed by all or most group members.[32]

Carson Strong builds on this account to claim that when we invoke "dependent moral status" we "misapply the concept of moral status."[33, p. 52] This claim makes sense only on the unquestioned assumption that the only kind of moral status is independent moral status. That this equation is commonly made is evidenced in the subtle but unargued conflation of moral status and personhood, i.e., possession of independent moral status: "There is no need to consider fetuses as independent patients or patients in their own right (i.e., apart from the patients in whom they develop) unless their status as patients is determined on the grounds that they are persons who therefore have an independent moral status."[34]

To be sure, this assumption is deeply ingrained in contemporary moral philosophy. This is not the case for the history of moral philosophy, e.g., Confucius's concept of filial piety based on the moral status of the relationship between father and son, a form of dependent moral status described in Chapter 1. The assumption that independent moral status is the only valid form of moral status does not withstand historical scrutiny. Furthermore, given the serious metaphysical difficulties and profound disagreement about the properties an entity must possess in order to generate independent moral status, as described in Section 2.4.2.2, the assumption that independent moral status is the only valid form of moral status does not withstand close philosophical scrutiny.

The ethical concept of the fetus as a patient well withstands historical scrutiny. The ethical concept of dependent moral status has a long history in the global history of moral philosophy that seeks reliability, not certainty, from Confucius to Hume and the Scottish moral scientists whose work profoundly influenced Gregory and Thomas Percival (1740–1804) (See Chapter 1). The ethical concept of the fetus as a patient also withstands philosophical scrutiny because it need not invoke endlessly contended metaphysical concepts such as being a person that, as we explained in Section 2.4.2.2, are disabled by unresolvable lack of agreement on the constitutive properties that make an individual a person. Reducing moral status to independent moral status and the discourse of rights that it generates, known as rights-based reductionism,[35] should be regarded as failed philosophical projects. Invoking contentious metaphysical claims of any kind, furthermore, is alien to clinical reasoning.

2.5.3 The Ethical Concept of the Fetus as a Patient Avoids Rights-Based Absolutism

Right-based absolutism adds to rights-based reductionism the claim that either (1) the pregnant woman's right to control what happens to her body is an absolute right or (2) the fetus has an absolute right to life. Howard Minkoff, Mary Faith Marshall, and Joan Liaschenko[36] defend the view that what they call "negative autonomy" is absolute: "the future interests of a child should not constrain a pregnant woman's negative autonomy (the right to refuse any intervention intended for the putative benefit of the fetus.)"[36, p. 1102] Any interests that a fetus might be thought to have, on the basis of being an unborn child, should never limit the pregnant woman's autonomy, which can be asserted only if one treats autonomy-based rights as absolute. George Annas has held that "the moral and legal primacy of the competent, informed pregnant woman in decision making is overwhelming."[37] Some have advocated to an absolute, autonomy-based right to have a clinically non-indicated cesarean delivery.[38]

The burden of proof to establish the negative absolute rights of the pregnant woman cannot be met because there are two types of negative right in the clinical setting. The first type is the right to refuse treatment coupled with the right to cease being a patient, as occurs when a pregnant woman leaves an obstetrician's practice after refusing to cooperate with prenatal care plans. The second type is the right to refuse treatment coupled with remaining a patient. In effect this creates an accompanying positive right to the pregnant woman's preferred alternative, even if that alternative is not medically reasonable.[39] For example, a pregnant woman may refuse cesarean delivery for well-documented, intrapartum complete placenta previa, in effect exercising a positive right to assistance with vaginal delivery. In such circumstances, vaginal delivery is ethically impermissible under the ethical principle of nonmaleficence in professional ethics in obstetrics and incompatible with the professional virtue of integrity. Such positive rights therefore cannot be understood in professional ethics in obstetrics to create an ethical obligation to implement them. There are ethically justified limits on patient's requests when the request is for clinical management that fails the test of being medically reasonable.

A similar absolutism is asserted but in favor of the fetus' rights. The right to life is claimed as an absolute right by conservative opponents of abortion rights. The view that there is never a justification to cause fetal death entails an absolute positive right of the fetus to continue to be supported in the uterine environment – to use the pregnant woman's body – until natural in utero fetal demise or live birth occurs. The burden of proof to establish this inextricably linked set of absolute rights is very steep, if not impossible, as is the case for all claims for absolute positive rights.

Grant, for the sake of argument only, that the burden of proof for absolute negative rights of the woman and linked absolute negative–positive rights of the fetus can be met. There is a further problem: no single perspective has emerged from which the various theological and philosophical claims about the absolute rights of the fetus and the philosophical claims about the absolute rights of the pregnant woman can be resolved, despite more than two millennia of attempts to do so. The reason is simple: the existence of a perspective that would have authority for all of the world's major religions and fiercely competing philosophical methods in the quest for certainty is inconceivable.

It should come as no surprise therefore that rights-based absolutism has resulted in clinical and ethical gridlock and is doomed to do so forever. The ethical concept of the fetus as a patient avoids this conceptual dead-end because beneficence-based obligations to the fetal patient do not invoke the discourse of rights. Indeed, rights discourse, as noted in Section 2.5.1, distorts beneficence-based ethical reasoning beyond recognition. We cannot emphasize enough that the ethical concept of the fetus does not and need not invoke the discourse of fetal rights. The ethical concept of the fetus as a patient also avoids this conceptual dead-end because autonomy-based ethical obligations to the pregnant woman are all prima facie; none is absolute.

2.5.4 The Fetus Is a Separate Patient: A Failed Critique of the Ethical Concept of the Fetus as a Patient

A prominent critique of the ethical concept of the fetus as a patient is that it implies that the fetus is a separate patient.[34,40] This critique claims that the concept of the fetus as a separate patient encourages "a tendency to ignore the pregnant woman."[34, p. 156] This is because, the critique continues, the ethical concept of the fetus as a separate patient has the implication that the obstetrician's ethical obligations to the fetal patient can be determined solely by reference to the fetal patient, i.e., without taking into account the obstetrician's ethical obligations to the pregnant patient. The critique considers this narrow, fetus-only focus of clinical obstetrics judgment to be unacceptable.

The first step in a critical appraisal of a published position is to undertake scholarly due diligence by providing textual evidence for such alleged implications: do they appear in the texts subject to critique? Critics of the ethical concept of the fetus as a patient often do not acknowledge the need for this step, leaving it uncompleted. This is an egregious violation of the scholarly due diligence requirement in a critical appraisal. The next step in a critical appraisal is governed by argument-based ethical reasoning: an argument to show that the alleged implications are indeed implications of the ethical concept of the fetus as a patient. This step, too, is uncompleted, with the result that the implications are merely asserted, not argued. This is an egregious violation of the intellectual discipline of argument-based ethical reasoning. These two egregious failures have an inescapable consequence for the critique: it should be judged completely irrelevant to the ethical concept of the fetus as a patient. The critique should be dismissed as a failure.

The introduction of the ethical concept of the fetus as a patient more than three decades ago makes clear that the beneficence-based obligations of the obstetrician to the fetal patient are but one chapter in a three-chapter story. The other two chapters, beneficence-based ethical obligations and autonomy-based ethical obligations to the pregnant woman, must also *always* be included.[22] Failure to do so results in conceptual and therefore clinical inadequacy. To insist that the ethical concept of the fetus as a patient implies that the fetus is a separate patient is an egregious misrepresentation if not outright distortion of the ethical concept of the fetus as a patient.

A 2016 statement from Committee on Ethics of the American College of Obstetricians and Gynecologists (ACOG) on refusal of recommended treatment during pregnancy adopts this failed critique of the ethical concept of the fetus as a patient.[41] This statement criticizes the ethical concept of the fetus as a patient on the grounds that it entails that "fetal patients are independent patients with treatment options and decisions separate from those of pregnant women."[41, p. e177] The statement goes on to claim that this is an unacceptable implication: "the pregnant woman and her medical interests, health needs, and rights can become secondary to those of the fetus."[41, p. e177] The statement treats this implication as unacceptable on the grounds that such restrictions on a woman's autonomy are not justified because the obstetrician has only a "beneficence-based motivation towards the fetus."[41, p. e177]

The statement fails to fulfill the requirement of scholarly due diligence in a critical appraisal to provide textual evidence that the ethical concept of the fetus as a patient supports the implication that the fetus is a separate patient. Indeed the textual evidence is to the contrary. The statement also violates argument-based ethical reasoning by appealing to an implicit, i.e., unstated, premise. This is an error in logical reasoning known as the suppressed premise and renders a line of reasoning invalid. This is the suppressed premise: the ethical principle of respect for the pregnant woman's autonomy is the controlling ethical consideration in obstetric ethics. Because this premise is suppressed, no argument is made to justify it.

The statement then compounds this error in logical reasoning. The suppressed premise makes sense if and only if there are no prima facie beneficence-based obligations of the obstetrician to the fetal patient. No argument is made to this effect. Instead, beneficence-based ethical obligations to the fetus are simply transmuted into "beneficence-based motivations."

This sleight of hand masquerading as ethical reasoning commits two egregious methodological errors. The first is an error in ethical reasoning: psychologizing ethical concepts. Psychologizing ethical concepts neuters ethical concepts, because psychological states have no implications for ethically justified decision making and behavior. Psychologizing ethical concepts may appear to be ethical reasoning to the unwary reader. The wary reader appreciates that psychologizing ethical concepts ignores the requirements of argument-based ethical reasoning. The appeal to psychologizing ethical concepts is therefore deceptive, which is incompatible with the intellectual integrity of argument-based professional ethics in obstetrics. The second is an error in scientific reasoning. Psychology is an evidence-based clinical science. The statement offers no evidence about the existence of such motivations. Like the critique that it echoes, this critique, too, fails.

This 2016 ACOG statement appeared five years *after* a joint statement by ACOG and the American Academy of Pediatrics (AAP) on maternal–fetal intervention.[42] The 2016 statement makes a nod to the 2011 statement by using "beneficence-based motivations." However, the 2011 statement begins by invoking the ethical concept of "a beneficence-based obligation to the fetus."[42, p. 405] The obstetrician has a beneficence-based ethical obligation to the fetus. The 2007 ACOG guidance on decision making allows for beneficence-based obligations to the fetus.[43] The pregnant woman has a parallel beneficence-based ethical obligation: "... most women will agree to the [maternal–fetal] treatment out of a beneficence-based obligation to their fetuses."[42, p. 406] The statement is silent on the origin of these two beneficence-based obligations but they are undeniably implications of the ethical concept of the fetus as a patient. The 2011 statement can be read as implicitly invoking this concept as a basis for its ethical reasoning. There is nothing in the text of the statement to block this interpretation. The 2016 statement simply ignores this content of the 2011 statement, as well as the 2007 guidance on decision making. This will not do, however, because the 2011 joint ACOG–AAP statement on fetal intervention is incompatible with the 2016 ACOG refusal of recommended treatment during pregnancy. The result is to further undermine the 2016 critique that the concept of the fetal patient has the implication that the fetus is a separate patient by ignoring its proper implication, recognized in the 2011 joint statement, the beneficence-based ethical obligations – not psychological motivations – of the obstetrician.

The critique that the ethical concept of the fetus as a patient has the implication that the fetal patient is a separate patient fails. This critique should no longer be made and, if repeated, should not be regarded as a serious contribution to professional ethics in obstetrics.

The moral logic of the ethical concept of the fetus as a patient excludes beginning and ending with beneficence-based obligations to the fetal patient. This is conceptually simplistic and therefore clinically inapplicable. In stark contrast, the moral logic of the ethical concept of the fetus as a patient in professional ethics in obstetrics is clinically and ethically nuanced and therefore clinically applicable. It begins in all cases with identifying beneficence-based and autonomy-based ethical obligations to the pregnant woman and then identifying beneficence-based ethical obligations to the fetal patient. It ends with evidence-based and argument-based judgments about the priority among these obligations when clinical circumstances or the informed decisions of the pregnant woman make the three ethical obligations incompatible.

2.6 Delivery Makes a Difference: Professional Ethics in Perinatal Medicine

Perinatal medicine combines Obstetrics with Neonatology, a subspecialty of Pediatrics. Pediatric ethics is based on the ethical concept of the best interests of the child when the child is a patient.[43,44] This is a beneficence-based concept. In professional ethics in perinatal medicine the best interests of the child standard creates the prima facie beneficence-based obligations of the pediatrician and other healthcare professionals to protect the health-related interests of the pediatric patient. Unlike the three-chapter story of professional ethics in obstetrics, professional ethics in pediatrics has but one chapter. This means that the pediatrician's prima facie beneficence-based obligations to the pediatric patient can be understood by focusing solely on the pediatric patient, which requires no reference to beneficence-based or autonomy-based obligations to parents.

There is a further reason why this is the case. In the professional ethics of pediatrics, the best interests of the child standard also applies to parents: they have beneficence-based obligations to protect the health-related interests of their child when their child is a patient. Like all other patients, a child becomes a patient when that child is presented to a physician and there exist forms of clinical management that in deliberative clinical judgment are reliably predicted to result in net clinical benefit for the child. Parental consent is not required. In professional ethics in pediatrics, parents have a beneficence-based obligation to their child who is a patient to authorize medically reasonable clinical management without reference to health risks of doing so to the parents. This is in striking contrast with professional ethics in obstetrics, in which the pregnant patient does not have such an ethical obligation; she is ethically obligated to take only reasonable risk to herself in her current and future pregnancies, a limit on beneficence-based obligations to the fetal patient that does not exist with respect to beneficence-based obligations to the neonatal patient. There is therefore a constraint on parental autonomy: their prima facie beneficence-based ethical obligation to protect and promote their child's health-related interests when their child is a patient. This is the basis for the AAP's proposal to replace "parental consent" with "parental permission" in the professional ethics of pediatrics.[43,44]

This account of perinatal ethics based on professional ethics in obstetrics and in pediatrics differs from a recently proposed approach based on a variant of shared decision making[45] in which respect for the autonomy of the patient or the patient's surrogate becomes the controlling consideration.[46] In this approach to neonatal ethics parental autonomy is not constrained by the best interests of the child standard.[44] This is best understood as pediatric ethics based on bioethics[47] rather than pediatric ethics based on professional ethics in pediatrics, which is the approach taken in this book.

Professional ethics in obstetrics and professional ethics in pediatrics combine to create professional ethics in perinatal medicine. This means that when the interdisciplinary team of obstetrician and neonatologist (or other pediatric subspecialist depending on the diagnosis of the fetal patient) counsel a pregnant woman about decision making for the clinical management of her pregnancy, professional ethics in obstetrics guides the process, in which the pediatrician will need to think like an obstetrician. When the interdisciplinary team of obstetrician and neonatologist (or other pediatric subspecialist) counsels the pregnant woman and the other prospective parent (partner or spouse) about planning for the clinical management of the future neonatal patient, professional ethics in pediatrics guides the process, in which the obstetrician will need to think like a pediatrician. Developing the habit of thinking in the professional ethics in another specialty is essential for professionally responsible clinical practice, innovation, and research in perinatal medicine.

References

1. Gregory J. Lectures on the duties and qualifications of a physician. London: W. Strahan and T. Cadell, 1772. Reprinted in McCullough LB, ed. John Gregory's Writings on Medical Ethics and the Philosophy of Medicine. Dordrecht, the Netherlands: Kluwer Academic, 1998: 161–248.
2. McCullough LB. John Gregory and the Invention of Professional Medical Ethics and the Profession of Medicine. Dordrecht, the Netherlands: Springer, 1998.
3. Coulehan J. On humility. Ann Intern Med 2010; 153: 200–201.
4. Faden RR, Beauchamp TL. A History and Theory of Informed Consent. New York: Oxford University Press, 1986.
5. Beauchamp TL, Childress JF. Principles of Biomedical Ethics, 7th ed. New York: Oxford University Press, 2013.
6. Liley AW: The fetus as personality. Austr N Zeal J Psych 1972; 6: 99–105.

7. Williams JW, Hellman LM, Pritchard JA. Williams Obstetrics, 14th ed. New York: Appleton-Century-Crofts, 1971.

8. Harrison MR, Golbus MS, Filly RA. Management of the fetus with a correctable congenital defect. JAMA 1981; 246: 774–777.

9. Harrison MR, Adzick NS. The fetus as a patient: surgical considerations. Ann Surg 1991; 213: 279–291.

10. Fletcher JC. The fetus as a patient: ethical issues. JAMA 1981; 246: 772–773.

11. Harrison MR, Golbus MS, Filly RA, eds. The Unborn Patient: Prenatal Diagnosis and Treatment. Philadelphia: Saunders, 1984.

12. Cunningham FG, Leveno KJ, Bloom SL, et al. J Preface. In Cunningham FG, Leveno KJ, Bloom SL, et al., eds. Williams Obstetrics, 25th ed. New York: McGraw-Hill Education, 2018. Available at https://accessmedicine.mhmedical.com/content.aspx?bookid=1918&sectionid=185041505 (accessed March 1, 2019; may be behind paywall).

13. Cunningham FG, Leveno KJ, Bloom SL, et al., eds. Williams Obstetrics, 25th ed. New York: McGraw-Hill Education, 2018.

14. International Academy of Perinatal Medicine. Available at https://iaperinatalmedicine.org/ (accessed March 1, 2019).

15. Bianchi D, Crombelhome TM, D'Alton ME. Fetology: Diagnosis and Management of the Fetal Patient. New York: McGraw-Hill Professional, 2000.

16. Bianchi D, Crombelhome TM, D'Alton ME, Malone F. Fetology: Diagnosis and Management of the Fetal Patient, 2nd ed. New York: McGraw-Hill Professional, 2010.

17. Harrison M. The Unborn Patient: The Art and Science of Fetal Therapy, 3rd ed. New York: Saunders, 2001.

18. Adzick NS. Prospects for fetal surgery. Early Hum Dev 2013; 89: 881–886.

19. Miller NM, Smith RP, Fisk NM. The fetal patient. In Myers LB, Bulich L, eds. Anesthesia for Fetal Intervention and Surgery. Hamilton, Ontario, Canada: D.C. Decker, 2010: 1–16.

20. Cannio M, Jani J. Fetal magnetic resonance imaging. In Cody AM, Brower S, eds. Twining's Textbook of Fetal Malformations, 3rd ed. London: Churchill Livingstone, 2015: 561–582.

21. Grady D. To mend a birth defect, surgeons operate on the patient within a patient. New York Times, October 23, 2017. Available at www.nytimes.com/2017/10/23/health/fetal-surgery-spina-bifida.html (accessed March 1, 2019).

22. Chervenak FA, McCullough LB. Perinatal ethics: a practical method of analysis of obligations to mother and fetus. Obstet Gynecol 1985; 66: 442–446.

23. Porter R, Teich M, eds. The Enlightenment in National Context. Cambridge: Cambridge University Press, 1981.

24. Kant I. Groundwork of the Metaphysics of Morals. Gregor M, Timmerman J, trans. and ed. Cambridge: Cambridge University Press, 2012.

25. Chervenak FA, McCullough LB. Ethical issues in periviable birth. Semin Perinatol 2013; 37: 422–425.

26. Skupski DW, Chervenak FA, McCullough LB, Bancalari E, et al. Ethical dimensions of periviability. J Pertinat Med 2010; 38: 579–583.

27. Chervenak FA, McCullough LB, Levine MI. An ethically justified, clinically comprehensive approach to periviability: gynaecologic, obstetric, perinatal, and neonatal dimensions. J Obstet Gyneacol 2007; 27: 3–7.

28. American College of Obstetricians and Gynecologists. Society for Maternal-Fetal Medicine. Obstetric Care consensus no. 6: Periviability. Obstet Gynecol 2017; 130: e187–e199.

29. Tyson JE, Parikh NA, Langer J, et al. Intensive care for extreme prematurity – moving beyond gestational age. N Engl J Med 2008; 358: 1672–1681.

30. Eunice Kennedy Shriver National Institute of Child Health and Human Development. NICHD Neonatal Research Network (NRN): Extremely preterm birth outcome data. Available at www1.nichd.nih.gov/epbo-calculator/Pages/epbo_case.aspx (accessed March 1, 2019).

31. Skupski DW, McCullough LB, Levene M, Chervenak FA. Improving obstetric estimation of outcomes of extremely premature neonates: an evolving challenge. J Perinat Med 2010; 38: 19–22.

32. Warren MA. Moral Status: Obligations to Persons and other Living Things. New York: Oxford University Press, 1997.

33. Strong C. Moral status and the fetus: continuation of a dialogue. Am J Bioeth 2011; 11: 52–54.

34. Lyerly AD, Mahowald MB. Maternal-fetal surgery for the treatment of myelomeningocele. Clin Perinatol 2003; 30: 155–165.

35. Chervenak FA, McCullough LB, Brent RL. The professional responsibility model of obstetric ethics: avoiding the perils of clashing rights. Am J Obstet Gynecol 2011; 205: 315.e1–5.

36. Minkoff H, Marshal MF, Liashenko J. The fetus and the "potential child," and the ethical obligations of obstetricians. Obstet Gynecol 2014; 123: 1100–1103.

37. Annas GJ. Protecting the liberty of pregnant patients. N Engl J Med 1987; 316: 1213–1214.

38. Högberg U, Lynöe N, Wulff M. Cesarean by choice? Empirical study of public values. Acta Obstet Gynecol Scand 2008; 87: 1301–1308.

39. Chervenak FA, McCullough LB. Justified limits on refusing intervention. Hastings Cent Rep 1991; 21: 12–18.

40. Lyerly AD, Little MO, Faden RR. A critique of the "fetus as a patient." Am J Bioeth 2006; 8: W42–W6.

41. American College of Obstetricians and Gynecologists. Committee on Ethics. Committee Opinion 664. Refusal of medically recommended treatment during pregnancy. Obstet Gynecol 2016; 127: e175–e1182.

42. American College of Obstetricians and Gynecologists. Committee Opinion No. 390. Ethical decision making in

obstetrics and gynecology. Obstet Gynecol 2007; 110: 1479–1487.

43. American Academy of Pediatrics. Committee on Bioethics. Informed consent, parental permission, and assent in pediatric practice. Pediatrics 1995; 95: 314–317.

44. Katz AL, Webb SA. Committee on Bioethics. American Academy of Pediatrics. Informed consent in decision-making in pediatric practice. Pediatrics 2016; 138: pii: e20161485. doi:10.1542/peds.2016-1485.

45. Kon AA. The shared decision-making continuum. JAMA 2010; 304: 903–904.

46. Lantos JD. Ethical problems in decision making in the neonatal ICU. New Engl J Med 2018; 379: 1851–1860.

47. Lantos JD, Lauderdale DS. Preterm Babies, Fetal Patients, and Childbearing Choices. Cambridge, MA: MIT Press, 2015.

Chapter 3: Decision Making By, With, and For Patients

GOAL
This chapter provides an ethical framework for decision making by, with, and for patients on a continuum of simple consent, informed consent, assisted decision making, assent, and surrogate decision making.

OBJECTIVES
On completing study of this chapter, the reader will:

Identify simple consent

Identify informed consent

Identify and list the seven components of decision-making capacity

Identify legal and ethical obligations in informed refusal

Describe the concept of an advance directive

Describe the concept of assisted decision making and its clinical application

Describe the concept of assent and its clinical application in pediatrics and geriatrics

Describe surrogate decision making

Describe the substituted judgment standard of surrogate decision making

Describe the best interests standard of surrogate decision making

Describe an ethically justified approach to decision making in medical emergencies

Apply the continuum of decision making by, with, and for patients in clinical practice

TOPICS

3.1 Decision Making By, With, and For Patients	47
3.2 A Decision Made *By* and *With* the Patient: Simple and Informed Consent	47
3.2.1 The Presumption of Decision-Making Capacity in Adult Patients	47
3.2.2 The Presumption of Decision-Making Capacity in Minors with Legal Authority over Themselves	47
3.2.3 "Competence" and "Capacity": Two Names for the Same Clinical Phenomenon	48
3.2.4 Seven Components of Decision-Making Capacity	48
3.2.5 Consent: Simple and Informed	49
3.2.5.1 Simple Consent	49
Legal Origin?	49
3.2.5.2 Informed Consent Process	51
Beneficence-Based Obligations	51
Autonomy-Based Obligations	52
How Much Information Should Be Provided?	52
Satisfying Legal Standards of Disclosure	52
Supporting Patient Autonomy	52

Section 1: Professional Ethics in Obstetrics and Gynecology

Voluntary Decision Making	53
The Role of Directive Counseling	53
The Role of Shared Decision Making	53
Recommendations Support Patient Autonomy	54
The Patient's Role in Evaluating Information	54
Outcomes of the Informed Consent Process	54
Respectful Persuasion	54
The Female Patient and Pregnant Patient as the Ultimate Decision Maker in the Clinical Practice of Gynecology and Obstetrics	55
3.3 Informed Refusal: A Strict Legal Obligation with a Preventive Ethics Component	55
3.3.1 The Strict Legal Obligation	55
3.3.2 The Preventive Ethics Component	56
3.4 How Attitudes Can Distort Clinical Judgment	56
3.5 Who Should Obtain Simple Consent?	57
3.6 Who Should Lead the Informed Consent Process?	57
3.7 Projecting Decision Making into the Future: Advance Directives	57
3.8 A Decision *By* the Patient *With* the Obstetrician-Gynecologist and Others Who Assist in the Decision-Making Process: Assisted Decision Making	58
3.8.1 Assessment of Decision-Making Capacity	58
3.8.2 Risk-Adjusted Assessment of Decision-Making Capacity: Proceed with Great Caution	58
3.8.3 Decision-Making Capacity Is Task Specific and Time Specific	58
3.8.3.1 Task-Specific Decision-Making Capacity	58
3.8.3.2 Time-Specific Decision-Making Capacity	59
3.8.3.3 Ulysses Contract	59
3.8.4 When One or More Components of Decision-Making Capacity Are Diminished	59
3.9 A Decision *By* Others but *With* the Patient: Pediatric and Geriatric Assent	59
3.10 A Decision *By* Others *For* the Patient but *Not With* the Patient: Surrogate Decision Making	61
3.10.1 Two Standards for Surrogate Decision Making	61
3.10.1.1 Substituted Judgment Standard	61
3.10.1.2 The Best Interests Standard	62
3.11 Clinical Ethical Topics in Decision Making for Patients	62
3.11.1 Variants of Impaired Autonomy	62
3.11.1.1 Chronic and Variable Impairment of Autonomy	62
3.11.1.2 Chronic and Invariable Impairment of Autonomy	63
3.11.1.3 Chronic and Progressive Impairment of Autonomy	63
3.11.1.4 Chronic and Decreasing Impairment of Autonomy	63
3.12 Surrogate Decision Making about Termination of Pregnancy	64
3.13 Surrogate Decision Making about Prevention of Pregnancy	64
3.14 Managing Doubts about the Reliability of a Surrogate Decision Maker	65
3.15 Managing Refusal of a Family Member to Accept the Legally Designated Surrogate	65
3.16 Medical Emergencies	66

Chapter 3: Decision Making By, With, and For Patients

Key Concepts

Advance directive
Assent
Assisted decision making
Best interests standard of surrogate decision making
Competence
Decision-making capacity
Geriatric assent
Impaired autonomy
Informed consent process
Informed refusal process
Medical emergency
Pediatric assent
Presumption of decision-making capacity of adult patients
Professional community standard
Reasonable person standard
Respectful persuasion
Shared decision making
Simple consent
Substituted judgment standard of surrogate decision making
Surrogate decision making
Voluntary

3.1 Decision Making By, With, and For Patients

In clinical practice, innovation, and research, decision making always has the goal of a decision *for* the patient. Most of the time decision making has the additional goal of a decision *by* and *with* the patient. This is the goal for female patients and pregnant patients who have the capacity to participate in decision making, i.e., most patients.

For other patients, the goal of a decision *by* and *with* the patient is not clinically realistic. Female patients and some pregnant patients who have not attained legal majority, or who have seriously impaired decision-making capacity, may not have the legal authority to make decisions for themselves. Adolescents, under applicable federal and state laws governing emancipated minors or pregnant minors, may have legal decision-making authority over themselves, but a conscientious obstetrician-gynecologist may have justified clinical concerns about the maturity of judgment of some of these patients. Adult patients may have mental illnesses and disorders that adversely affect their capacity to participate in decision making about the clinical management of their conditions, a problem that can become exacerbated when a patient has struggled to manage a mental illness or disorder or has not received treatment for it. Adolescent and adult patients may have cognitive disabilities that adversely affect their capacity to participate in decision making. Geriatric patients, especially older geriatric patients, may be at risk for dementing disorders that can, sometimes subtly and sometimes overtly, affect their capacity to make decisions or to adapt and carry out decisions or both.

This wide range of capacity for decision making requires a clinically comprehensive set of goals for decision making *for* the patient. There are four such goals: (1) a decision made *by* and *with* the patient – simple and informed consent – the most common goal, as noted in Section 3.1; (2) a decision made *by* the patient *with* others who assist in the decision-making process – assisted decision making; (3) a decision made *by* others but *with* the patient – pediatric and geriatric assent; and (4) a decision made *by* others but *not with* the patient – surrogate decision making.

3.2 A Decision Made *By* and *With* the Patient: Simple and Informed Consent

3.2.1 The Presumption of Decision-Making Capacity in Adult Patients

All patients who have attained the age of legal adulthood (18 in the United States) are presumed in health law and professional ethics in obstetrics and gynecology to have the intellectual and affective capacity to participate in decision making about the clinical management of their condition and about participation in innovation (an experiment performed on an individual patient for the benefit of that patient; see Chapter 17) and research (an experiment performed on a group of patients to create generalizable knowledge; see Chapter 17).[1]

3.2.2 The Presumption of Decision-Making Capacity in Minors with Legal Authority over Themselves

In the United States legal minors do not have legal authority over themselves for decision making about clinical management of their diagnoses but there are

47

exceptions. A minor female or pregnant patient who has had the "disabilities" of being a minor removed by a court and thus has become an emancipated minor has the same authority over herself that an adult female or pregnant patient has. The law in some states provides for emancipation by virtue of being pregnant. The law in other states grants full authority for decision making about pregnancy and conditions related to pregnancy. The law in still other states grants authority for decision making about pregnancy but not for other clinical conditions. Some states restrict the scope of decision-making authority. Parental notification laws about induced abortion for a minor pregnant patient have the effect of restricting the minor's scope of decision-making authority. Federal law grants legal decision-making authority to minors about reproductive medicine in federally supported programs.

Organizational policy on when a female or pregnant patient who is a minor has decision-making authority over herself should be comprehensive and based on applicable federal and state law and be as clear as possible. Questions or concerns about whether a minor female or pregnant patient has legal decision-making authority over herself or the clinical scope of that authority should be addressed to organizational legal counsel.

The fact that a minor female or pregnant patient by law has decision-making authority over herself means that legally she is an adult patient or the functional equivalent of an adult patient. The presumption that she has decision-making capacity applies, as a matter of heath law. However, depending on the patient's developmental stage, the obstetrician-gynecologist may have justified concerns about whether this presumption applies, as a matter of professional ethics in obstetrics and gynecology. In such clinical circumstances, the obstetrician-gynecologist should engage the patient in the assent process with the goal of supporting the patient to make adult-like decisions. (See Section 3.9.) With the patient's permission, her parents should be asked to become involved in the role of supporting their daughter, not making decisions for her. The assisted decision-making process should be followed. Organizational policy should identify the process to be followed if these clinical measures do not result in the patient exhibiting adult-like decision-making capacity.

3.2.3 "Competence" and "Capacity": Two Names for the Same Clinical Phenomenon

Some make a sharp distinction between decision-making capacity and competence by pointing out, correctly, that only a court of law can determine whether an individual is no longer competent. This is because in statutory and common law "competence" carries with it legal rights and obligations that a judicial finding of incompetence can remove, in whole or in part. A court can find an individual to be incompetent to manage all aspects of his or her life or incompetent to manage some aspects, e.g., complex financial matters and decisions about medical care, but competent to manage others, e.g., to continue to live at home with some supervision of self-care activities.

To be competent means that one has the capacities required for making decisions, caring for oneself, and managing one's personal and family matters. To have decision-making capacity means that a patient can complete the seven components of decision-making capacity described in Section 3.2.4 and therefore participate in the informed consent process. On this account "competence" and "capacity" are but two names for the same clinical phenomenon. The difference is that incompetence is determined by a judge in a court of law whereas diminished or absent capacity is determined by the obstetrician-gynecologist or psychiatrist in the clinical setting without court review and following organizational policy for doing so.

3.2.4 Seven Components of Decision-Making Capacity

Decision-making capacity comprises seven iterative components: the success of completing each component, starting with the second, depends on successful completion of the previous component(s). (See Table 3.1.) We therefore list the components to reflect their iterative nature.[2,3] In its clinical application, this list should not be read as a rigid set of rules for the order of the patient's decision-making process. Patients' actual decision-making processes may vary but nonetheless should include all seven steps.

1. The patient pays attention to the information that is provided to her.
2. The patient absorbs, retains, and recalls this information as needed in subsequent components.

Table 3.1 Seven components of decision-making capacity.

Attention	The patient pays attention to the information that is provided.
Information intake and use	The patient absorbs, retains, and recalls this information as needed in subsequent components.
Cognitive understanding	The patient can reason from present events (clinical management) to their future likely consequences (clinical outcomes).
Appreciation	The patient believes that these consequences could happen to her (in gynecology) or to her or her fetus or her future child should the pregnancy continue to delivery (in obstetrics).
Evaluative understanding	The patient assesses these consequences on the basis of her values and beliefs.
Explicit authorization	The patient explicitly authorizes clinical management that has been offered or recommended or refuses to do so in a voluntary fashion, i.e., free of control by external factors (other people, including family and healthcare team members) or internal factors (such as unreasoning fear or auditory hallucination).
Communicating reasons	The patient can, when requested, explain her authorization or refusal of authorization on the basis of her cognitive and evaluative understanding.

3. The patient can reason from present events (clinical management) to their future likely consequences (clinical outcomes), which is called cognitive understanding.[4]
4. The patient believes that these consequences could happen to her (in gynecology) or to her or her fetus or her future child should the pregnancy continue to delivery (in obstetrics). This is called appreciation.[5]
5. The patient assesses these consequences on the basis of her values and beliefs, which is called evaluative understanding.[4]
6. The patient explicitly authorizes clinical management that has been offered or recommended or refuses to do so in a voluntary fashion, i.e., free of control by external factors (other people, including family and healthcare team members) or internal factors (such as unreasoning fear or auditory hallucination).[6,7]
7. The patient can, when requested, explain her authorization or refusal of authorization on the basis of her cognitive and evaluative understanding.[2,3]

The presumption of decision-making capacity means that the burden of proof is on the physician to establish in deliberative clinical judgment that the patient's decision-making capacity is diminished in a clinically significant way or absent altogether, i.e., one or more of these seven components is impaired or absent.

3.2.5 Consent: Simple and Informed

Consent takes two forms, simple consent and informed consent. We provide an account of each in turn. (See Table 3.2.)

3.2.5.1 Simple Consent

"Simple consent" means that the patient has agreed to clinical management that has been offered or recommended. Of the seven components of decision making only the sixth occurs, in simplified form: the patient agrees or disagrees with offered or recommended treatment expressly or through her behavior. Simple consent is appropriate for clinical management that in deliberative clinical judgment is medically reasonable, noninvasive, low-risk, and either of well-established clinical benefit or highly probable clinical benefit.[8] An example of the first is antibiotic therapy for a vaginal tract infection with a bacterium documented to respond to a specific class of antibiotics for a patient with no history of allergic reaction to antibiotics. An example of the second is intake of folic acid during pregnancy for a patient with no contraindications. Simple consent can be explicit and is signaled by the patient by saying "yes" or one of its cognates. Simple consent can be implicit when a patient presents her arm for venipuncture or follows the prescribed regimen for self-care after an uncomplicated hysterectomy.

Legal Origin?

The creation of simple consent as an accepted standard for these types of decisions, until recently, was

Table 3.2 Simple consent, informed consent, assent, assisted decision making, surrogate decision making.

Simple consent	Decision making by and with the patient	The patient has agreed to clinical management that has been offered or recommended.
Informed consent	Decision making by and with the patient	A process that requires the obstetrician to present to the patient a description of the patient's condition or diagnosis, the *medically reasonable alternatives* for its clinical management, the clinical benefits and risks of each medically reasonable alternative and to support the patient in her completion of the seven components of decision-making capacity.
Assisted decision making	Decision making by the patient with others	A clinical response to impaired decision-making capacity that begins with a clinical assessment of the patient's decision-making capacity, identification of impaired components, and clinical management designed to reverse these impairments to an acceptable threshold so that the patient can exercise her autonomy in the informed consent process.
Assent	Decision making by others with the patient	A process in which decision making for patient with impaired decision-making capacity refractory to assisted decision making occurs *with* the patient but *by* others who should take into account the results of the assent process. The authority of the patient's preferences is a function of the patients' cognitive and affective developmental status.
Surrogate decision making	Decision making by others for the patient	Decision making by the legally designated individual for a patient who has lost decision-making capacity and for whom assisted consent and assent cannot be employed. Surrogate decision making is guided, in priority order, by the substituted judgment standard and the best interests standard.

commonly understood to have been invented by the American common law early in the twentieth century, in a New York State civil case, *Schloendorff v. Society of New York Hospital*.[9] This case, decided in 1914, was about alleged failure to ask a patient undergoing hysterectomy for a suspected fibroid tumor in 1908 whether she wanted the recommended surgery to be performed. In the trial court, the plaintiff's attorney requested a directed verdict by the judge against the hospital. The judge declined and the case was referred to the Court of Appeals, the highest civil court in New York State. Following the accepted legal procedure, the Court of Appeals heard the case on the grounds most favorable to the plaintiff and therefore without review of the trial transcript.

The origin of simple consent is taken to be found in these stirring words of Judge Benjamin Cardozo (1870–1938), a distinguished jurist who later served as associate justice of the Supreme Court of the United States (1932–1938):

> Every human being of adult years and sound mind has the right to determine what shall be done with his body; and a surgeon who performs an operation without his patient's consent, commits an assault for which he is liable in damages ... except in cases of emergency where the patient is unconscious and where it is necessary to operate before consent can be obtained.[9]

This may be the most frequently quoted passage from American common law in the ethics of consent literature.

More recent scholarship has produced two pertinent results. The case was not directly about consent, because the court assumed it had not been given by the patient. Instead, as Paul Lombardo has shown, the issue before the court was the immunity of a hospital as a charitable organization from the actions of physicians who provided patient care in the hospital.[10] The court upheld this immunity and Mrs. Schloendorff lost her case, an outcome that is not as well known as Judge Cardozo's stirring words underscoring a fundamental freedom in American history, evoking the era of legal slavery that had been ended by the Civil War and the Thirteenth Amendment only five decades earlier.

In addition, a close examination of the patient's hospital record in the archives of New York Hospital and the original trial court record discovered that the patient's agreement to the surgery is documented in her record.[11] Judge Cardozo did not invent the idea of simple consent because it was already a clinical practice. Given the routine nature of the entries in her record and the testimony of the physicians to the trial court, the practice of simple consent was common. Unwittingly in all likelihood, Judge Cardozo added a legal endorsement to what was already common clinical practice.

Simple consent has been a physician-originated clinical practice for more than a century. This means that respect for autonomy in the form of obtaining simple consent predated the invention of bioethics, with its strong emphasis on respect for patient autonomy. (See Chapter 1.) Bioethics came six decades later. Simple consent should be deployed to obtain the patient's agreement of offered or recommended clinical management when in deliberative clinical judgment that clinical management is medically reasonable, non-invasive, low-risk,[8] and either of well-established clinical benefit or of highly probable clinical benefit.

3.2.5.2 Informed Consent Process

Informed consent is required for clinical management that in deliberative clinical judgment is medically reasonable and of high risk,[8] with the evidence base for benefit ranging from weak to strong. Informed consent is not limited to invasive clinical management because noninvasive management such as radiation for the treatment of various cancers can be high risk and of uncertain benefit. Obviously, gynecologic surgery and cesarean delivery are invasive and therefore require an informed consent process. Informed consent is also required whenever a healthcare organization requires it.[6]

We use "informed consent process" to emphasize the difference between simple and informed consent. In simple consent, the patient says yes or no. In informed consent the patient's authorization or refusal to authorize is the outcome of a process of communication of information to the patient and her response to that information in the seven steps described in Section 3.2.4. This process should not be equated with a completed and signed organizational form, which provides evidence of the patient's authorization of clinical management and only secondarily the process that should precede it.

Beneficence-Based Obligations

Beneficence-based ethical obligations play an essential role in the informed consent process.[12] The informed consent process begins with the obstetrician-gynecologist fulfilling two beneficence-based obligations to the female patient or pregnant patient. First, the obstetrician-gynecologist should deploy deliberative clinical judgment to characterize the patient's condition, keeping always in mind that, in obstetrics, pregnancy is a condition and not a disease. Pregnancy, however, is a condition that can pose biopsychosocial risks arising from maternal or fetal complications.

"Biopsychosocial" is a term introduced by George Engel a half-century ago to emphasize that health and disease, as well as conditions such as pregnancy, have a biomedical dimension (the "bio" part), a psychological dimension (the "psycho" part), and a social dimension (the "social" part).[13] Deliberative clinical judgment about gynecologic disorders and diseases, as well as conditions such as pregnancy, becomes inadequate when it reduces diseases or conditions to their biomedical dimensions and ignores the psychosocial dimensions, which become especially important, e.g., when gynecologic surgery will eliminate reproductive capacity or a fetal anomaly is diagnosed. The obstetrician's deliberative clinical judgment about the patient's condition or diagnosis should be presented to the patient and explained to her at a level at which the patient can be expected to understand, i.e., as clearly and simply as possible to convey the key clinical points and prevent information overload. She should be encouraged to ask questions, an especially important consideration for patients who may tend to defer to a physician's authority. Her questions should be answered clearly, with a focus on the key clinical points related to formation of cognitive and evaluative understanding.

Having characterized the condition or diagnosis (or differential diagnosis) the obstetrician-gynecologist should deploy deliberative clinical judgment to identify the medically reasonable alternatives for the management of the patient's condition or diagnosis. One of three outcomes will occur. There is only one medically reasonable alternative for the management of the patient's diagnosis, e.g., cesarean delivery to manage well-documented, intrapartum, complete placenta previa. There are two or more medically reasonable alternatives and one is clinically superior in deliberative clinical judgment, e.g., a form of contraception is recommended based on marginal improvement of safety given the patient's condition and history. There are two or more medically reasonable alternatives but they are equivalent in the sense that in deliberative clinical judgment the evidence base for each is equivalent in strength, e.g., planned cesarean delivery versus trial of labor after low-transverse cesarean (TOLAC) in hospitals that meet accepted standards.

Autonomy-Based Obligations

The next phase of the informed consent process should be guided by the ethical principle of respect for autonomy. As explained in Chapter 2, this ethical principle creates an ethical obligation to empower the female patient to make informed and voluntary decisions about the management of her clinical condition.

How Much Information Should Be Provided?

A patient's decision is informed when she has an adequate understanding of the nature of her condition or diagnosis, the medically reasonable alternatives for its clinical management, the strength of evidence supporting the clinical judgment of medical reasonableness, and the nature and probability of the clinical benefits and risks of each medically reasonable alternative for her (in gynecology) or for her, the fetal patient, and the future neonatal patient (in obstetrics). In short, these are the clinically salient aspects of deliberative clinical judgment and therefore should be provided to the patient so that she can replicate for herself what the obstetrician-gynecologist thinks is clinically important about her condition and its clinical management.[12]

Satisfying Legal Standards of Disclosure

During the middle of the twentieth century, standards of disclosure of information by the physician in the informed consent process developed in common law (made by appellate courts) and statutory law (made by legislatures with the approval of the chief executive).[6] Adopting the approach just described for providing information will satisfy both legal standards for disclosure of information.

The dominant legal standard in the United States is the reasonable person standard: providing information to the patient that any patient in her clinical circumstances needs to know. This does not call for a level of information tailored to each individual patient's informational needs at a particular time (known as the subjective standard) but to the informational needs of *any* patient in the patient's clinical circumstances. All patients need to know what is clinically important in forming cognitive and evaluative understanding.

The second legal standard in the United States is the professional community standard: providing information that any experienced and qualified obstetrician-gynecologist would provide. This standard was once based on local practice patterns. With the advent of evidence-based medicine, local standards are giving way to evidence-based standards. In effect, the professional community standard reflects standards of patient safety and quality. This standard can effectively be met by following the reasonable person standard. In our view, the professional community standard in the context of patient safety and quality has merged into the reasonable person standard. In short, by making the reasonable person standard routine in clinical practice, the legal standard for disclosure under applicable law will be routinely satisfied.

The reasonable person standard takes a very substantial step toward meeting the informational needs of the individual patient. Beyond this foundational information for the informed consent process, the informational needs of individual patients will vary. One way to determine what these are is to encourage the patient to ask questions and answer them to her satisfaction. Experienced obstetrician-gynecologists have become familiar with the range of questions that are important to individual patients. On this basis, a list of frequently asked questions could be prepared and provided to patients in electronic or print format, as the patient prefers. This will signal to patients that their questions are welcome, which can help reduce the unwillingness of some patients to ask questions. Patients with chronic disease or end-stage disease should be encouraged to ask questions, to help them cope with life-altering diagnoses.

Supporting Patient Autonomy

When patients indicate the need for support in processing this clinical information or seem to be challenged by this task, e.g., because of complex cognitive demands or because of posttraumatic distress from rape, incest, or other forms of sexual abuse, the ethical principle of respect for autonomy creates the ethical obligation to offer the female patient psychosocial support, especially from team members and consultants with mental health expertise.

Voluntary Decision Making

A patient's decision making is voluntary when it is not controlled by internal or external controlling influences.[6,7] The physician should be alert to such influences and act to blunt them. To prevent external controlling influences (pressure from well-meaning family members) or internal controlling influences (the sometimes compelling commitment to do anything for fetal and neonatal benefit), the obstetrician should make clear – and, as needed, repeat for emphasis – that the pregnant patient is not ethically obligated to take any and all risks to herself but only risks judged to be reasonable in deliberative clinical judgment. (See Chapter 2.)

The Role of Directive Counseling

Fulfilling the autonomy-based ethical obligation to empower the female patient or pregnant patient includes recommending clinical management, under two conditions. First, deliberative clinical judgment supports the conclusion that there is only one medically reasonable alternative for the management of the patient's condition or diagnosis. Second, of two or more medically reasonable alternatives one is supported in deliberative clinical judgment as superior, e.g., the evidence base for it is stronger (for two medically reasonable alternatives) or strongest (for more than two medically reasonable alternatives). The recommendation should be presented to the patient and explained to her. She should be encouraged to ask questions, an especially important consideration for patients who may tend to defer to a physician's authority. Her questions should be answered clearly, with a focus on the key clinical points related to formation of cognitive and evaluative understanding.

Making recommendations supported in deliberative clinical judgment is a form of directive counseling. This means that directive counseling has an important but limited role in the informed consent process. This role does not extend to include the informed consent process when two or more medically reasonable alternatives are supported in deliberative clinical judgment but none has clearly stronger evidence, e.g., planned cesarean versus TOLAC. When this is the case, all of the medically reasonable alternatives should be presented, along with their risks and benefits, and a clear statement that none is considered to be clearly clinically superior. The patient's values and beliefs become decisive and she should be supported in developing her cognitive and evaluative understanding of each alternative and identifying the one she prefers.

The Role of Shared Decision Making

Shared decision making is a phrase without a fixed meaning in the ethics literature.[14,15] Some take the view that the informed consent process should start with the identification of the patient's values and beliefs that should then guide the subsequent decision-making process as the controlling consideration. This implements the ethical principle of respect for autonomy in medical ethics and bioethics: "To respect autonomous agents is to acknowledge their right to hold views, to make choices, and to take actions based on their values and beliefs."[7, p. 106] This specification of respect for autonomy, however, is incompatible with the specification of respect for autonomy in professional ethics in obstetrics and gynecology: to empower the female patient or pregnant patient with information about medically reasonable alternatives. The specification of respect for autonomy in medical ethics and bioethics omits the crucial role of the obstetrician-gynecologist in identifying the medically reasonable alternatives and recommending one when it is justified to do so in deliberative clinical judgment. This difference in the specification of respect for autonomy means that shared decision making – understood as starting with and being guided by the patient's values and beliefs as the controlling consideration[14,15] – should not be considered applicable as a universal model for the informed consent process in professional ethics in obstetrics and gynecology.

A different account of shared decision making is compatible with the account of the informed consent process that we set out in Section 3.2.5.2. When there are two or more clinically equivalent medically reasonable alternatives, the patient's values and beliefs do indeed become the controlling consideration in evaluating which medically reasonable alternative is superior, because beneficence-based deliberative judgment remains indecisive in this respect. In addition, when decision making is about matters that are primarily psychosocial and not primarily biomedical, such as whether to continue pregnancy, shared decision making should be used. This account of shared decision making, we emphasize, means that shared decision making is but one variant of the informed consent process in specific, clinical circumstances:

when the medically reasonable alternatives are in evidence-based equipoise or when decision making is primarily psychosocial. Shared decision making therefore cannot be understood to be a universal model of the informed consent process.[16]

Recommendations Support Patient Autonomy

Recommending clinical management is considered by some to limit a patient's choice and thus not compatible with respect for patient autonomy.[17] Such an objection makes an implicit assumption: recommendations are more than influential but experienced by patients as controlling, resulting in an involuntary decision by the female or pregnant patient. No evidence is presented to support this assumption, because there is none. Worse, this assumption demeans, even infantilizes women, which is completely incompatible with a position that understands itself to be advocating for the autonomy of female and pregnant patients.

The Patient's Role in Evaluating Information

The informed consent process continues with the patient forming her evaluation of what has been recommended or offered to her. Patients may welcome support in this stage, especially when the cognitive demands are high, e.g., interpreting the results of genome sequencing of a gynecologic cancer. The obstetrician-gynecologist can be helpful by asking a question that has been successful in eliciting the patient's values in geriatric long-term care[18]: As you consider what I have recommended/offered, what is important to you? The obstetrician-gynecologist should support the patient in achieving an as-clear-as-possible expression of her values. When her expressed values support a medically reasonable alternative, the obstetrician should point this out and ask the patient whether she agrees. If so, then the obstetrician should suggest she consider that medical alternative seriously. If the patient does not agree, the process should be repeated.

Outcomes of the Informed Consent Process

There are four outcomes of the informed consent process. The patient authorizes the medically reasonable alternative that has been recommended. Clinical management should proceed. In the situation in which there are two or more medically reasonable alternatives and one has been recommended on the basis of deliberative clinical judgment, the patient may refuse to authorize what has been recommended but authorize another medically reasonable alternative that was presented. Clinical management should proceed, because the patient has authorized a medically reasonable alternative; the best should not be the enemy of the good. In the situation in which there are two or more medically reasonable alternatives but none is clinically superior, the patient authorizes one of them. Clinical management should proceed.

The fourth outcome occurs when the patient refuses to authorize any of the medically reasonable alternatives, which is a rare event in clinical practice. The discipline of deliberative clinical judgment should guide the obstetrician's professional response. The professional response excludes taking the patient's refusal personally or thinking less of the patient. The professional response also excludes the clinical hypothesis that the patient has impaired decision-making capacity, because refusal to authorize any medically reasonable alternative is not evidence in and of itself that one or more of the iterative components of decision-making capacity is impaired or absent.

Respectful Persuasion

Respectful persuasion, the effort to support the patient to make a decision based on her beliefs and values, should be the obstetrician-gynecologist's next response. Respectful persuasion is designed to prevent paternalism: interference with the patient's decision-making process based on the obstetrician-gynecologist's deliberative judgment about what is in the patient's health-related interests.[7] Respectful persuasion is based on the assumption, borne out in clinical practice, that the patient almost always has what she considers to be a good reason for her refusal, based on her beliefs and values. The goals should be to discover those reasons and determine whether they support a medically reasonable alternative. The patient should be asked, "What is important to you in refusing?" The obstetrician-gynecologist should listen for incomplete or false beliefs and respectfully correct them, to support the patient in developing an accurate and therefore reliable cognitive understanding of her condition or diagnosis and its clinical management. The obstetrician-gynecologist should be alert to expressed values that support a medically reasonable alternative and ask her to consider it. It is ethically permissible to recommend this alternative to her and explain that the recommendation is supported both by the obstetrician-gynecologist's clinical judgment and the patient's expressed values and beliefs.

Respectful persuasion can be enhanced by making recommendations, especially those supported by the patient's values and beliefs of which support the patient may not have become aware in clinically stressful circumstances.[19] The obstetrician-gynecologist should aim to elucidate the patient's values and goals, to express them clearly, and identify their implications for creating a plan of care. This can be accomplished with patients with clinically manageable mental disorders such as depression or anxiety. For these patients, the obstetrician should call attention to the positive effect that clinical management could have on her pregnancy and ability to parent or become a successful survivor of gynecologic cancer. The obstetrician can also explain norms that patients frequently endorse and follow, for example, patients with depression that can be safely managed during pregnancy welcome learning about this aspect of pharmacologic management and taking it into account.[20]

Using phrases such as "low risk" or "high risk" can confuse patients and impair the respectful persuasion process, because they are imprecise. Confusion can be prevented by stating absolute measures of effects as percentages or percent ranges and then explaining what this means in terms of the number needed to treat. For example, 20% means that, for every five patients treated, one will benefit and the other four will not benefit and not be put at serious risk. This is known as "intentional framing" that aims to support clear thinking by the patient.[19]

Respectful persuasion rules out paternalism, which is interference with the patient's autonomy based on the obstetrician-gynecologist's beneficence-based clinical judgment about what the patient ought to do.[7] Paternalism can unduly influence the patient's decision making by creating a controlling influence that impairs or even eliminates voluntariness. The use of negative incentives, deception in the form of withholding information about medically reasonable alternatives, or threats are prima facie incompatible with respectful persuasion.[19] There are rare exceptions when a pregnant woman refuses cesarean delivery that will benefit both her and the fetal patient. (See Chapter 12.)

The Female Patient and Pregnant Patient as the Ultimate Decision Maker in the Clinical Practice of Gynecology and Obstetrics

The ethical principle of respect for autonomy in professional ethics in obstetrics and gynecology has two implications that cannot be overemphasized. The female patient is the ultimate decision maker about the clinical management of her condition. The pregnant patient is the ultimate decision maker about the clinical management of her pregnancy. Others – spouse, partner, other family members – may have a stake in her decisions. However, having a stake in a patient's decision does not make one a decision maker for that patient. Sometimes well-meaning, or not so well-meaning, others may attempt to assert a controlling role in the female patient's or pregnant patient's decision-making role. This is an attempt to deny her a voluntary decision-making process, which the ethical principle of respect for autonomy makes ethically impermissible.[6,7] The female patient and the pregnant patient have the autonomy-based right to involve whomever they want in their decision-making process. The obstetrician-gynecologist has the autonomy-based ethical obligation to make clear to these other individuals that their support of the patient and her decision-making process is welcome but that the female patient and the pregnant patient are the ultimate decision makers. It sometimes happens that the obstetrician-gynecologist must also fulfill the autonomy-based ethical obligation to prevent others from denying the patient a voluntary decision-making process, if necessary, by excluding them from the decision-making process with the agreement of the female or pregnant patient.

In clinical research for fetal benefit in the United States, federal research regulations in the United States require paternal consent. See Chapter 17 for more detail on this requirement.

3.3 Informed Refusal: A Strict Legal Obligation with a Preventive Ethics Component

3.3.1 The Strict Legal Obligation

If the patient continues to refuse, then the obstetrician-gynecologist has a strict legal obligation to complete and document the informed refusal process. This legal obligation originates in the patient's right to learn about the clinical risks of her refusal and the legitimate self-interest of the obstetrician-gynecologist and of his or her healthcare organization to prevent unnecessary exposure to professional liability. The legal obligation of informed refusal was first set out in 1970 in the case of *Truman v. Thomas*, which occurred when Dr. Thomas did not explain to a patient who refused a Pap smear that he was concerned about the risk of nonsymptomatic cervical cancer, from which she died.[21]

The obstetrician-gynecologist should follow organizational policy for informed refusal. There are two main components. The obstetrician-gynecologist must inform the patient about the clinical risks that she is taking by refusing to authorize any form of medically reasonable clinical management, including increased probability of disease or complications that could compromise her health and lost functional status and, when clinically applicable, increased probability of death. The details of this disclosure must be documented in the patient's record, in accordance with organizational policy for doing so. Completing this process means that the patient has consented to accept these risks.

Consent confers immunity to professional liability. As explained in Chapter 1, Friedrich Hoffmann's concept of *medicus politicus* provides the basis for identifying the legitimate self-interests as self-interests aligned with the health-related interests of the patient. Fulfilling the legal obligation of informed refusal aligns the physician's self-interests with the patient's interests in her health and life. Thus, reducing the risk of professional liability by completing the informed refusal process is a legitimate self-interest of the obstetrician-gynecologist.

For example, an adult female patient who is not pregnant and is a member of the Jehovah's Witnesses may refuse the administration of blood products that are prohibited in this faith community. Such a patient is invoking a moral commitment that is common to many faith communities: preservation of one's life is not always of paramount value when it is in conflict with divine commands. There is also a secular counterpart: some things are worth dying for, as in the ancient belief of death before dishonor. The professional virtues of self-effacement and self-sacrifice create the prima facie ethical obligation not to disparage such beliefs but treat them with respect. As long as her refusal is voluntary, i.e., free of controlling influences of others, her refusal should be respected. Without commenting on her beliefs, the informed refusal process should be followed. Clinical experience has taught the surgical community that many patients survive bloodless surgery, which means that the patient's refusal should not be considered uniformly to result in a disastrous outcome. In almost all cases, when a pregnant woman refuses blood products as a component of cesarean delivery, fetal and neonatal benefit are not unacceptably compromised. Honoring her refusal of blood products and with her consent to cesarean delivery, it should be performed.

3.3.2 The Preventive Ethics Component

The obstetrician-gynecologist's legal obligations end at this point. Professional ethics in obstetrics and gynecology requires one further step: preventive ethics. Preventive ethics is the use of the informed consent process to avert preventable conflict between the patient and her obstetrician-gynecologist.[22] Taking advantage of the potential effect of the informed refusal process to focus the patient's mind on the clinical seriousness for her well-being of her refusal, the obstetrician-gynecologist should ask her to reconsider. If she expresses an interest in reconsidering, the respectful persuasion process should be reactivated. If she does not express such an interest, the obstetrician-gynecologist should emphasize the symptomatic changes of which she should be aware and that she should not hesitate to contact the obstetrician-gynecologist for a follow-up appointment if she has any concerns or questions. Restating the obstetrician-gynecologist's professional commitment to the patient's health and, when applicable, life does not end when the process of informed refusal has been completed. A reasonable effort to follow-up with the patient should be made.

3.4 How Attitudes Can Distort Clinical Judgment

The informed consent process is intended mainly to manage risk,[8] sometimes considerable risk. Moreover, patients may struggle with the burden of high-risk decisions and even make decisions that appear to be in tension with or even inconsistent with their expressed values. Patients may also make requests that the obstetrician-gynecologist believes are imprudent in that their implementation would unnecessarily put the patient's health-related interests and safety at risk. These clinical situations can provoke strong feelings that can become strong enough to turn the attention of the obstetrician-

Table 3.3 Professional integrity-based responses to strong feelings that can distort the informed consent process.

Identify and recognize the potential for strong feelings in the informed consent process for high-risk clinical management.

Prevent strong feelings by adhering to the discipline of evidence-based clinical reasoning.

Prevent strong feelings by adhering to the discipline of argument-based ethical reasoning.

Expand the agenda of team meetings to seek mentorship and to debrief.

---

gynecologist away from the patient and toward him- or herself in an effort to mitigate those feelings. This understandable response can undercut the professional virtues, especially self-effacement and self-sacrifice. The result is distorted clinical judgment that can distort the informed consent process should the obstetrician-gynecologist unduly influence the patient's decision making.

The professional virtue of integrity should guide the response of the obstetrician-gynecologist. In the informed consent process about high-risk clinical management the obstetrician-gynecologist should be alert to the possibility of strong feelings occurring and prevent their emergence by refocusing on the patient's interests, needs, and concerns. Keeping a steady focus on evidence-based clinical reasoning and argument-based ethical reasoning should discipline these feelings and prevent them from becoming so strong as to develop into potentially distorting feelings. Team meetings, especially to seek mentorship and to debrief, have become an essential component of patient safety. The agenda of team meetings should include reporting strong feelings and group reflection on why they emerged and group support for their successful management in the future, using the responses just described.

3.5 Who Should Obtain Simple Consent?

By its very nature, simple consent does not require provision of complex clinical information about the patient's condition, the medically reasonable alternatives for its management, or prognosis with and without treatment. Simple consent requires only a concise and accurate description of the clinical intervention, e.g., "We need to draw some of your blood to send to the laboratory for analysis." A medical education is not required for this simple communication. Simple consent can therefore be obtained by any member of the healthcare team with the training and experience to perform the intervention.

3.6 Who Should Lead the Informed Consent Process?

The informed consent process, by contrast, does require provision of complex clinical information about the patient's condition, the medically reasonable alternatives for its management, and prognosis with and without treatment. Only a relevantly trained and experienced physician can provide this information. The obstetrician-gynecologist therefore has the professional responsibility to lead in the informed consent process in the care of female and pregnant patients. When other specialty physicians are involved, e.g., consideration of appendectomy in a pregnant patient, the obstetrician remains responsible for the patient's care and therefore should initiate the informed consent process and then ask the general surgeon to lead the informed consent process for the appendectomy. Both physicians should then respond to the patient's questions, maintaining respect for professional boundaries. For example, the general surgeon should defer to the obstetrician for questions about the implications of appendectomy for continued pregnancy, while the obstetrician should defer to the general surgeon for questions about complications of the surgical wound that might occur after the patient has been discharged.

3.7 Projecting Decision Making into the Future: Advance Directives

The ethical principle of respect for autonomy grounds the right of a patient to make healthcare decisions that will apply in the future should the patient lose the capacity to make decisions for herself. The law in all jurisdictions in the United States supports this projection of autonomous decision making into the future in the form of advance directives: a patient with decision-making capacity can make decisions about setting limits on life-sustaining treatment (Living Will or Directive to Physicians) and about appointing someone to make decisions for them, a surrogate decision maker (Medical Power of Attorney or Durable Power of Attorney for Health Care).[23] Sometimes the phrase "advance directives" is used, which is a misnomer and therefore should not be used. See Chapters 14 and 15 for a more detailed discussion of advance directives.

3.8 A Decision *By* the Patient *With* the Obstetrician-Gynecologist and Others Who Assist in the Decision-Making Process: Assisted Decision Making

3.8.1 Assessment of Decision-Making Capacity

If, during the informed consent process, the patient has exhibited signs of diminished ability to complete one or more of the seven components of decision-making capacity, the hypothesis that the patient has experienced impaired decision-making capacity becomes clinically justified. (See Table 3.2.) The obstetrician-gynecologist should test this hypothesis with an assessment of the patient's decision-making capacity. There is no requirement in the law or in the professional ethics of obstetrics and gynecology to have this assessment performed by a consultation-liaison psychiatrist or other qualified and experienced mental health professional. Indeed, in the outpatient setting such colleagues are not always readily available.

The obstetrician-gynecologist should evaluate each of the seven components of decision-making capacity, keeping in mind that an acceptable threshold for each should, as a rule, be set low, to prevent unjustified usurpation of the patient's autonomy. When the obstetrician-gynecologist elects to involve a psychiatrist or other mental health professional, there should be a clear division of labor and a plan to meet to review the results of the evaluation and perform a critical appraisal of the evaluation and its results, again to protect the patient's autonomy from unjustified usurpation.

3.8.2 Risk-Adjusted Assessment of Decision-Making Capacity: Proceed with Great Caution

Some have argued that it is ethically permissible to risk-adjust assessment of decision-making capacity. This means that, when the risk of not treating increases, the higher is the threshold for each component of decision making. Put another way, the greater the risk of nontreatment the greater is the burden on the patient to demonstrate decision-making capacity.[24] At first, it makes intuitive sense to risk-adjust thresholds of decision-making capacity as the risk of morbidity and mortality increases.

However, this approach risks introducing uncontrolled variation into setting the threshold for decision-making capacity, because different physicians will assess and respond to increased risk of nontreatment differently. This is not acceptable inasmuch as uncontrolled variation in any component of the processes of patient care is the definition of poor quality. Engaging in a poor process of patient care, especially when there is an alternative, is incompatible with professional integrity and is therefore ruled out.

The alternative is that the assessment of decision-making capacity should be independent of risk. The assessment of risk has a different and important role: The assessment of risk comes to bear concerning how much weight should be given to a patient's refusal and reengaging the patient in respectful persuasion in response.

3.8.3 Decision-Making Capacity Is Task Specific and Time Specific

3.8.3.1 Task-Specific Decision-Making Capacity

Decision making is task specific, especially with respect to the amount and complexity of the information provided to the patient. As both the amount and complexity of information increase, the demands on the patient's cognitive understanding and evaluative understanding increase. In such cases, an acceptable threshold for successfully completing these components of the decision-making process may need to be increased and efforts intensified to support the patient in meeting the increased cognitive and affective demands. The adjusted threshold should not be based on the mastery of cognitive demands of deliberative clinical judgment by the obstetrician-gynecologist. The adjustment should be autonomy based, oriented to what the patient signals is her level of mastery.

This provides a further objection to risk-adjusting the threshold: doing so invokes a beneficence-based rather than autonomy-based adjustment of the threshold. The goal therefore is not to set an increased threshold that leads to a judgment of impaired capacity. The goal, instead, is to empower the patient's autonomy by supporting her to meet an autonomy-based threshold.

3.8.3.2 Time-Specific Decision-Making Capacity

Decision-making capacity is also time specific, which becomes clinically relevant for patients whose capacity waxes (and meets acceptably low thresholds) and wanes (and does not meet such thresholds). This waxing and waning may be reversible and therefore should be worked up with appropriate consultation. If the waxing and waning is reversible, during its waxing phase this should be explained to the patient and she should be asked to authorize clinical management of it in the informed consent process. If the waxing and waning does not respond or is otherwise considered irreversible, the goal should be to obtain simple consent (when that is all that is needed) and to support the informed consent process when the patient is waxing. The patient should be informed that treatment will continue during the waning phases even if the patient expresses rejection verbally or physically. These expressions should be considered a function of diminished capacity to participate in the informed consent process and therefore should not alter the plan of clinical management provided that it can be continued safely.

3.8.3.3 Ulysses Contract

A preventive ethics approach to the challenges of waxing and waning capacity is called a Ulysses contract.[25,26] This is based on the episode in the *Odyssey* in which Ulysses and his crew were about to sail near the island of the Sirens. The Sirens were notorious for using their lovely song to entice crews to sail to their island, only for their ship to founder in hidden reefs and the crew to drown. To prevent these outcomes, Ulysses instructed his crew to stuff their ears with wax so that they would not hear the Sirens' song or his order to sail to the Sirens' island when he fell under their sway. He also ordered them to lash him to the mast so that when he lost cognitive and affective control, he could not endanger himself or the crew. A Ulysses contract is a species of advance directive: A patient who currently has decision-making capacity either requests or refuses treatment in advance of the time when she loses decision-making capacity. Some states in the United States recognize Ulysses contracts in the form of Mental Health Directives that can be used in advance to authorize or refuse to authorize specific forms of clinical management should the patient later decompensate.

3.8.4 When One or More Components of Decision-Making Capacity Are Diminished

When this assessment supports the deliberative clinical judgment that one or more components of decision making is impaired or absent, the next step is to deploy assisted decision making, i.e., decision making *by* the patient *with* the support of the obstetrician-gynecologist and appropriate consultations, as needed. The working assumption should be that this condition is reversible and efforts should be made to reverse the diminished or absent components of decision-making capacity, with the goal of returning the patient's capacity to threshold. Assisted decision making is especially clinically applicable when the female patient or pregnant patient has a mental disorder or illness. The obstetrician-gynecologist, in concert with psychiatry, should consider a series of responses. Psychosocial interventions such as communication skills training and problem-solving strategies should be considered, especially when the deficit concerns cognitive or evaluative understanding. Targeted education can also restore cognitive understanding to an acceptable threshold. Medications that can be safely administered during pregnancy should be considered, if there is time for them to take effect.[2,3,20,27]

3.9 A Decision *By* Others but *With* the Patient: Pediatric and Geriatric Assent

Some patients have impaired but not absent decision-making capacity, for whom assisted decision making is not successful in helping them attain an acceptable threshold for all of the components of decision making. (See Table 3.2.) This population includes adolescent patients who have not attained legal majority and do not have maturely developed components of decision making; patients with mental disorders and diseases that impair but do not eliminate the components of decision making; patients with cognitive disabilities that result in perhaps irreversible impairments of components of decision making but not their elimination; and patients with dementing disorders that result in components of decision making that have diminished below an acceptable threshold but have not disappeared altogether. These patients may be able to participate in the decision-making process to a level that requires the obstetrician-gynecologist, team members, and family members – especially those who seek to completely control the decision-making process – to attend to the patient's cognitive and evaluative understanding and take account of them in the decision-making process.

The first effort to articulate a clinical ethical concept to capture the phenomenon of diminished but not absent decision-making capacity was made in the pediatric ethics literature in the 1980s by a pediatric oncologist, Sanford Leikin.[28,29] Leikin proposed the concept of pediatric assent. The word "assent" appeared at that time in the federal regulations for research involving children and meant that a child who was a potential research subject had to be asked if he or she wanted to participate. If the child said "no," assent was not satisfied and the child could not be enrolled in the study. Leikin argued that this simple refusal – a variant of simple consent – was not sufficient. Assent should also mean that the child should, in a developmentally appropriate fashion, be informed about his or her condition, proposed clinical management of it, and the experience he or she would have during and after clinical management. The more adult-like the child's decision-making process is, the more weight that should be given to his or her decision making. It follows that the more adult-like the patient's decision making is, the stronger the obstetrician-gynecologist should advocate for it and ask the parents to consider the importance of the patient's decision to her. At the same time, the patient should be encouraged to listen to her parents' concerns. Sometimes this process of joint listening defuses tension and allows agreement to be reached.

The American Academy of Pediatrics has endorsed pediatric assent as one of the core concepts of pediatric ethics.[30,31] The Academy interpreted pediatric assent to ethically obligate the pediatrician to undertake the assent process with adolescent patients by completing the following steps:

1. Helping the patient achieve a developmentally appropriate awareness of the nature of his or her condition
2. Telling the patient what he or she can expect with tests and treatment(s)
3. Making a clinical assessment of the patient's understanding of the situation and the factors influencing how he or she is responding (including whether there is inappropriate pressure to accept testing or therapy)
4. Soliciting an expression of the patient's willingness to accept the proposed care. Regarding this final point, we note that no one should solicit a patient's views without intending to weigh them seriously. In situations in which the patient will have to receive medical care despite his or her objection, the patient should be told that fact and should not be deceived.[30, pp. 315–316]

Put more generally, the clinical ethical concept of assent requires that decision making occur *with* the patient but *by* others who should take into account the results of the assent process. The more adult-like that process is considered in deliberative clinical judgment to be, the more seriously should those making the decision *for* the patient take the patient's cognitive and evaluative understanding and preference(s) based on them.

These four steps can be reframed to serve as a clinically comprehensive guide to decision making with the populations of patients to whom the clinical ethical concept of assent applies: diminished but not absent components of decision making that cannot be restored to an acceptable threshold:

1. Helping the patient achieve a developmentally appropriate awareness of the nature of his or her condition by supporting the most complete possible development of his or her cognitive and evaluative understanding
2. Telling the patient what he or she can expect with tests and treatment(s) and addressing the patient's questions, to further support development of his or her cognitive and evaluative understanding
3. Making a clinical assessment of the patient's cognitive and evaluative understanding and the factors influencing the voluntariness of how he or she is responding, including whether there is potentially controlling pressure to accept or refuse testing or therapy
4. Soliciting an expression of the patient's willingness to accept the proposed care. No obstetrician-gynecologist should solicit a patient's views without intending to weigh them seriously and without supporting the

decision maker in weighing them seriously. In situations in which the patient will have to receive medical care despite her objection, the patient should be told that fact and should not be deceived.

This assent process should be understood in the professional ethics of obstetrics and gynecology to acknowledge and respect the remaining autonomy of the patient: her values and beliefs to the extent that she can express them. The ethical principle of respect for autonomy, which does apply in the informed consent process and results in a decision *by* and *with* the patient, does not apply to patients who exhibit irreversibly impaired autonomy. Applicable law and organizational policy should be followed for the identification of what is known as a surrogate decision maker. (See Section 3.10.) Following the assent process will satisfy the substituted judgment standard for surrogate decision making, which is explained in Section 3.10.

3.10 A Decision *By* Others *For* the Patient but *Not With* the Patient: Surrogate Decision Making

In some cases, informed consent, assisted decision making, and assent fail clinically, despite best efforts to achieve them by the obstetrician-gynecologist. (See Table 3.2.) Some patients are reliably assessed to have lost decision-making capacity: impairments of the components of decision making are so clinically severe that the patient cannot reliably complete them. Unlike patients for whom assisted decision making results in components of decision making restored to an acceptable threshold, these impairments are irreversible; decisions cannot be made *by* such patients. Unlike patients who have the capacity for assent, these patients cannot meaningfully express cognitive or evaluative understanding; decisions cannot be made *with* such patients. Decision making *by* such patients is not clinically, ethically, or legally meaningful. Decisions must be made *by* and *with* others *for* such patients. These individuals are known as surrogate decision makers.

Applicable law designates the surrogate decision maker, usually in a listed priority. Typically the priority list starts with a court-appointed guardian or the person named in the patient's medical power of attorney. Next in order come the patient's spouse, adult children, other family members, or a close friend (as in Veterans Health Affairs), in descending priority. Most jurisdictions identify a surrogate of last resort, when no one on the priority list exists, is willing to become the surrogate decision maker, or cannot be found, e.g., the attending physician and one other physician not previously involved in the patient's care. Court review of assessment of decision-making capacity and of surrogate decision-making process is usually not required. The obstetrician-gynecologist should follow organizational policy for the identification of the legally designated decision makers. Questions about the interpretation of organizational policy as to who should become the patient's surrogate decision maker should be directed to organizational legal counsel, because such questions are about the interpretation of applicable law.

Some states restrict the scope of decision-making authority of the surrogate decision maker. Of particular note is the fact that some states do not permit the surrogate decision maker to authorize termination of pregnancy or discontinuation of life-sustaining treatment for a pregnant patient with a terminal or irreversible condition. (See Section 3.1.2.)

3.10.1 Two Standards for Surrogate Decision Making

In health law and professional ethics in medicine generally, there are two standards, *in priority order*, that should guide the surrogate decision maker in the informed consent process for the clinical management of the patient's condition: first, the substituted judgment standard and then the best interests standard.

3.10.1.1 Substituted Judgment Standard

The substituted judgment standard is an autonomy-based standard, which explains its priority. The informed consent process includes the beneficence-based ethical obligation to identify the medically reasonable alternatives for the management of the patient's condition and the autonomy-based obligation to empower the patient to interpret and evaluate this information and make an informed decision. The goal of the substituted judgment standard is to empower the surrogate decision maker to make a decision that is reliably based on the patient's values and beliefs and thus in this sense respect the patient's autonomy. These values and beliefs become the basis for the surrogate's evaluative understanding and in this way implement respect for the patient's past autonomy.

How reliable does the surrogate's substituted judgment have to be? There are two standards in the law for the reliability of substituted judgment, i.e., acting with confidence that the surrogate has made a good-faith effort to represent the patient's values and beliefs. In the majority of states in the United States, the standard for reliability is preponderance of the evidence: the surrogate's substituted judgment is more likely than not to reliably represent the patient's judgment. In other states, the standard is clear and convincing evidence, or a 75% probability of reliably representing the patient's judgment. No legal standard requires 100% reliability for the practical reason that such a standard is not attainable and, even if it were, there is no way for an obstetrician-gynecologist to reliably determine whether such a standard has been satisfied by a surrogate, who is doubly under stress by being concerned about the well-being of the patient and coping with the weighty responsibility of making clinically significant decisions for the patient. Certainty is not required. Insisting on certainty is a formula for undermining the substituted judgment standard.

Some surrogate decision makers know the patient well enough, e.g., from conversations in which the patient stated her preferences explicitly, that the surrogate can simply report what the patient would want were she still able to speak for herself. Research indicates that in such circumstances the surrogate does not experience decision making as a decision but as making a report, because the surrogate has very high confidence in meeting the substituted judgment standard.[32] It may be useful to ask surrogates who have been in long-standing relationships with a patient whether the patient had ever expressed her preferences explicitly. In that case, the surrogate can make a report and perhaps reduce the risk of biopsychosocial stress from having to make a decision by reconstructing the patient's preference.[33]

3.10.1.2 The Best Interests Standard

When the surrogate decision maker is not able to reliably make a substituted judgment, he or she should base his or her decisions on a considered judgment of which course of clinical management is reliably predicted to protect and promote the patient's health-related interests. The best interests standard is a beneficence-based standard.

The beneficence-based obligation of the obstetrician-gynecologist to identify the medically reasonable alternatives for the management of the patient's condition should guide the application of the best interests standard. The justification for this proposal is that all medically reasonable alternatives, by definition, are reliably predicted to protect and promote the health-related interests of patients. The obstetrician should explain this clinical ethical reality to the surrogate decision maker and present the medically reasonable alternatives. Just as in the informed consent process, the obstetrician-gynecologist should recommend a medically reasonable alternative when it is the only one or when in deliberative clinical judgment it is clinically superior to the other medically reasonable alternative(s). The surrogate fulfills the best interests standard by accepting such a recommendation, which should reduce the biopsychosocial stress of surrogate decision making. When in deliberative clinical judgment there are competing medically reasonable alternatives, i.e., none is clinically superior, all should be presented and explained. The surrogate should be assured that authorizing any one of these medically reasonable alternatives will satisfy the best interests standard.

As noted in Section 3.10.1.1, there is some evidence that when a surrogate needs to make a decision in the absence of knowing what the patient would want and simply reporting it the surrogate can experience clinically significant biopsychosocial stress.[32,33] The process of assuring the surrogate decision maker that authorizing a medically reasonable alternative always satisfies the best interests standard may help reduce such unwelcome stress.

3.11 Clinical Ethical Topics in Decision Making for Patients

3.11.1 Variants of Impaired Autonomy

Impaired autonomy is not invariant. Instead, like all human traits, it displays variation. There are clinical differences among the variants of impaired autonomy that have distinctive ethical implications for the roles of simple and informed consent, assisted decision making, assent, and surrogate decision making.

3.11.1.1 Chronic and Variable Impairment of Autonomy

Mental disorders and illnesses can have a chronic and variable effect on autonomy.[2,3,20,27,34] The chronicity of the impairment relates to the chronicity of mental illness and is one of its distinctive characteristics, inasmuch as remission is not usually accomplished. Instead, long-term management is undertaken with the goals of secondary and tertiary prevention. This means that the impairment of the components of decision-making capacity is long lasting, requiring periodic reassessment and, if necessary, a revised plan of clinical management. Mental illness and disorders can have a distinctive impairing effect on these components. Psychosis can distract the patient, affecting her ability to pay attention and thus adversely affecting the remaining six components. Patients with even well-managed depression tend to accent the negative consequences of current events, which can result in incomplete cognitive understanding if positive potential outcomes are not believed to have the potential to occur. This accenting of the negative can distort evaluative judgment. Paranoia can affect cognitive understanding by introducing counterfactual causal reasoning. Impulsiveness can reduce the voluntariness of decision making.

These impairments may be ameliorable, which calls for assisted decision making as the first response. If assisted decision making is not successful in restoring the seven components to an acceptable threshold, assent becomes the second response. If both assisted decision making fails to produce a decision made *by* and *with* the patient and if assent fails to produce a decision made *by* others and *with* the patient, then surrogate decision making is required. This means that a deliberative clinical judgment that a mental disorder or illness has caused chronic and variable impairment of autonomy does not support turning immediately to surrogate decision making.

3.11.1.2 Chronic and Invariable Impairment of Autonomy

Some conditions, such as cognitive disabilities of various kinds, can impair one or more of the components of decision-making capacity and this impairment may prove refractory to clinical management aimed at restoring an acceptable threshold of decision-making capacity. When after thorough evaluation and trial of accepted clinical management, deliberative clinical judgment supports the assessment that the patient's autonomy is chronically and invariably impaired, assisted decision making will not succeed. However, invariable impairment of one or more of the components of decision-making capacity, especially cognitive understanding in the case of cognitive disabilities, does not mean that the component(s) have been eliminated. This means that assent remains an approach to decision making *with* the patient but *by* others that should be implemented and assessed. Only if assent fails to produce a decision *with* the patient but *by* others is it ethically permissible to turn to surrogate decision making.

3.11.1.3 Chronic and Progressive Impairment of Autonomy

Dementing disorders that do not respond to clinical management, e.g., those resulting from vitamin B_{12} deficiency, are chronic. Many of them are progressive, which means that the impairing effects on the components of decision-making capacity increase over time. It is not meaningful to respond to chronic impairments of autonomy that are refractory to clinical management and that are progressive with assisted decision making. The appropriate response should be guided by the clinical reality that dementing disorders take a great toll on cognitive understanding and do so before adversely affecting evaluative understanding. This means that many patients retain the capacity to express their values in response to the question, "What is important to you?"[18] As long as family members and others confirm that the expressed values sound like those the patient has lived by, then assent based on such evaluative understanding remains a viable option. The first response to chronic and progressive impairment of autonomy should be to attempt to make decisions *with* the patient but *by* others. This is known as geriatric assent.[35]

3.11.1.4 Chronic and Decreasing Impairment of Autonomy

Adolescence is marked by the progressive diminution of the "disabilities of minority," as they are known in the law, and the progressive emergence of adult-like and then adult decision-making capacity. This emergence displays variation, e.g., some older adolescents with chronic diseases such as cystic fibrosis display adult-like cognitive and evaluative understanding or notable progress toward these over time. The impairments of autonomy of children are chronic but not permanent and they progressively decrease until they disappear. This means that assent should be the primary approach to decision making *with* adolescent patients but *by* their parents or guardians. This is known as pediatric assent.

The obstetrician-gynecologist should start preparing during the patient's eighteenth year for her transition to adulthood, i.e., the transition from pediatric assent to decision making *by* the patient in simple consent and in the informed consent process. The patient's parents, especially when they have served as primary caregivers at home, should also be prepared for this transition. The patient who remains dependent on her parents for care also needs to become aware that adults take responsibility for the impact of their decisions on others. This means that the patient needs to develop a sustained awareness of the burden of her decisions on her parents and other family caregivers and recognize when these individuals might justifiably judge such burdens to be unacceptable.

3.12 Surrogate Decision Making about Termination of Pregnancy

Like all surrogate decision making, surrogate decision making about termination of pregnancy should be based, in priority order, on the substituted judgment standard and best interests standard. The goal should be a decision that reliably respects the patient's past autonomy.

Health law about termination of pregnancy is a complicating legal factor that cannot be ignored. Some jurisdictions legally restrict the scope of a surrogate decision maker to authorize termination of pregnancy in their statutes governing decision making for patients who have lost decision-making capacity. Some states also exclude the application of an advance directive when a patient with a terminal or irreversible condition also is pregnant. To date, this restriction has not been legally challenged.

Organizational policy should be based on surrogate decision making and its two standards, as well as applicable law. Organizational policy should be comprehensive and provide clear guidance for the obstetrician-gynecologist on how to proceed, to prevent unnecessary exposure of the obstetrician-gynecologist and organization to legal risk. Uncertainty about the clinical implementation of such policies should be managed by consulting the organization's legal counsel. (See Chapter 9.)

3.13 Surrogate Decision Making about Prevention of Pregnancy

Sometimes the parent(s) or guardian of a patient who requires a surrogate decision maker may request clinical management to prevent pregnancy. Such requests may be made for an adolescent patient with a cognitive disability. There may be concern about the biopsychosocial risks of unwanted pregnancy resulting from sexual activity, including sexual predation. There may be concern about the biopsychosocial risks of pregnancy for their disabled daughter or her ability to become an adequate parent. There may be concern about the biopsychosocial burdens on them of an unwanted pregnancy or the caregiving responsibilities to a grandchild, especially when the parent(s) have clinically significant health issues of their own. There may be concern about the biopsychosocial burdens on their daughter of menorrhagia. The parent(s) or a guardian may request prevention of pregnancy for a patient with a mental disorder or disease that has reduced the patient's self-care capacity or her ability to protect herself from unwanted and unprotected sexual intercourse. These are especially compelling requests because such patients are known to be at risk of abuse by sexual predators.

In the professional ethics of obstetrics and gynecology one prima facie autonomy-based ethical obligation and three prima facie beneficence-based ethical obligations provide a framework to guide the response of the obstetrician-gynecologist. There is a prima facie autonomy-based ethical obligation to prevent unwanted pregnancy.

There is a general, prima facie beneficence-based ethical obligation to provide clinical management that will protect and promote the patient's biopsychosocial interests. The focus should not be solely on just one of these three dimensions, to prevent distortion of clinical judgment that reduction to one or two dimensions causes. There is a prima facie beneficence-based ethical obligation to prevent sexual exploitation of patients whose capacity for self-care and self-protection is diminished. There is also a prima facie beneficence-based ethical obligation to preserve fertility.

There is potential for conflict among these prima facie ethical obligations, to which a preventive ethics approach should be taken. The goal should be to transform the initial request into a deliberative judgment of the parent(s) or guardian as the outcome of the informed consent process that is based on a comprehensive clinical evaluation of the patient and identification of the implications of each of the four prima facie ethical obligations for whether prevention of pregnancy is ethically permissible and, if so, which forms of prevention of pregnancy are ethically permissible. The three prima facie beneficence-based ethical obligations and the prima facie autonomy-based ethical obligation should guide a deliberative judgment about the ethical permissibility of preventing pregnancy. All four prima facie ethical obligations should guide a deliberative judgment about the ethical permissibility of technically possible forms of prevention of pregnancy.

Obstetrician-gynecologists should advocate for and follow organizational policy to guide professionally responsible responses to such requests. Such a policy should establish a committee to review all proposals by physicians to implement such parental requests and state the four prima facie ethical principles that should guide the informed consent process. Such a policy should begin with the requirement that the patient has had a thorough evaluation by relevant specialists, including their assessment of the patient's capacity to manage pregnancy or disorders such as menorrhagia. Such a policy also should be based on applicable law; define clearly a process for reaching a deliberative clinical judgment about the justification of such requests; and identify the forms of clinical management that are acceptable and the clinical circumstances in which a trial of contraception, including implantable long-term contraception, should be undertaken before sterilization. Such a policy should also define the role of pediatric assent with the patient, so that her values and beliefs, if she can express them, can be identified and taken into account. Finally, such a policy should define clearly the documentation required for committee review. (See Chapter 7.)

3.14 Managing Doubts about the Reliability of a Surrogate Decision Maker

Questions are raised about the reliability of some surrogate decision makers when they do not comport themselves according to the substituted judgment standard or the best interests standard. An especially important situation is when there is concern that the surrogate decision maker is basing decisions on his or her self-interest and not on the values and beliefs of the patient, as required by the substituted judgment standard, or the patient's interests, as required by the best interests standard. This may be an innocent mistake, resulting from the surrogate experiencing the burden of decision making as very difficult to manage and naturally substituting his or her values for those of the patient. The obstetrician should express a respectful reminder that everyone is bound by the ethical obligation to identify, respect, and implement decisions based on the patient's values and beliefs as the first goal. If that goal cannot be achieved, then the *patient's* best interest should guide everyone. Surrogates who are family members will usually recall that their relationship to the patient is one of respect for and deference to the patient's values and interests and return to the role of responsible surrogate decision maker.

In rare instances, the surrogate continues to make decisions on the basis of his or her interests and not the values and interests of the patient. There are two worst case scenarios. The surrogate may make decisions for which there is evidence that the substituted judgment standard is not being followed, i.e., when from other reliable sources the patient's values and beliefs have been reliably identified. The surrogate may also make decisions that, if implemented, would result in net clinical harm in violation of the best-interests standard. In such circumstances the obstetrician-gynecologist must consult with organizational legal counsel. Organizational policy should support legal counsel in informing the surrogate that decisions about clinical management of the patient's condition will be made by the obstetrician-gynecologist and implemented by him or her and the patient's care team until the status of the surrogate has been determined in the appropriate legal venue.

3.15 Managing Refusal of a Family Member to Accept the Legally Designated Surrogate

Refusal of a family member to accept the legally designated surrogate decision maker is not common. Refusal may be motivated by complex family dynamics or by concern that the surrogate decision maker is not willing to fulfill the substituted judgment and best interests standard or has impaired or absent decision-making capacity. The response to the first situation should be to involve consultation-liaison psychiatry and other disciplines such as social work and chaplaincy as needed to gain a clinically grounded understanding of the family dynamics. The obstetrician should point out that everyone, including him- or herself and all of the other members of the patient's care team, have ethical and legal obligations to the patient to accept decisions made *by* the surrogate *for* the patient and to support the surrogate in this important role. Respectfully, it should be pointed out that family members have the same obligations.

Concerns about the decision-making capacity of the surrogate should be explored in detail with the family member who has them and then by observation of the surrogate. If there is clinical concern that one or more of the seven components of decision making is impaired or absent in the surrogate, formal evaluation of decision-making capacity should be undertaken with the consent of the surrogate. Otherwise, an observational assessment should be considered and, if pursued, should include a psychiatrist.

If a family member continues to refuse to accept the legally designated surrogate of if there are clinically grounded concerns about the surrogate's decision-making capacity, then the obstetrician-gynecologist must consult with organizational legal counsel and hospital policy to identify the legally permitted forms of challenging the status of the surrogate decision maker by another individual in a class of persons that appears on the list of eligible surrogate decision makers in applicable law and organizational policy. The results should be explained to family members, who are then free to pursue legal recourse. Meanwhile the surrogate should continue in his or her role until removed and replaced according to the provisions of applicable law. In some jurisdictions a healthcare organization may have standing to challenge a surrogate on the ground that he or she has impaired or absent decision-making capacity.

3.16 Medical Emergencies

A medical emergency exists when there is an immediate threat to the patient's life or threat of immediate serious, far-reaching, and irreversible loss of health entailing immediate clinical management of the patient's condition to prevent these outcomes. There is therefore no time for the informed consent process or the informed refusal process. There is also no time for the surrogate decision-making process. Appropriate clinical management should begin without any delay.

The ethical justification for providing immediate emergency medical care is beneficence based and nonmaleficence based, to prevent unacceptable outcomes. The justification is also autonomy based, appealing to the assumption that any patient wants to prevent these unacceptable outcomes.

There is one important exception: the patient has an applicable advance directive that refuses life-sustaining treatment, which includes cardiopulmonary resuscitation and admission to a critical care unit. Hospital policy should be clear that advance directives will be honored, so that emergency medical teams will be supported when they do so. Some patients leave the hospital with a form of advance directive known as an Out-of-Hospital Do-Not-Resuscitate Order (OOH DNR Order) that instructs rescue teams in the field not to resuscitate the patient, to provide comfort care, and transport the patient to the hospital. Hospital policy should require communication by the rescue crew that they are transporting a patient with an OOH DNR Order. Hospital policy should also provide, should the patient arrive in the emergency department alive, for hospice and palliative care starting in the emergency department with prompt admission to the appropriate in-hospital service.

Once the patient has been stabilized there are two possible decision-making pathways. The patient recovers decision-making capacity, in which case the informed consent process should be followed. Or, the patient does not recover decision-making capacity, in which case the surrogate decision-making process should be followed.

When initiating emergency responses, there may be time to tell the patient what is being done, to which the patient may agree or disagree. Agreement does not count as simple consent, much less informed consent. Disagreement has no authority because there is no time for the informed refusal process. Nonetheless, this brief disclosure represents an important form of respect for the patient.

References

1. American College of Obstetricians and Gynecologists. ACOG Committee Opinion No. 439: Informed consent. Obstet Gynecol 2009; 114 (2 Pt 1): 401–408.
2. McCullough LB, Coverdale JH, Chervenak FA. Ethical challenges of decision making with pregnant patients who have schizophrenia. Am J Obstet Gynecol 2002; 187: 696–702.

3. Coverdale JH, Chervenak FA, McCullough LB, Bayer T. Ethically justified, clinically comprehensive guidelines for the management of the depressed pregnant patient. Am J Obstet Gynecol 1996; 171: 169–173.

4. White BC. Competence to Consent. Washington, DC: Georgetown University Press, 1994.

5. Grisso T, Appelbaum PS. Assessing Competence to Consent to Treatment: A Guide for Physicians and Other Health Professionals. New York: Oxford University Press, 1998.

6. Faden RR, Beauchamp TL. A History and Theory of Informed Consent. New York: Oxford University Press, 1986.

7. Beauchamp TL, Childress JF. Principles of Biomedical Ethics, 7th ed. New York: Oxford University Press, 2013.

8. Whitney SN, McGuire AL, McCullough LB. A typology of shared decision making, informed consent, and simple consent. Ann Intern Med 2003; 140: 54–59.

9. *Schloendorff v. Society of New York Hospital*, 211 N.Y. 125, 129–130 (1914).

10. Lombardo PA. Phantom tumors and hysterical women: revising our view of the Schloendorff case. J Law Med Ethics 2005; 33: 791–801.

11. Chervenak J, McCullough LB, Chervenak FA. Surgery without consent or miscommunication? A new look at a landmark legal case. Am J Obstet Gynecol 2015; 212: 586–590.

12. Wear S. Informed Consent: Patient Autonomy and Physician Beneficence within Clinical Medicine. Dordrecht, the Netherlands: Springer, 1993.

13. Engel GL. The need for a new medical model: a challenge for biomedicine. Science 1977; 196: 129–136.

14. McCullough LB. The professional medical ethics model of decision making under conditions of uncertainty. Med Care Rev Res 2013; 70(1 Suppl): 141S–58S.

15. Kon AA. The shared decision-making continuum. JAMA 2010; 304: 903–904.

16. Chervenak FA, McCullough LB. The unlimited rights model of obstetric ethics threatens professionalism: a commentary. BJOG 2017; 124: 1144–1147.

17. Ecker J. Minkoff H. Home birth: what are physicians' ethical obligations when patient choices may carry increased risk? Obstet Gynecol 2011; 117: 1179–1182.

18. McCullough LB, Wilson NL, Teasdale TA, Kolpakchi AL, Skelly JR. Mapping personal, familial, and professional values in long-term care decisions. Gerontologist 1993; 33: 324–332.

19. Blumenthal-Barby JS, Coverdale JH, McCullough LB. A typology and ethical considerations of methods of influence on decision making in patients with psychiatric disorders. Harv Rev Psychiatry 2013; 21: 275–279.

20. Coverdale JH, McCullough LB, Chervenak FA, Bayer T. Clinical implications and management strategies when depression occurs during pregnancy. Aust N Z J Obstet Gynaecol 1996; 36: 424–429.

21. *Truman v. Thomas*, 27 Cal.3d 285 (1980).

22. Chervenak FA, McCullough LB. Clinical guides to preventing ethical conflicts between pregnant women and their physicians. Am J Obstet Gynecol 1990; 162: 303–307.

23. American College of Obstetricians and Gynecologists. ACOG Committee Opinion Number 617: End-of-life decision making. Obstet Gynecol 2015; 125: 261–267.

24. Drane JF. Competency to give informed consent: a model for making clinical assessment. JAMA 1984; 252: 925–927.

25. Winston ME, Winston SM, Appelbaum PS, Rhoden N. Can a subject consent to a 'Ulysses Contract'? Hastings Cent Rept 1982; 12: 26–28.

26. Spellecy R. Reviving Ulysses contracts. Kennedy Inst Ethics J 2003; 13: 373–392.

27. McCullough LB, Coverdale JH, Chervenak FA. Is pharmacologic research on pregnant women with psychoses ethically permissible? J Perinat Med 2015; 43: 439–444.

28. Leikin S. Minors' assent, consent, or dissent to medical treatment. J Pediatr 1983; 102: 169–176.

29. Leikin S. Minors' assent, consent, or dissent to medical research. IRB 1993; 15: 1–7.

30. American Academy of Pediatrics. Committee on Bioethics. Informed consent, parental permission, and assent in pediatric practice. Pediatrics 1995; 95: 314–317.

31. Katz AL, Webb SA. Committee on Bioethics. American Academy of Pediatrics. Informed consent in decision-making in pediatric practice. Pediatrics 2016; 138 (2): e20161485.

32. Braun UK, Naik AD, McCullough LB. Reconceptualizing the experience of surrogate decision making: reports vs genuine decisions. Ann Fam Med 2009; 7: 249–253.

33. Braun UK, McCullough LB, Beyth RJ, Wray NP, Kunik ME, Morgan RO. Racial and ethnic differences in the treatment of seriously ill patients: a comparison of African American, Caucasian, and Hispanic veterans. J Natl Med Assoc 2008; 100: 1041–1051.

34. Coverdale JH, Bayer TL, McCullough LB, Chervenak FA. Respecting the autonomy of chronic mentally ill women in decisions about contraception. Hosp Community Psychiatry 1993; 44: 671–674.

35. Coverdale JH, McCullough LB, Molinari V, Workman R. Ethically justified clinical strategies for promoting geriatric assent. Int J Geriatr Psychiatry 2006; 21: 151–157.

Chapter 4
Confidentiality

GOAL
This chapter provides an ethical framework for the prima facie ethical obligation of confidentiality to patients.

OBJECTIVES
On completing study of this chapter, the reader will:

Identify the historical transition from an absolute ethical obligation of confidentiality to a prima facie ethical obligation of confidentiality

Identify ethical challenges to the prima facie ethical obligation of confidentiality

Demonstrate how ethical challenges to the prima facie ethical obligation of confidentiality should be responsibly managed

Apply the ethical framework of the prima facie ethical obligation of confidentiality to patients in clinical practice

TOPICS

4.1	Confidentiality in Professional Ethics in Obstetrics and Gynecology	69
	4.1.2 History of the Obligation	69
	4.1.2.1 The Hippocratic Oath	69
	4.1.2.2 Friedrich Hoffmann on the Politic Physician as Taciturn	69
	4.1.2.3 John Gregory on Keeping Patients' Secrets	70
	4.1.2.4 Thomas Percival on Keeping Patients' Secrets	71
	4.1.2.5 The Shift from an Absolute to Prima Facie Ethical Obligation	71
	4.1.2.6 Confidentiality: A Prima Facie Ethical Obligation	72
4.2	Setting Ethically Justified Limits on the Prima Facie Ethical Obligation of Confidentiality in Obstetrics and Gynecology	72
4.3	Ethical Challenges to Fulfilling the Prima Facie Ethical Obligation of Confidentiality	73
	4.3.1 Emergency Medical Care	73
	4.3.2 Disclosure to Family Members during and after Procedures Requiring Sedation or Anesthesia	73
	4.3.3 Inquiries by the Patient's Employer	74
	4.3.4 Insurance Claims	74
	4.3.5 Electronic Medical Record	75
	4.3.6 Implications of Genetic and Genomic Information for Individuals Other than the Patient	75
	4.3.7 Patients with Sexually Transmitted Disease Engaging in Behavior Known to Transmit Disease	76
	4.3.8 Health Insurance Portability and Accountability Act	76
	4.3.9 Electronic Communication with Patients	77
	4.3.10 Use of Social Media	77

Chapter 4: Confidentiality

> **Key Concepts**
>
> Absolute ethical obligation of confidentiality
> Confidentiality
> Enlightened self-interest
> Harm principle
> Medical emergency
> Prima facie ethical obligation of confidentiality
> Right to privacy
> Surrogate decision making
> *Tarasoff v. Regents of the University of California*

4.1 Confidentiality in Professional Ethics in Obstetrics and Gynecology

Confidentiality names the ethical obligation in the professional ethics of medicine of all physicians and other healthcare professionals involved in a patient's care to maintain, as inaccessible, information about the patient by preventing access to that information by those without authorization to have access to it. Confidentiality is now understood as a prima facie ethical obligation that is both beneficence based and autonomy based. The history of the obligation of confidentiality is crucial to understanding how and why this double justification is taken for granted, because the understanding of confidentiality was different in the past. The obligation started out based on the physician's honor, and then on the physician's prudence as an expression of enlightened self-interest, and became explicitly beneficence based, to protect the patient from psychosocial harm. In the twentieth century an autonomy-based account emerges: the appeal to the patient's right to privacy. The obligation also started out as an absolute ethical obligation until later in the twentieth century justified limits on the obligation were recognized.

4.1.2 History of the Obligation

4.1.2.1 The Hippocratic Oath

The ethical obligation of confidentiality is perhaps the oldest ethical obligation in the history of Western medical ethics. For example, the Hippocratic oath treats confidentiality as an absolute (i.e., no exceptions) ethical obligation: "8. i. And about whatever I may see or hear in treatment, or even without treatment, in the life of human beings – things that should not ever be blurted out outside –I will remain silent, holding such things to be unutterable [sacred, not to be divulged]."[1]

The ethical obligation was absolute. Inasmuch as there were no permanent records, an absolute obligation could be maintained. The scope is very broad and includes psychosocial consequences for the sick individual of violating confidentiality. The justification appeals to "things that should not ever be blurted out outside" that therefore become "unutterable."

One plausible interpretation is that ancient Greek societies were cultures based on maintaining one's honor and integrity. One sees this line of reasoning, for example, in *Crito*, in which Plato (ca. 427–ca. 348 BCE) has Socrates defend not escaping from, but accepting, his death sentence because as a good citizen of Athens he is obligated to obey the law.[2] Honor is a cluster concept – it has several components, not all of which have to apply in every usage. These components include a kind of proper self-regard that is warranted when one is self-disciplined in one's adherence to values that an individual should regard as important and one experiences the excellence of achievement from doing so. In this meaning of it, honor is an expression of intellectual and moral integrity. Honor is not mere self-regard or *amour propre*, as it came to be known later: a preening self-regard based on inconsequential values and no achievement.[3] Sharing information about someone, no matter whether from learning about their intimacies in clinical care or from general, social awareness, is to "blurt" out what should remain inaccessible to others, i.e., secret. Blurting anything out is an unacceptable loss of self-discipline. Blurting out is gossip, another unacceptable loss of self-control, a flawed behavior in which serious-minded people (another component of honor) do not ever indulge themselves. Violating confidentiality is to speak the "unutterable" and thus always and everywhere ethically impermissible.

4.1.2.2 Friedrich Hoffmann on the Politic Physician as Taciturn

In the early eighteenth century Friedrich Hoffmann (1660–1742) wrote *Medicus Politicus* (*The Politic Physician*), a guide for medical students entering a world of medical practice in which payers had far more power than physicians.[4] (See Chapter 1.) To protect their legitimate self-interests, including some level of job security, physicians should cultivate the virtue of prudence: the habit of identifying and acting to protect and promote one's legitimate self-interests. Hoffmann's distinctive contribution to the history of Western medical ethics was to interpret the physician's legitimate self-interests as enlightened self-interests: the physician should define his self-interests in terms of the legitimate interests of the sick individual. Prudence requires the physician, out of enlightened self-interest, to keep information about the sick individual secret because doing so protects the patient's health-related self-interest. Maintaining confidentiality never gives the sick individual pause that the physician might be a gossip and thus untrustworthy. Maintaining confidentiality thereby prevents the physician from being dismissed from service, without being paid to boot. The self-interest of the physician and that of the sick individual align. This is enlightened self-interest, i.e., the self-interest of the physician is understood to align with the self-interests of the sick individual and therefore become the physician's legitimate self-interest.

"Taciturn" is the word Hoffmann uses. Under the heading "Concerning the peculiar virtues of utmost necessity for conserving public opinion," he writes: "Rule 1: The physician should be humble, not arrogant." This includes not bragging about one's clinical accomplishments that, in the small community of the well-to-do who could afford physicians' fees, might easily be linked to the individual who received the benefits of such accomplishments. He adds: "Rule 2: The physician should be taciturn," an explicit admonition to maintain confidentiality. Under the heading "On the duties of the physician in obstetrics and the care of women," Hoffmann puts taciturnity in the company of other prudence-based virtues of the midwife, i.e., man-midwife as obstetricians were once called: "Rule 1: The midwife above all should be pious, chaste, sober, not timid, taciturn, and experienced."[4] Enlightened self-interest dictates that there should be no exceptions to the physician's prudence-based taciturnity.

4.1.2.3 John Gregory on Keeping Patients' Secrets

Later in the eighteenth century, John Gregory (1724–1773), coinventor with Thomas Percival (1740–1804) of the ethical concept of medicine as a profession (see Chapter 1), goes into detail about keeping patients' secrets, especially those of female patients:

> A physician, by the nature of his profession, has many opportunities of knowing the private characters and concerns of the families in which he is employed. Besides what he may learn from his own observation, he is often admitted to the confidence of those, who perhaps think they owe their life to his care. He sees people in the most disadvantageous circumstances, very different from those in which the world views them; – oppressed with pain, sickness, and low spirits. In these humiliating situations, instead of wonted chearfulness, evenness of temper, and vigour of mind, he meets with peevishness, impatience, and timidity. Hence appears how much the characters of individuals, and the credit of families, may sometimes depend on the discretion, secrecy, and honour of a physician. Secrecy is particularly requisite where women are concerned. Independent of the peculiar tenderness with which a woman's character should be treated, there are certain circumstances of health, which, though in no respect connected with her reputation, every woman, from the natural delicacy of her sex, is anxious to conceal; and, in some cases, the concealment of these circumstances may be of consequence to her health, her interest, and to her happiness.[5, pp. 26–27]

A patient's reputation for steadiness and reliability could be ruined by reports about how he behaves when ill enough to summon the physician. "Credit" means financial credit or borrowed money that lenders could call in before the due date if the lender became concerned that the debtor might not live to pay off a debt.[3] In other words, maintaining confidentiality protects the patient from psychosocial harm, echoing the broad scope of confidentiality in the Hippocratic oath.

Gregory goes on to address confidentiality regarding female patients. Gregory in his lectures on professional ethics in medicine championed "women of learning and virtue" as moral exemplars that his medical students, who were all men, should emulate.[3,5] "Delicacy" is the tender regard for others and models the physician–patient relationship. It is a serious error to read this text through twenty-first-century sensibilities in which the use of "delicacy" to characterize women would be understood as condescending or sexist. This is the error that historians call presentism.[6]

The last sentence refers, obliquely, to a dark side of obstetrics at that time. The birth of a bastard child (the woman's husband is not the biological father of her child) was a social calamity for women in the upper classes, the only social group that could afford the fees of a physician. Man-midwives (forerunners of modern obstetricians) used forceps – the advanced intrapartum technology of the time – for difficult deliveries. As all obstetricians know, the aggressive use of forceps can cause death. To prevent bastardy from being discovered, women would ask their obstetrician to cause stillbirth, which could be accomplished by dismissing attendants from the woman's bedchambers to devote uninterrupted attention to a challenging delivery. This was accepted practice,[3] although condemned by female midwives.[7] If later the husband dismissed the obstetrician from service or did not pay, some obstetricians apparently blackmailed their female patients out of economic self-interest. Gregory is addressing – and condemning – this practice as an ethically impermissible breach of confidentiality. Gregory continues the tradition of absolute confidentiality and provides an ethical justification for it in professional ethics in medicine, which is based on sympathetic regard for the patient, especially the female patient. (See Chapter 1.)

4.1.2.4 Thomas Percival on Keeping Patients' Secrets

Percival, coinventor with Gregory of the ethical concept of medicine as a profession (See Chapter 1.), addresses the challenges of maintaining confidentiality in the architecturally open spaces of a hospital.

> V. In the large wards of an infirmary the patients should be interrogated concerning their complaints, in a tone of voice which cannot be over*heard. Secrecy,* also, when required by peculiar circumstances, should be strictly observed. And females should always be treated with the most scrupulous *delicacy.* To neglect or to sport with their feelings is cruelty, and every wound thus inflicted tends to produce a callousness of mind, a contempt of decorum, and an insensibility to modesty and virtue. Let these considerations be forcibly and repeatedly urged on the hospital pupils [emphasis in original].[8, pp. 72–73]

Percival adopts Gregory's account of respect for the "delicacy" of female patients. Percival therefore emphasizes the psychosocial harms that any breach of secrecy should be expected to cause. Like Gregory, Percival is committed to an absolute ethical obligation of confidentiality in professional ethics in medicine.

4.1.2.5 The Shift from an Absolute to Prima Facie Ethical Obligation

In the twentieth century the tradition of an absolute obligation came to an end. With the adoption of written records courts of law could obtain them, thus violating confidentiality for the purpose of meting out justice in civil and criminal cases. There emerged a striking shift away from an obligation without exception, an absolute ethical obligation, to an obligation with exceptions, a prima facie ethical obligation. In the mid-twentieth century, the World Medical Association remained committed to the former view: "A doctor owes to his patient absolute secrecy on all which has been entrusted to him or which he knows because of the confidence entrusted to him."[9]

Under pressure from legal institutions, the British Medical Association (BMA) just a little more than two decades later signaled the shift. "If, in the opinion of the doctor, disclosure of confidential information to a third party seems to be in the best interest of the patient, it is the doctor's duty to make every effort to allow the information to be given to a third party, but where the patient refuses, that refusal must be respected."[10]

The final clause is autonomy based, introducing the second basis of the ethical obligation of confidentiality: the patient's right to privacy. Each patient has a justified claim that information about her obtained or developed in the course of clinical management of her condition not be shared with others because it is private. The right to privacy is claimed by the patient to protect herself from predators who would use this information to cause biopsychosocial harm. The right to privacy creates a prima facie ethical obligation to obtain the patient's consent to release of information protected by her right.

The American Medical Association (AMA) had already made the important contribution of identifying two justified limits on confidentiality: "A physician may not reveal the confidences entrusted to him in the course of medical attendance, or the deficiencies he may observe in the character of his patients, unless he is required to do so by law or unless it becomes necessary in order to protect the welfare of the individual or of the society."[11]

The first exception is justified because in American democracy we secure our freedom, person, and property by submitting to the rule of law. Physicians and patients are no exception, creating a powerful limit on professional and personal autonomy, respectively. The subsequent statement of the AMA is more compact: "A physician shall respect the rights of patients, of colleagues, and of other health care professionals, and shall safeguard patient confidences within the constraints of the law."[12] Notice that the right to privacy is not absolute, as it was in the 1971 BMA statement. This view is compatible with the view that respect for autonomy, the basis of patients' rights, is a prima facie and not absolute ethical principle, as explained in Chapters 1 and 2.

4.1.2.6 Confidentiality: A Prima Facie Ethical Obligation

There emerges from this history the view that in professional ethics in obstetrics and gynecology confidentiality is a prima facie ethical obligation. Obstetrician-gynecologists should prevent unauthorized access to information obtained or developed in the course of patient care unless ethical reasoning establishes that another prima facie ethical obligation should take precedence.

The ethical obligation of confidentiality is beneficence based: to promote the clinical good of maintaining only authorized access to information about the patient. The patient is more likely to be forthcoming about her condition or disease, its clinical management, and any health-related concerns that she may have if confidentiality is maintained. This is an especially important ethical consideration when the patient has experienced rape, sexual exploitation or abuse, domestic violence, or trafficking. This ethical obligation is autonomy based: to respect the patient's right to privacy. Finally, Hoffmann's approach provides a buttressing, i.e., not main but supporting, prudence-based ethical justification that appeals to enlightened self-interest: Having an earned reputation for being trustworthy is in the patient's interest and is a legitimate self-interest of the obstetrician-gynecologist, two interests that strongly align.

4.2 Setting Ethically Justified Limits on the Prima Facie Ethical Obligation of Confidentiality in Obstetrics and Gynecology

Given the strength of the combined beneficence-based and autonomy-based ethical justification for the prima facie ethical obligation in professional ethics in obstetrics and gynecology, fulfilling the prima facie ethical obligation is the default position in professional ethics in obstetrics and gynecology. Setting ethically justified limits on the basis of competitor prima facie ethical obligations *in all cases* bears the burden of proof in ethical reasoning.

Meeting this burden of proof requires completion of demanding steps. The first step is to assiduously avoid the errors in ethical reasoning identified in Chapter 1, an especially important consideration when the clinical stakes are high.

The second step is to make the case that prevention of harm to identifiable others requires breaching confidentiality. A landmark ruling of the California Supreme Court addressed a case in which an endangered third party was not warned about the violent intentions of a patient, who subsequently murdered her. In 1976 the Court in *Tarasoff v. Regents of the University of California* defined a concept for setting ethically justified limits: "the protective privilege ends where the public peril begins."[13] This is an appeal to the ethical principle of nonmaleficence, which creates an ethical obligation to prevent predictable, potential harm to others, especially potentially serious, far-reaching, and irreversible harm. The appeal to nonmaleficence thus provides for "peril" a clinically applicable meaning. Death is certainly a serious, far-reaching, and irreversible harm to others. Morbidity that can cause chronic functional loss or long-term disability also counts as a potentially serious, far-reaching, and irreversible harm. Preventing harms that are less than serious, far-reaching, and irreversible faces a much steeper burden of proof in setting ethically justified limits on the prima facie ethical obligation of confidentiality in professional ethics in obstetrics and gynecology.

The third step is to respect the patient's right to privacy, which is autonomy-based. When the patient is asked to authorize the release to others of confidential clinical information about her, her right to privacy is voluntarily waived and therefore not violated. Obtaining consent to release confidential information is a major preventive ethics tool for protecting the right to privacy. When there is a nonmaleficence-based ethical justification to breach confidentiality, the patient's right to privacy will be violated. In such circumstances, the right to privacy requires that the patient be so informed and also advised why the breach will occur.

The final step is to consider Hoffmann's prudence-based approach to confidentiality, because breaches of confidentiality, even when they have a strong nonmaleficence-based ethical justification, risk preventable damage to the earned reputation of the obstetrician-gynecologist as trustworthy. There is a corollary risk of harm to the patient: diminished trust or loss of trust altogether in her obstetrician-gynecologist and in other physicians and healthcare professionals when she experiences dis-alignment of her interests and those of the obstetrician-gynecologist. This loss of trust is at risk for becoming long term for women with a history of experiencing sexual violence and abuse as well as major mental illnesses and disorders.

4.3 Ethical Challenges to Fulfilling the Prima Facie Ethical Obligation of Confidentiality

We turn now to clinical circumstances that create ethical challenges in fulfilling the prima facie ethical obligation of confidentiality. For each, we identify the nature of the challenge and an argument-based response.

4.3.1 Emergency Medical Care

Medical emergencies can make breach of confidentiality a clinical necessity. The concept of a medical emergency can be clearly stated: The patient's life is in imminent danger or when the patient's health is at immediate risk of serious, far-reaching, and irreversible loss; and clinical management must be initiated immediately in order to prevent death or unacceptable loss of health. There is therefore no time for the informed consent or informed refusal processes with the patient described in Chapter 3. Simple consent and refusal are clinically inadequate substitutes.

It is commonly the case that patients who survive medical emergencies do not recover their decision-making capacity immediately. Surrogate decision making, as explained in Chapter 3, is required for the authorization to continue clinical management. The ethical challenge is to responsibly manage the violation of confidentiality that surrogate decision making requires. Surrogate decision makers are not the patient's physician or other clinician and so they are not bound by the professional ethical obligation of confidentiality in professional ethics in obstetrics and gynecology. Common practice is to assume that surrogate decision makers will understand that information about the patient that is provided to them in their decision-making role is confidential and may not be shared with others, including other family members, without the patient's consent. This ethical obligation should be made explicit, so that the patient's confidentiality and right to privacy are not violated. Some surrogates may welcome the suggestion that they can respond to inquiries by other family members by stating that the patient's physician instructed them to respect the patient's confidentiality and therefore respond only in general terms that do not reveal clinical details about the patient's condition and its clinical management.

4.3.2 Disclosure to Family Members during and after Procedures Requiring Sedation or Anesthesia

Families are complex social institutions. This means that is impossible to predict what information the patient will want disclosed to her family members, e.g., during a surgical procedure requiring sedation or general anesthesia. There is an autonomy-based prima facie ethical obligation to respect the patient's right to privacy by working with her before such procedures to identify the level of information to be provided to family members intraoperatively. This is especially important when updating family members that a procedure is taking longer than anticipated.[14]

The preventive ethics approach to respecting the patient's privacy and meeting baseline informational needs is to ask the patient for her preferences for family notification before and after the procedure. The approach preferred by the patient should be explained to the family before the procedure begins. When the patient prefers that information be withheld until she has recovered, the physician can say to the family that one's professional practice is to be guided by the patient's preferences and that everyone – physician, care team, and family members alike – should respect the patient's preferences. The disclosure plan should be documented in the patient's record. When it becomes necessary for a procedure to require more time than expected, it is common practice for a team member to visit with waiting family members. Their informational needs can be met by communicating that the procedure is taking more time than anticipated and stating the predicted amount of additional time that will be required.[14]

The ethical justification for this preventive ethics approach to the ethical challenges of informing family members of patients about procedures is that meeting only the baseline informational needs of family members, even if intensely felt, lasts only until the patient recovers. This approach does not result in serious, far-reaching, or irreversible psychological harm to family members. Breaching confidentiality by violating the patient's preferences puts her at risk of psychological harm and violates her right to privacy. The latter ethical concerns far outweigh the former.

4.3.3 Inquiries by the Patient's Employer

The patient's employer may have a legitimate interest in learning about her condition and its clinical management. The employer, however, has no right to obtain such information, as providing it violates the obstetrician-gynecologist's ethical obligation to prevent the risk of potentially serious biopsychosocial harm to the patient and the ethical obligation to respect the patient's right to privacy. The latter ethical concerns far outweigh the former.

The ethical challenges in such cases should be managed by appealing to professional ethics in occupational medicine.[15] Physicians who are employed or contracted for services by the patient's employer must deal with this ethical challenge on a daily basis. The American College of Occupational and Environment Medicine provides ethical guidance: the employer should be informed only about when the patient will be ready to return to work and about the reasonable accommodations (including those required by the 1990 Americans with Disabilities Act[16]) that will need to be made.[15] The ethical justification is that the legitimate interests of the patient's employer are limited to these two domains of information, in order to satisfy the employer's legitimate interest in planning for the absence of the patient and what changes, if any, she will need in her workplace so that she can continue to be a productive employee. There is significant potential biopsychosocial harm to the patient from managers and coworkers learning the details of her condition and its clinical management, especially when some of these individuals might be her competitors at work and thus could become predators on her health-related interests. Providing detailed information also violates the patient's right to privacy. The latter ethical concerns far outweigh those related to the employer's interest in the patient's condition.

There should be organizational policy, shaped by these ethical considerations and by legal counsel, to guide responses to employers who inquire – formally or informally – about a patient's condition and its clinical management. Obstetrician-gynecologists who are in the role of an occupational physician should be clear to the employer from the outset that the patient's employer is paying them and is therefore a client; they should also be clear to the employer about the aforementioned limits on confidentiality. No disclosure should occur unless explicitly authorized by the patient and only for information consistent with applicable law.

Disclosure of genetic or genomic information about a patient has been covered by federal legislation for more than a decade: the Genetic Information Nondiscrimination Act (GINA) of 2008.[17,18] This legislation provides for strong protection of the patient's right to privacy and for penalties if this information is used to discriminate against employees and in hiring. Organizational policy should therefore be based on this legislation.

4.3.4 Insurance Claims

A viable business model requires that payment to which a physician is entitled be collected. Third-party payers require documentation of claims, to prevent fraud and to create databases that they need for actuarial purposes. Information about a patient must be provided in claims. In this system of payment, the patient gains the biopsychosocial benefit of access to clinical care but risks violation of her right to privacy. The health insurance industry, so far as we know, has a solid track record of protecting its vast databases from hacking and other breaches. However, there may have been serious breaches that have not been made public.

It is an error in ethical reasoning to conclude that, in a context of manageable risk of harm and considerable benefit, the patient's right to privacy can be ignored. The ethical logic of rights is that they cannot be ignored. They must either be justifiably overridden or explicitly waived. The aforementioned ethical considerations do not override a patient's right to privacy because we do not know how the patient assesses the risk of violation of her privacy by breaches of insurance company databases. She must therefore assess this risk for herself. If she accepts it, she is free to waive her right to privacy by authorizing access by the payer to otherwise protected health information. This is the ethical reasoning that supports a policy of requiring the patient to sign a waiver or permission form authorizing release of information required to document a claim.

The patient is free to refuse to do so. The ethics of informed refusal, as explained in Chapter 3, should guide the response. The patient must be informed that she takes the risk of requiring making the payment herself, perhaps not at the discounted rate that the payer has negotiated. The financial consequences could be considerable and should be made clear to the patient in detail.

4.3.5 Electronic Medical Record

The creation and maintenance of an electronic medical record is becoming increasingly important for documenting insurance claims. By providing for continuity of care through continuity of information and also by becoming a source of reliable data about the processes and outcomes of care, the electronic medical record has become an essential component of patient safety and quality. In addition, each obstetrician-gynecologist has the confidentiality-based prima facie ethical obligation to protect the security of a patient's record. The cost of doing so is considerably more than the cost of maintaining and storing paper records. In the era of increasingly proficient hacking of computer systems, reliably predicting this cost and providing for its recovery become essential components of the business model of a clinical practice. Reasonable limits on this cost must, however, be set. This means that absolute confidentiality of electronic medical records cannot be guaranteed. To respect the right to privacy, each patient should be informed that security measures to protect the electronic medical record are in place but have their limits.

Casual violations of the confidentiality of the electronic medical record can be prevented at little or no cost and therefore are ethically impermissible. Each clinician should log out of the patient's record before leaving a work station, so that those who do not have authorized access do not have the opportunity to be what the British call "nosy parkers." This group includes well-meaning or perhaps not-so-well-meaning family members. Curiosity, even intense curiosity, disconnected from responsibility for patient care never justifies violation of the patient's right to privacy.

This line of ethical reasoning also makes impermissible accessing the medical record of a patient for whose clinical care the clinician or other individual with authorized access to the medical records system is not responsible. There have been incidences of such violations of the right to privacy of public personalities and also of brother or sister trainees.[19] Again, wanting to be a nosy parker fails to establish that the patient's right to privacy can be ignored and thereby egregiously violated. This line of ethical reasoning explains why nosy-parker violations of the right to privacy should be subject to severe penalty, including termination of employment or dismissal from medical school, residency training, or fellowship.

4.3.6 Implications of Genetic and Genomic Information for Individuals Other than the Patient

The results of genetic and genomic analysis are reported from laboratories using the complex and difficult-to-understand technical discourse of genomic medicine. However, the results can be sorted into the following, already very familiar clinical categories: diagnosis, risk assessment, a combination of diagnosis and risk assessment, variants of unknown clinical significance (previously unreported alleles of genes known or suspected to be pathological), and pharmacogenomics that can bear directly on drug selection and dosing.[20] These results apply not only to the proband (the patient tested) but also to genetic kinfolk who may or may not be patients of the obstetrician-gynecologist who ordered the testing.

Current law emphasizes respect for the privacy of the patient, resulting in the view that the physician may share the results of genomic testing with family members only with the consent of the patient.[21] This view is grounded in the ethical principle of respect for autonomy, which, in turn, grounds the patient's right to privacy. Given the strength of the grounding of the right to privacy, the burden of proof is on establishing ethically justified exceptions to release genetic or genomic testing results only with consent. There is ethical controversy about whether exceptions to the right to privacy in this context meet the burden of proof.

There is no agreement in the genomic ethics literature on whether the burden of proof has been met to share results without the consent of the patient. The burden of proof would have to address the following considerations. Genomic analysis has not yet become routine in patient care. Patients may have such analysis performed in research projects aimed at establishing efficacy and safety. Patients may also have testing ordered on the basis of their current condition. Not informing other family members that they should consider genomic analysis does not deny them access to routine clinical evaluation. Given the noted complexity of families, there is no reliable basis for predicting the sense of obligation that the patient may or may not have toward potentially at-risk family members. Sharing results without the patient's permission may put her at nontrivial biopsychosocial risk.

The American College of Human Genetics has published a statement in which they argue that the burden of proof for disclosure can sometimes be met. The first set of clinical circumstances comprises serious genetic conditions the disclosure of which to at-risk family members is not predicted to result in more harm than benefit. Disclosure without consent is ethically permissible but it is not an ethical obligation.[22] There is ongoing controversy about this matter.

Existing consensus should guide the obstetrician-gynecologist in the context of sustained ethical controversy. The obstetrician-gynecologist should inform the patient that her results may have potential clinical significance for her family members. She should be asked for permission to notify them. Her consent or refusal to consent to such sharing of her results should be considered determinative. If in the deliberative clinical judgment, the results pertain to serious, far-reaching, and without treatment irreversible conditions, this should be pointed out to the patient and she should be asked to reconsider.

If she refuses, the obstetrician should explain that some results of genomic analysis have potentially serious, far-reaching, and irreversible consequences. For example, the diagnosis of a serious but treatable condition may be made. Or, the results may reveal an increased relative risk of a later-onset serious condition for which there is effective prevention. These are surely compelling beneficence-based and autonomy-based reasons to share results with the patient and identify a treatment plan. They are also compelling reasons to include the patient's family members. Should she repeat her refusal it should be respected. These conversations should be documented in the patient's record.

Genomic analysis of fetal cells or tissue is often performed in a "trio" analysis that includes the pregnant woman and prospective father. The results of such analysis will therefore be returned to each prospective parent and fall into the aforementioned clinical categories. The prospective parents should be informed that these are the kinds of results they will receive and that there may be results that are unexpected, e.g., increased risk of a later-onset condition for which there are currently no signs or symptoms or nonpaternity. There is also ongoing controversy about the issue. A preventive ethics approach is to explain that nonpaternity may be discovered and explore with the prospective parents whether they wish to take this psychosocial risk for their relationship.

4.3.7 Patients with Sexually Transmitted Disease Engaging in Behavior Known to Transmit Disease

In beneficence-based and nonmaleficence-based judgment in ethics generally there is agreement that no one is free to put others at risk of serious, far-reaching, and potentially irreversible harm without sufficient reason. This is known as the "harm principle." The harm principle provides the ethical justification for the public health requirement to report communicable diseases that carry such risk. The patient should be reported following legally applicable procedures for doing so, including report of sexual contacts. Respect for autonomy requires that the patient be informed and also be advised that contact tracing is routinely accomplished without revealing the name of the index case, the patient.

In some states it is legally permissible for the physician to inform the patient's spouse, with immunity from civil action. The scope of this protected permission does not include other sexual partners. The ethical justification appeals to the harm principle that grounds the obstetrician-gynecologist's public health obligation. The physician is not at legal risk for not disclosing. The permission does not extend to a patient's sexual partner who is not her spouse.

4.3.8 Health Insurance Portability and Accountability Act

When federal legislation known as the Health Insurance Portability and Accountability Act (HIPAA) and its implementing regulations took effect in 2003, there was considerable uncertainty about what the regulations required.[23] Patients learn about HIPAA and other privacy protections when they are provided the required "privacy notice" to read and sign when they make their initial visit. To respect her right to privacy, HIPAA requires authorization by the patient for release of individually identifiable information to others who do not have authorized access to this information. This requirement is an obvious implication of the right to privacy. We emphasize that it is redundant to extend the scope of the right to privacy to clinicians or others with authorized access to patient information: their access to and use of such information is subject to the stringent requirements of the ethical obligation of confidentiality, as explained in Section 4.1.

4.3.9 Electronic Communication with Patients

All forms of electronic communication with patients, including email, texting, and remotely accessed records, must be stringently secured from unauthorized access in order to fulfill the ethical obligation of confidentiality and the patient's right to privacy. Patients should be cautioned to take adequate security measures to prevent unauthorized access by family members, employers, friends, etc., by not sharing access to their email and not sharing their user name and password with others unless the patient has complete confidence in their discretion.

4.3.10 Use of Social Media

The use of social media to maintain contact with patients is fraught with ethical peril, despite such benefits as creating online support groups of patients with chronic disorders and diseases. The ethical obligation of confidentiality is easy to violate in the casual, permissive environment of virtual reality. This tendency can be reinforced when people, especially younger people, have come to accept what older demographic groups may consider a perilous disregard for personal privacy. There is also the persistent concern about the adequacy of security measures taken by online platforms.

Online criticism of an obstetrician-gynecologist can provoke a strong personal response. However, a clinically compelling response usually requires revealing protected health information, which is a violation of HIPAA with nontrivial consequences. The obstetrician should also keep in mind that, when an identified individual makes libelous statements, there are remedies in civil law. Pursuit of them should be considered in consultation with competent, experienced legal counsel. Physician leaders may consider responding to libelous statements with civil action for corporate libel.

With a nod to Rudyard Kipling,[24] the obstetrician should keep his or her head – by remaining highly self-disciplined and therefore professional – while others are losing theirs by abandoning self-discipline in virtual reality. To prevent unauthorized access to information about patients, the obstetrician-gynecologist should be guided by strict adherence to the ethical obligation of confidentiality and respect for the patient's right to privacy, reinforced by prudential self-interest in not risking unnecessary loss of reputation that is the inevitable result of leaping into the maelstrom of social media. The AMA has provided useful general guidance: "Physicians should be cognizant of standards of patient privacy and confidentiality that must be maintained in all environments, including online, and must refrain from posting identifiable patient information online."[25,26]

We propose the following provision of explicit guidance that will fulfill the ethical obligation and prudence-based protection of legitimate self-interest: "Don't disclose confidential patient Protected Health Information. Do not make public comment about the care of any patient or participation of any research volunteer. This is a federal offense and basis for immediate dismissal." This is based on the policy of the medical school of one of us (JHC). It will also serve one well to remember and apply the admonition to the people of London during the blitz against that great city during World War II: Keep calm and carry on – with fulfilling one's professional ethical obligation of confidentiality with a strong burden of proof on making an exception.

References

1. von Staden H. "In a pure and holy way:" personal and professional conduct in the Hippocratic Oath. J Hist Med Allied Sci 1996; 51: 404–437.
2. Plato. Crito. In Cooper JM, Hutchinson DS, eds. Plato Complete Works. Indianapolis, IN: Hackett, 1997: 37–48.
3. McCullough LB. John Gregory and the Invention of Professional Medical Ethics and the Profession of Medicine. Dordrecht, the Netherlands: Springer, 1998.
4. Hoffmann F. Medicus politicus; sive, regulae prudentiae secundum quas medicus juvenis studia sua & vitae rationem dirigere debet. (The Politic Doctor, or Rules of Prudence according to which a Young Physician Should Direct his Studies and Reason of Life). Leiden: Philip Bonk, 1738.
5. Gregory J. Lectures on the Duties and Qualifications of a Physician. London: W. Strahan and T. Cadell, 1772. Reprinted in McCullough LB, ed. John Gregory's Writings on Medical Ethics and the Philosophy of Medicine. Dordrecht, the Netherlands: Kluwer Academic, 1998: 161–248.
6. Pernick MS. Bioethics and history. In Baker RB, McCullough LB, eds. The Cambridge World History of Medical Ethics. New York: Cambridge University Press, 2009: 16–20.
7. Baker RB. Before Bioethics: A History of American Medical Ethics from the Colonial Period to the Bioethics Revolution. New York: Oxford University Press, 2013.
8. Percival T. Medical Ethics; or, A Code of Institutes and Precepts, adapted to the Professional Conduct of Physicians and Surgeons. London: Johnson & Bickerstaff, 1803.
9. World Medical Association. International Code of Medical Ethics. 1949. Available at www.wma.net/wp-content/uploads/

10. British Medical Association. Medical ethics. Brit Med J Spec Suppl 1971; 3465: 143.

11. American Medical Association. Principles of Medical Ethics. 1957. In Baker RB, Caplan AL, Emanuel LL, Latham SR, eds. The American Medical Ethics Revolution: How the AMA's Code of Ethics *Has* Transformed Physicians' Relationships to Patients, Professionals, and Society. Baltimore, MD: The Johns Hopkins University Press, 1999: 356.

12. American Medical Association. AMA Principles of Medical Ethics. 2001. Available at www.ama-assn.org/sites/ama-assn.org/files/corp/media-browser/principles-of-medical-ethics.pdf (accessed March 1, 2019).

13. *Tarasoff v. Regents of the University of California*, 17 Cal. 3d 425, 551 P.2d 334, 131 Cal. Rptr. 14 (Cal. 1976).

14. Jones JW, McCullough LB. Disclosure of intraoperative events. Surgery 2002; 132: 531–532.

15. American College of Occupational and Environmental Medicine. Confidentiality of medical information in the workplace. 2012. Available at www.acoem.org/Confidentiality_Medical_Information.aspx (accessed March 1, 2019).

16. Americans With Disabilities Act of 1990, Pub. L. No. 101–336, 104 Stat. 328 (1990).

17. Hudson KL, Holohan MK, Collins FS. Keeping pace with the times – the Genetic Information Nondiscrimination Act of 2008. N Engl J Med 2008; 358: 2661–2663.

18. Annas GJ, Roche PW, Green RC. GINA, genism, and civil rights. Bioethics 2008; 22: ii–iv.

19. Moran C. Harris County Hospital District fires 16 over privacy. Houston Chron November 25, 2009. Available at www.chron.com/news/houston-texas/article/Harris-hospital-district-fires-16-over-privacy-1736905.php (accessed March 1, 2019).

20. McCullough LB, Brothers KB, Chung WK, Joffe S, et al. In behalf of the Clinical Sequencing Exploratory Research (CSER) Consortium Pediatrics Working Group. Professionally responsible disclosure of genomic sequencing results in pediatric practice. Pediatrics 2015; 136: e974–982.

21. Wolf SM, Branum R, Koenig BA, Petersen GM, et al. Returning a research participant's genomic results to relatives: analysis and recommendations. J Law Med Ethics 2015; 43: 440–463.

22. The American Society of Human Genetics Social Issues Subcommittee on Familial Disclosure. ASHG Statement. Professional disclosure of familial genetic information. Am J Human Genet 1998; 62: 474–483.

23. Lo B, Dornbrand L, Dubler NN. HIPAA and patient care: the role of professional judgment. JAMA 2005; 293: 1766–1771.

24. Kipling R. If: a father's advice to his son. Available at www.goodreads.com/quotes/143729-if-you-can-keep-your-head-when-all-about-you (accessed March 1, 2019).

25. American Medical Association. Professionalism in the use of social media. N.d. Available at www.ama-assn.org/delivering-care/ethics/professionalism-use-social-media (accessed March 1, 2019).

26. Kind T. In the literature: professional guidelines for social media use: a starting point. AMA J Ethics 2015; 17: 441–447.

Chapter 5

Conflicts of Interest and Conflicts of Commitment

GOAL
This chapter provides an ethical framework for the identification and responsible management of conflicts of interest and conflicts of commitment.

OBJECTIVES
On completing study of this chapter, the reader will:

Identify the concept of conflict of interest

Identify the concept of conflict of commitment

Identify conflicts of interest in initiating romantic or sexual relationships with patients and demonstrate how they should be responsibly managed

Identify conscientious objection as a conflict of commitment and demonstrate how it should be responsibly managed

Apply the ethical framework for the identification and responsible management of conflicts of interest and conflicts of commitment in clinical practice

TOPICS

5.1	Conflicts of Interest and Conflicts of Commitment in Historical Perspective	80
5.2	Conflicts of Interest	80
	5.2.1 Entrepreneurial versus Professional Relationships	80
	5.2.2 Conflict of Interest Defined	81
	5.2.3 John Gregory on Conflicts of Interest	81
	5.2.4 Thomas Percival on Conflicts of Interest	82
	5.2.5 Conceptual Confusion about Conflicts of Interest	83
	5.2.6 Professionally Responsible Management of Conflicts of Interest	83
	5.2.6.1 Use of Imaging	83
	5.2.6.2 Payment for Clinical Practice	83
	5.2.6.3 Cosmetic Procedures	84
	5.2.6.4 Research	84
5.3	Conflicts of Commitment	85
	5.3.1 Conflict of Commitment Defined	85
	5.3.2 Percival on Conflicts of Commitment	85
	5.3.3 Professionally Responsible Management of Conflicts of Commitment	85
	5.3.4 Preventing Conflation of Conflicts of Interest with Conflicts of Commitment	86
5.4	The Ethics of Romantic and Sexual Relationships with Patients	86
	5.4.1 An Historical Perspective	86

Section 1: Professional Ethics in Obstetrics and Gynecology

5.4.2 Contemporary Perspective		88
5.5 Conscientious Objection: A Conflict of Commitment		89
5.5.1 Conscientious Objection Defined		89
5.5.2 A Useful Historical Analogy		89
5.5.3 Conscientious Objection in Residency Training		89
5.5.4 Conscientious Objection to Contraception		89
5.5.5 Conscientious Objection to Referral for Induced Abortion and Feticide		90
5.5.5.1 Invoking Individual Conscience Bears the Burden of Proof		90
5.5.5.2 Beneficence-Based and Autonomy-Based Indications		90
5.5.5.3 Beneficence-Based Direct Referral		90
5.5.5.4 Autonomy-Based Indirect Referral		91
5.5.5.5 Polarized Positions Are Unnecessary		91

Key Concepts

Conflict of commitment
Conflict of interest
Conscientious objection
Ethical concept of medicine as a profession

Ethical principle of beneficence in professional ethics in gynecology
Ethical principle of beneficence in professional ethics in obstetrics

Ethical principle of respect for autonomy in professional ethics in gynecology
Ethical principle of respect for autonomy in professional ethics in obstetrics
Public trust

5.1 Conflicts of Interest and Conflicts of Commitment in Historical Perspective

The professionally responsible management of conflicts of interest and conflicts of commitment is essential for sustaining the three commitments of the ethical concept of medicine as a profession (see Chapter 1) and therefore for professional integrity. The physician-ethicists John Gregory (1724–1773) and Thomas Percival (1740–1804), who originated the ethical concept of medicine as a profession (see Chapter 1), addressed both conflicts of interest and conflicts of commitment.

5.2 Conflicts of Interest

5.2.1 Entrepreneurial versus Professional Relationships

Gregory and Percival originated the ethical concept of medicine because the medicine of their day was entrepreneurial, as it had been since the time of ancient Greece. Clinical care was based on a contractual agreement between the ill person and the physician, surgeon, apothecary, or other practitioner. A contractual agreement is based on the self-interests of both parties, and the goal of each is to maximize his or her self-interest. Inasmuch as there is no ethical obligation to protect and promote the interests of the other party, each party is free to injure the interests of the other.

In such circumstances the virtue of prudence should guide judgment and the behavior based on it. Prudence schools an individual in identifying his or her interests, especially his or her legitimate interests in such matters as protecting one's health and the security of one's person, money, and reputation, and then in acting to protect and promote these interests. Prudence becomes the basis for the well-known admonition to all who engage in commercial transactions: *caveat emptor*, or "let the buyer beware." The buyer must beware because neither party in a market exchange has an ethical obligation to protect the other party's interests, including his or her legitimate ones. Indeed, each party is free to become a predator on the other party's interests if doing so will advance his or her own interests. For example, a passenger on a commercial flight may discover that the passenger next to him or her paid 75% less for the same kind of seat. In a commercial transaction the passenger who paid four times as much as the person in the next seat can have no ethically justified objection, because in a commercial transaction the seller has no ethical obligation to protect the financial interests of the buyer.

In an entrepreneurial, market exchange relationship protecting the interests of the two parties is the primary motivation of each. A conflict of interest can exist only after one party has made the commitment to protect and promote the interests of the other party. When a physician makes the commitment to the ethical concept of medicine as a profession, he or she becomes a professional with the commitment to protect and promote the health-related interests of the patient as his or her primary concern and motivation rather than self-interest.

5.2.2 Conflict of Interest Defined

A conflict of interest can exist only for a professional physician, not for an entrepreneurial physician. A conflict of interest therefore exists when fulfilling ethical obligations to a patient becomes incompatible with satisfying individual self-interest and group or guild self-interest. Conflicts of interest occur at two levels. Prioritizing individual self-interest over ethical obligations to the patient is not compatible with the ethical concept of medicine as a profession, which requires making protection and promotion of the patient's health-related interests the physician's primary concern and motivation. Prioritizing individual self-interest is therefore prima facie ethically impermissible in the professional ethics of obstetrics and gynecology. Prioritizing guild self-interest over ethical obligations to patients is also not compatible with the ethical concept of medicine as a profession, because such prioritization does not make protection and promotion of the patient's health-related interests the primary concern and motivation of physicians as a group. Prioritizing guild self-interest is therefore prima facie ethically impermissible in the professional ethics of obstetrics and gynecology.[1] This means that prioritizing either individual or guild self-interest bears the burden of proof, which is very steep because of the unacceptable consequence – deprofessionalizing obstetrics and gynecology – of such prioritization.

5.2.3 John Gregory on Conflicts of Interest

Gregory, who witnessed the rampant distrust that defined the entrepreneurial relationship between an ill person and a practitioner,[2] was keenly aware of the ethical dangers that individual self-interest and group self-interest pose to the commitments of the ethical concept of medicine as a profession. He was concerned that there were too many physicians who were "men of interest" (there were no women physicians at that time in Britain) who put self-interest ahead of professional responsibility to and for patients.[3,4]

> Physicians, considered as a body of men, who live by medicine as a profession, have an interest separate and distinct from the honour of the science. In pursuit of this interest, some have acted with candour, with honour, with the ingenuous and liberal manners of gentlemen. Conscious of their own worth, they disdained every artifice, and depended for success on their real merit. But such men are not the most numerous in any profession. Some impelled by necessity, some stimulated by vanity, and others anxious to conceal ignorance, have had recourse to various mean and unworthy arts, to raise their importance among the ignorant, who are always the most numerous part of mankind.[3, p. 4]

Self-interest is built into the practice of medicine, for the simple reason that physicians need to earn a living. But this economic interest is "separate" from the commitment to the ethical concept of medicine as a profession. Some physicians, Gregory says, pursue this commitment, confident that self-interest in an adequate income and an earned reputation for trustworthiness will therefore be protected. Some physicians, Gregory cautions, take a different path: the pursuit of individual self-interest as their primary concern and motivation.

Notice the shift in vocabulary in the foregoing passage. Self-interested physicians exhibit vices, traits of character or habits that morally deform physicians. Systematically putting self-interest ahead of ethical obligations to patients had become a functional norm for most physicians and surgeons in the late eighteenth century and for the "corporations" of physicians and surgeons, the Royal Colleges. Men of interest thus pursued individual and guild self-interest as their primary concern and motivation. In effect, they turned the ethical concept of medicine on its head. Instead of making the protection of the patient's health-related interests the physician's primary concern and motivation, "men of interest" put the pursuit of individual self-interest first, and physicians imbued with what Gregory called the "corporation spirit" put the group or guild interests of physicians first. Acting on such self-interest caused the clinical judgment and practice of these physicians to become distorted by unrecognized and therefore unmanaged bias. Bias, of course, is antithetical to the commitment to the ethical concept of medicine, because it is incompatible with scientific and clinical excellence. Turning the ethical concept of medicine as a profession on its head replaced the discipline of scientific reasoning with rampant bias that put the health and lives of patients at preventable risk. The ethical principles of beneficence and nonmaleficence in professional ethics in medicine make this ethically impermissible. (See Chapters 1 and 2.)

Patients' health and lives came to be imperiled. The intellectual virtue of what Gregory called "candour" – being open to new information and critically appraising it as required by the ethical concept of medicine as a profession – was undermined. The result was an intellectual arrogance and indifference to medical errors: "To this species of pride, a pride incompatible with true dignity and elevation of mind, have the lives of thousands been sacrificed."[3, p. 29] He meant this to be a literal truth, not a metaphor, and it is some of the strongest language that he uses in his book on professional ethics in medicine.

Gregory provides a vivid example, the physician whose practice ages badly:

> We sometimes see a remarkable difference between the behaviour of a physician at his first setting out, and afterwards, when he is fully established in reputation and practice. In the beginning he is affable, polite, humane, and assiduously attentive to his patients: but afterwards, when he has reaped the fruits of such a behaviour, and finds himself independent, he assumes a very different tone; he becomes haughty, rapacious, careless, and often somewhat brutal in his manners. Conscious of the ascendency he has acquired, he acts a despotic part, and takes a most ungenerous advantage of the confidence which people have in his abilities.[3, p. 25]

The use of *rapacious* was not metaphorical but literal, naming the most insidious behavior that occurs when a physician's "interest" dominates the relationship with female and pregnant patients and obliterates the commitment to the ethical concept of medicine as a profession.

5.2.4 Thomas Percival on Conflicts of Interest

Like Gregory, Percival was concerned about conflicts of interest, especially the conflict between ethical obligations to patients and guild self-interests. Putting guild self-interests first turns medicine into a politically and economically driven organization and therefore not a professional association.[1] The antidote, Percival holds, is to consider medicine a public trust.[5] He invokes this concept when he addresses the ethics of retirement from clinical practice. It is important to keep in mind that, when Percival wrote the following words, he had already retired from clinical practice because of severely impaired vision.

> The commencement of that period of senescence, when it becomes incumbent on a physician to decline the offices of his profession, is not easy to ascertain; and the decision on so nice a point must be left to the moral discretion of the individual. For, one grown old in the useful and honourable exercise of the healing art, may continue to enjoy, and justly to enjoy, the unabated confidence of the public. And whilst exempt, in a considerable degree, from the privations and infirmities of age, he is under indispensable obligations to apply his knowledge and experience, in the most efficient way, to the benefit of mankind.
>
> For the possession of powers is a clear indication of the will of our Creator, concerning their practical direction. But in the ordinary course of nature, the bodily and mental vigour must be expected to decay progressively, though perhaps slowly, after the meridian of life is past. As age advances, therefore, a physician should, from time to time, scrutinize impartially, the state of his faculties; that he may determine, *bona fide,* the precise degree in which he is qualified to execute the active and multifarious offices of his profession. And whenever he becomes conscious that his memory presents to him, with faintness, those analogies, on which medical reasoning and the treatment of diseases are founded; that diffidence of the measures to be pursued perplexes his judgment; that, from a deficiency in the acuteness of his senses, he finds himself less able to distinguish signs, or to prognosticate events; he should at once resolve, though others perceive not the changes which have taken place, to sacrifice every consideration of fame or fortune, and to retire from the engagements of business. To the surgeon under similar circumstances, this rule of conduct is still more necessary. For the energy of the understanding often

subsists much longer than the quickness of eye-sight, delicacy of touch, and steadiness of hand, which are essential to the skilful performance of operations. Let both the physician and surgeon never forget, that their professions are *public trusts*, properly rendered lucrative whilst they fulfill them; but which they are bound, by honour and probity, to relinquish, as soon as they find themselves unequal to their adequate and faithful execution [emphasis added].[5, pp. 109-111]

Obstetrician-gynecologists work very hard and long to become specialists in women's health and the clinical management of reproduction and pregnancy. They therefore have a strong ownership claim on their knowledge and skills. However, obstetrician-gynecologists do not have *exclusive* ownership of their knowledge and skills, because the use of these affects the health and lives of patients and therefore the well-being of society. Obstetrics and gynecology is therefore not a private guild based on group self-interest in economic success and social and political power.[1] It is, to quote the phrase first used by Percival, a "public trust." The fund of knowledge and clinical skills of obstetrics and gynecology, including their improvement, is held by obstetrician-gynecologists in trust for current patients and for future obstetrician-gynecologists and their patients.

5.2.5 Conceptual Confusion about Conflicts of Interest

The American College of Obstetricians and Gynecologists (ACOG) defines a conflict of interest as occurring "when a primary interest (usually the patient's well-being) is in conflict with a physician's secondary interest (such as his or her financial interest)."[6, p. 390] The National Academy of Medicine follows ACOG by conceptualizing a conflict of interest in terms of conflicting interests.[7]

ACOG's definition of conflict of interest is not the definition of conflict of interest associated with professional ethics in medicine. In the ACOG definition the professional obligations of physicians are transmuted into "primary interests." The problem is that interests can evanesce; professional obligations cannot. Interests therefore cannot be considered ethical obligations.

Before the pioneering work of Gregory and Percival, described in Chapter 1, the concept of conflicting interests did make sense. The relationship between the medical practitioner and the ill person was entrepreneurial. Entrepreneurial relationships are based on the self-interests of the two parties.

ACOG's definition is conceptually adequate only to this preprofessional era of medicine. Making the commitment to the ethical concept of medicine as a profession replaces the entrepreneurial relationship with a professional relationship based on the physician's commitment to the ethical concept of medicine as a profession. ACOG's definition is not adequate from the perspective of the ethical concept of medicine as a profession and should not be applied in professional ethics in obstetrics and gynecology.

5.2.6 Professionally Responsible Management of Conflicts of Interest

The most effective way to manage conflicts of interest is to eliminate them. Conflicts of interest in this category in clinical practice include having an ownership interest in an outside imaging facility or laboratory.

5.2.6.1 Use of Imaging

There is evidence that an ownership interest can result in overuse of imaging when compared to American Academy of Radiology standards.[8] Ownership interests in outside facilities thus pose the risk of preventable bias, which is ethically impermissible. There are also non–health-related investments that pose no conflicts of interest.

Imaging, especially ultrasound imaging, is an integral component of obstetric and gynecologic practice. Conflict of interest in the use of imaging cannot be eliminated and therefore must be managed with professional integrity. (See Chapters 1 and 2.) This includes intellectual integrity, which requires adherence to standards of scientific and clinical excellence. The use of ultrasound imaging should therefore follow evidence-based guidelines published by professional associations.[9,10] Usage patterns should be retrospectively reviewed routinely and corrected as necessary to prevent an incremental drift away from these guidelines.

5.2.6.2 Payment for Clinical Practice

Clinical practice is the provision of medically reasonable clinical management to the patient with his or her consent or the consent of his or her surrogate decision maker. The professional virtue of self-sacrifice in professional ethics in obstetrics and gynecology creates the prima facie ethical obligation to keep self-interest secondary in clinical practice by offering, recommending, and providing only medically reasonable clinical management to patients. (See Chapter 2.)

In clinical practice, the conflict of interest created by fee-for-service cannot be eliminated. This includes salaried obstetrician-gynecologists because their income will be a function of the billings that they generate. Professionally responsible management of such unavoidable conflicts of interest can be achieved by adhering without exception to the ethical concept of medicine as a profession and its requirement of maintaining scientific and clinical excellence. (See Chapters 1 and 2.) This is achieved by following the discipline of deliberative clinical judgment, especially by using and continuously improving clinical guidelines to reduce variability in the processes of patient care to a minimum consistent with beneficence-based ethical obligations to patients. Creating and sustaining an organizational culture of patient safety and quality aims at reducing biases, including those originating in self-interest in income, time, and convenience. Such an organizational culture should include retrospective review and using the results of such review to continuously improve the processes of patient care. Compensation should be tied to adherence to such processes of care.

5.2.6.3 Cosmetic Procedures

Providing cosmetic procedures can become a source of revenue in addition to that generated in clinical practice. As this revenue stream grows, it can activate financial self-interest. The professional virtue of self-sacrifice in professional ethics in obstetrics and gynecology creates the prima facie ethical obligation to keep such financial self-interest systematically secondary. This can be accomplished by fulfilling the prima facie ethical obligation, generated by the professional virtue of integrity in professional ethics in obstetrics and gynecology, to have both scientifically and ethically valid reasons to offer or perform a cosmetic procedure. The point of an integrity-based ethical obligation is to protect the patient from clinical management that lacks such reasons. When the following criteria have been satisfied there are scientifically and ethically valid reasons to offer or perform a cosmetic procedure. Focusing on satisfying these criteria functions as an antidote to ethically impermissible self-interest.

1. There is no pathology present. This means that there is no medical indication for the procedure.
2. The procedure has clinical validity in that there is an evidence base for its efficacy.
3. There is an evidence base for the minimization of the complications and risks of the procedure required by beneficence-based clinical judgment.
4. The indication for the procedure is the informed and voluntary consent of the patient. The informed consent process should include information about the biomedical risks but also its psychosocial risks, including the risk that the patient may become dissatisfied with the results. The informed consent process should therefore include information about whether there are valid procedures to modify or reverse the cosmetic alteration of the patient's anatomy and physiology, as well as the psychosocial risk that the patient may judge results of a cosmetic procedure to be unsatisfactory.

Each of these criteria is a necessary condition, which means that if even one criterion is not satisfied, the patient should be informed and the procedure should not be offered or performed. The four criteria jointly comprise a sufficient condition: when all four are satisfied, it is ethically permissible to offer or perform a cosmetic procedure. A cosmetic procedure is not medically reasonable because there is no expected clinical benefit. When the second and third criteria are satisfied, a cosmetic procedure is not medically unreasonable, because it is not net clinically harmful. In deliberative, beneficence-based clinical judgment, cosmetic surgery is compatible with beneficence. This means that it is ethically permissible to offer or perform a cosmetic procedure when all four criteria are satisfied but not to recommend it because its indication is purely autonomy based. This indication originates in the request from a patient for the procedure. Adhering to the requirement that all four criteria should be satisfied becomes the antidote to self-interest becoming the primary concern and motivation of the obstetrician-gynecologist who elects to provide cosmetic procedures to patients.

5.2.6.4 Research

In research, an inventor of a new device or drug should either not become involved in clinical investigation or abandon ownership, so that the testing phase is not tainted by the appearance of conflict of interest. Inventors who wish to retain ownership interest also have a prudential self-interest in not becoming involved in investigation: preventing even the appearance of bias in the research process. The alternative is for the inventor to give up his or her rights of ownership (and not transfer them to others such as family members) and for the research to be conducted without even the appearance of an economic conflict of interest.

5.3 Conflicts of Commitment

Conflicts of commitment are frequently conflated with conflicts of commitment. This is a conceptual error because the two are distinctively different, requiring different management strategies.

5.3.1 Conflict of Commitment Defined

A conflict of commitment occurs when fulfilling an ethical obligation to a patient becomes incompatible with fulfilling an ethical obligation to people other than patients in the obstetrician-gynecologist's life, including, spouse, children, parents and other family members, friends, faith community, and nation. Like self-interest that can be compromised, ethical obligations to others can be compromised but there is an additional burden of proof. Either the individual to whom the obligation is owed frees the obstetrician-gynecologist from it or the burden of proof is met to override the obligation to another.

5.3.2 Percival on Conflicts of Commitment

Percival addresses conflicts of commitment when he examines the conflict between ethical obligations to patients and ethical obligations to one's faith community, especially the ethical obligation to attend organized worship on the Sabbath. This conflict of commitment becomes clinically relevant when hospital rounds are held on the Sabbath. Percival makes it clear that sometimes the commitment to patients should justifiably take precedence over the commitment to one's faith-based obligations: "Hospital consultations ought not to be held on Sundays, except in cases of urgent necessity; and on such occasions an hour should be appointed, which does not interfere with attendance on public worship."[5, p. 83] In clinical circumstances that do not threaten a patient's life, the commitment to one's faith-based obligations may justifiably take precedence. This is the reasoning that justifies the long-standing practice of not scheduling a call that conflicts with an obstetrician-gynecologist's religious obligations.

> The observance of the Sabbath is a duty to which medical men are bound, so far as is compatible with the urgency of the cases under their charge. Visits may often be made with sufficient convenience and benefit, either before the hours of going to church, or during the intervals of public worship. And in many chronic ailments, the sick, together with their attendants, are qualified to participate in the social offices of religion; and should not be induced to forego this important privilege, by the expectation of a call from their physician or surgeon.[5, p. 108]

Percival's proposal to minimize conflicts of commitment by proposing to confine rounds on the Sabbath to the most serious cases fulfills the beneficence-based ethical obligation to see to it that the problems of the seriously ill are effectively managed in a timely fashion. This preventive ethics approach does not violate beneficence-based ethical obligations to less seriously ill patients for whom rounds will be held the next day or for whom home visits can be scheduled on days other than the Sabbath, and fulfills the physician's ethical obligation in his or her faith community.

5.3.3 Professionally Responsible Management of Conflicts of Commitment

The first management strategy for responsibly managing conflicts of interest, eliminating them, is not available because the physician is not free simply to abrogate ethical obligations to people in his or her life other than patients. In addition, there are no evidence-based guidelines, the strict following of which protects the first commitment of the ethical concept of medicine from biasing influences. Disciplined ethical judgment is required.

Two clinical ethical judgments should guide the professionally responsible management of conflicts of commitment. One comes from the history of medical ethics and the second is the corollary of this historical guidance.

One major reason to study the history of medical ethics is that even long-dead physician-ethicists may have identified an effective and responsible approach to ethical challenges in current clinical practice. Percival's approach to conflicts of commitment is an important example: when the clinical outcomes for patients of prioritizing commitments to people other than patients should, in deliberative clinical judgment, be considered serious, far-reaching, and irreversible, commitments to others become secondary in order to fulfill beneficence-based and nonmaleficence-based ethical obligations to the patient. (See Chapters 1 and 2).

Table 5.1 Conflict of interest and conflict of commitment.

Conflict of interest	Exists when fulfilling ethical obligations to patients or research subjects become incompatible with legitimate self-interests.
Conflict of commitment	Exists when the physician's *ethical obligations* to patients or research subjects become incompatible with the physician's ethical obligations to other people in his or her life, especially family members.

In cases that do not meet these criteria and are therefore of less-than-"urgent necessity," a corollary of Percival's guidance applies. Fulfilling commitments to people other than patients may justifiably be given priority but only when another qualified clinician is available to care for the patient in a timely manner.

5.3.4 Preventing Conflation of Conflicts of Interest with Conflicts of Commitment

As noted in Section 5.3, it is a conceptual error in ethical reasoning to conflate conflicts of interest with conflicts of commitment, because doing so violates the core requirement of ethical analysis: to become and remain clear about pertinent concepts. (See Table 5.1.) Failure to adhere to the discipline of clear thinking in ethical analysis means that ethical argument, identifying the implications of clearly expressed concepts, breaks down completely. Conflicts of interest are conflicts between fulfilling ethical obligations to patients and self-interest. Conflicts of commitment are conflicts between fulfilling ethical obligations to patients and fulfilling ethical obligations to people other than patients. Conflation of conflicts of interest with conflicts of commitment should be assiduously prevented.

5.4 The Ethics of Romantic and Sexual Relationships with Patients

When someone with power over others engages in sexual harassment and unwanted contact, the individual with power takes unfair advantage of that power to violate the ethical principle of respect for autonomy. The #MeToo movement has recently brought these issues to prominence and made them a matter of urgent social concern. The #MeToo movement has exposed a chronic problem of sexual morality that can no longer be ignored or tolerated. Many industries and professions have been exposed to the harsh light of public scrutiny.

At the time of our writing, we conducted a PubMed search using the term #MeToo, which produced 38 citations. These primarily concerned sexual behaviors within healthcare organizations.[11,12] There are few peer-reviewed reports on sexual contact with female and pregnant patients by obstetrician-gynecologists.[13,14] A 1996 report states that 4.5% of physicians, including obstetrician-gynecologists, dated a patient and "3.4% reported had sexual (genital-genital, oral-genital, or anal-genital) contact with a patient. Physicians more than 50 years of age and unmarried physicians were significantly more likely to have dated patients."[13] Although there are no recent studies on this matter, sexual abuse of patients by obstetrician-gynecologists has been reported in the lay press.[15,16] Inappropriate behavior on an anesthetized patient by a gynecologist, in which a medical student joined, has also been reported.[17] Such behavior has the potential to undermine professional ethics in obstetrics and gynecology and therefore should be prevented.

5.4.1 An Historical Perspective

Romantic and sexual relationships have been a vexed topic through the history of Western medical ethics. A brief review of this history will identify key elements of ethical reasoning about the permissibility of these relationships.

The Hippocratic oath addressed sexual relationships with the sick: "7. i. Into as many houses as I may enter, I will go for the benefit of the ill, ii. while being far from all voluntary and destructive injustice, especially from sexual acts both upon women's bodies and upon men's, both of the free and of the slaves."[18]

At first, this passage appears to invoke a beneficence-based regard for the ill individual. However, this is a presentist reading, i.e., a reading based on the false assumption that the oath is based on values that we take for granted.[19] The oath provides no justification for the admonitions in the oath. As noted in Chapter 1, the oath is based on preservation of the physician's reputation, a matter of considerable self-interest in the unforgiving, competitive marketplace for medical services in ancient Greece. Physicians with a reputation for entering houses of the sick to do them or other household members harm would not have survived in such a market. Those who entered to benefit the sick were more likely to do so. It is a presentist error to interpret "for the benefit of the ill" as a prima facie beneficence-based ethical obligation to patients to protect them from the physician's romantic or sexual interest in them. This admonition should be interpreted as a matter of prudential self-interest of the physician who wanted to maintain his reputation.

In ancient Greece slaves had little or no moral status and women, at best, had only slightly more. Free men did have moral status. The scope of the second admonition in this passage includes both free and enslaved individuals, with their quite different moral status, as well as heterosexual and homosexual relations with the ill who were men (at a time when the latter relationships were not judged unacceptable). The "injustice" to be done to them should be understood as a perception that, if it spreads throughout a community, will damage the physician's reputation. It is a presentist error to interpret "injustice" as a prima facie justice-based ethical obligation to patients to protect them from the physician's romantic or sexual interest in them. This admonition should be interpreted as a matter of prudential self-interest of the physician who wanted to maintain his reputation.

For the Hippocratic oath romantic and sexual relationships create conflicting interests, not conflicts of interest. The prudent physician prevents risk to reputation as a way to manage conflicting interests.

In the early eighteenth century Friedrich Hoffmann published a text in the tradition of *medicus politicus*.[20] (See Chapter 2.) This translates as the "politic" doctor, not the "political doctor." Not much in use now, "politic" means someone who is committed to the virtue of prudence, the habit of identifying and acting to protect one's self-interests when one is subject to the power of others. Prudence becomes an especially important virtue to cultivate when one is in a position of relative powerlessness. At that time physicians were in such a position because they were subject to the power of the purse – private patients, municipalities, and royal courts who employed them and could dismiss them without pay and with impunity. Taking this context seriously, Hoffmann proposed that the physician should understand the virtue of prudence, on which his entire text is based, as enlightened self-interest: the physician should understand his interest as aligned with the interest of the sick individual, which is known as enlightened self-interest. Hoffmann addresses the prudence-based duties of midwives, i.e., who were then known as "man-midwives" and now as obstetricians, under two headings. The first is from Chapter 3 of his *Medicus Politicus*, "On the duties of the physician in obstetrics and the care of women," which includes the following: "Rule 1: The midwife above all should be pious, chaste, sober, not timid, taciturn, and experienced." The second is from Chapter 5, "On the prudence of the physician regarding sick women," and includes: "Rule 1: "The physician should be chaste. The physician should be chaste in word and deed, when he is obliged to visit sick women; for this ought not to be the occasion for exciting the lust of the physician, especially concerning unchaste women, unless he wishes to violate the laws of conscience."[19] To be chaste means that the obstetrician-gynecologist has the self-discipline to enter into physically intimate relationships with women that are asexual. Asexual intimate physical contact with female and pregnant patients protects them from abuse. Being chaste thus prevents conflicting interests of the physician and sick individual.

As explained in Chapter 1, Gregory and Percival should be credited with inventing professional ethics in medicine. Gregory made what he called "women of learning and virtue" the moral exemplars of caring for others, which Rosemary Tong characterizes as "feminine ethics."[21] Gregory was therefore committed to a caring relationship of physicians to their female patients, to which maintenance of an asexual, yet physically intimate, relationship was essential.

> We sometimes see a remarkable difference between the behaviour of a physician at his first setting out, and afterwards, when he is fully established in reputation and practice. In the beginning he is affable, polite, humane, and assiduously attentive to his patients: but afterwards, when he has reaped the fruits of such a behaviour, and finds himself independent, he assumes a very different tone; he becomes haughty, rapacious, careless, and often somewhat brutal in his manners.[3, p. 25]

Gregory means "rapacious" not as a metaphor, but as rape, the violation of the woman's body and person, which is totally incompatible with an asexual relationship. So is being "somewhat brutal in his manners." Callous disregard is incompatible with a caring relationship with female patients. Gregory understood very well that initiating a romantic or sexual relationship was always motivated by self-interest that takes advantage of the physician's power when he is alone with a female patient in her bedchambers. In violation of the commitment to the ethical concept of medicine, the obstetrician-gynecologist gives the pursuit of self-interest primacy, making the fulfillment of professional responsibility systematically secondary. Such a physician becomes a "man of interest" and no longer a professional physician.

5.4.2 Contemporary Perspective

In the contemporary discourse of professional ethics in obstetrics and gynecology, such a physician – whether a man or a woman – irresponsibly manages a conflict of interest and therefore undermines his or her commitment to being a professional. Intellectual integrity is violated when the physician embraces self-deception of falsely believing that there are no ethical constraints on initiating a romantic or sexual relationship. Moral integrity is violated when the physician embraces the self-deception of falsely believing that the female patient will not be harmed by his having a romantic or sexual relationship with him or her, despite the abundant evidence that falsifies such a belief.

The elements of ethical reasoning from this historical review can now be identified. The pursuit of a romantic or sexual relationship with a current patient upends the commitment to the ethical concept of medicine as a profession: the pursuit of self-interest at known risk to the patient (prohibited in beneficence-based clinical ethical judgment), to which she has not consented (prohibited in autonomy-based clinical ethical judgment). Doing so comes at an unacceptable price: reverting to the contractual relationship between a medical practitioner and an ill individual. Honesty requires that all of a physician's patients be immediately informed that professional integrity no longer governs his or her practice. It is difficult to countenance that such a public announcement would advance the physician's reputation and might well imperil the viability of the business model of his or her practice. If the obstetrician-gynecologist is in a group practice, its directors might dismiss him or her for cause. Legitimate self-interest would thereby be imperiled, creating a buttressing argument against initiating romantic and, especially, a sexual relationship with a current patient.

The commitment to the ethical concept of medicine as a profession and legitimate self-interest combine to create a strong, prima facie ethical obligation not to pursue a romantic or sexual relationship with a female or pregnant patient. The burden of proof on doing so is therefore very high. As a matter of intellectual integrity, failure to meet this burden of proof is ethically permissible.

The American Psychiatric Association takes the position that this burden of proof can never be met for psychiatrists. In psychiatry the imbalance of power is considered to be durable beyond the termination of the professional relationship between psychiatrist and patient. The potential abuse of this imbalance of power, to the biopsychosocial harm of the patient, is ethically impermissible on the basis of the second commitment of the ethical concept of medicine as a profession. The American Psychiatric Association therefore prohibits initiation of a romantic or sexual relationship, current and former alike.[22]

In obstetrics and gynecology, it appears that the burden of proof can be met under strict conditions. It is not clear that there is durability of power imbalance after termination of the professional relationship. This explains why ACOG prohibits romantic and sexual relationship with current patients, but not past patients.[23] Terminating the professional relationship and only afterwards initiating a romantic or sexual relationship becomes ethically permissible. Otherwise initiating a romantic of sexual relationship is ethically impermissible. Prudence, the virtue grounded in the protection of legitimate self-interest, adds a buttressing consideration of caution. The trap of self-deception must be addressed and removed after rigorous self-scrutiny, which can best be accomplished in consultation with a skilled and experienced psychiatrist or other mental health professional. The prima facie beneficence-based ethical obligation to prevent biopsychosocial harm to the patient requires an equally rigorous assessment of the potential for such risk and its prevention, an assessment that is also made in consultation with a skilled and experienced psychiatrist or other mental health professional. The ethical obligation to earn and keep the trust of the patient in her obstetrician-gynecologist, as well as in other physicians and healthcare professionals, is essential. Loss of such trust is a very grave ethical matter, reinforcing the obligation, as a matter of intellectual integrity, to rigorously assess this risk as well. The burden of proof on initiating a romantic or sexual relationship with a female or pregnant patient is therefore very steep.

5.5 Conscientious Objection: A Conflict of Commitment

5.5.1 Conscientious Objection Defined

Conscientious objection is invoked to justify deliberate failure to fulfill professional responsibility to patients on the basis of conscience. Conscience should be understood to mean the fundamental convictions of an individual that shape his or her identity. Such convictions are rooted in sustained commitment to what an individual judges to be of paramount importance in his or life other than being an excellent obstetrician-gynecologist. Conscientious objection thus should be understood as a conflict of commitment between ethical obligations to patients and ethical obligations originating in conscience.

Conscientious objection should not be understood as a species of conflict of interest. An interest is a stake that an individual has in the past, present, or future. Interests can be temporary as well as durable. Interests usually do not define an individual's identity. Core commitments of one's life do so. Conceptualizing conscientious objection as a conflict of interest risks trivializing what is far from trivial in the life of an individual invoking conscientious objection.

5.5.2 A Useful Historical Analogy

The concept of conscientious objection originated outside of medicine, notably in the context of conscription for military service, also known as "the draft." The United States Selective Service System, for example, has allowed those subject to the draft to claim conscientious objection to bearing arms and to participating in warfare in any of its forms.[24] The basis for conscientious objection must be demonstrated by a fundamental, long-standing commitment to a faith community or other tradition that objects to bearing arms or to participating in warfare in any way. This commitment must be public, with evidence for it provided by others. In short, conscientious objection should not be an interest that an individual adopts as a way to avoid conscription. Matters of conscience are not matters of mere interest; matters of conscience spring from sustained commitment to a set of fundamental, defining values.

5.5.3 Conscientious Objection in Residency Training

Conscientious objection has been invoked by residents to refuse training in the procedures of induced abortion and feticide on religious grounds.[25] Some faith communities consider induced abortion and feticide to be ethically prohibited forms of killing innocent human beings. Other faith communities do not. Permitting residents who can document objection to induced abortion and feticide as a matter of conscience not to participate in these procedures does not result in any patient being denied access to them. The conflict of commitment may therefore justifiably be managed by permitting such residents to act on their sustained moral convictions about the ethical permissibility of induced abortion and feticide.

Respecting conscientious objection applies only to participation. All residents must have the fund of knowledge and clinical skills to manage the sequelae of induced abortion and feticide, because all obstetrician-gynecologists must have this fund of knowledge and clinical skills. Patients, including those with urgent sequelae, might be denied access to timely and effective diagnosis and treatment, an outcome that is not compatible with the commitment to the ethical concept of medicine as a profession.

All residents must also be prepared to counsel pregnant women about induced abortion and feticide. The decision-making process with patients, as described in Chapter 3, is based on the ethical principles of beneficence and respect for autonomy, secular ethical concepts that apply by their very nature to all obstetrician-gynecologists. Moreover, the outcome of this counseling process is controlled by the patient, not the obstetrician-gynecologist. There therefore can be no valid conscientious objection to mastering the fund of knowledge and skills required to fulfill the role of the obstetrician-gynecologist in decision making about the disposition of pregnancy, a role that is described in detail in Chapter 9.

5.5.4 Conscientious Objection to Contraception

Conscientious objection may also be invoked as the basis for not counseling women who want to prevent pregnancy or for prescribing contraception, on the grounds that the medications used are abortifacients. However, not all forms of contraception are abortifacients. For these forms of contraception, such as birth control pills, there cannot be a valid conscience-based objection because there is no evidence base for it. This means that the assertion of a conscience-based objection to a form of contraception as an abortifacient must be accompanied by a structured scientific review that critically appraises the evidence and reaches an evidence-based conclusion that a form of contraception is an abortifacient. In the absence of such evidence, the conscience-based objection lacks scientific merit and therefore has no intellectual or moral authority for the obstetrician-gynecologist or others.

In addition, healthcare professionals, including pharmacists, may invoke conscientious objection to writing or filling a prescription for a contraceptive medication because is it an abortifacient, which their religious or moral commitment considers unjustified killing of a human life form. The claim that contraception is an abortifacient is not evidence based. Even if it were, the claim alone is not sufficient to ethically justify refusal to write or fill a prescription. This is because the woman is solely and completely in control of the decision to take the medication as directed. There is no justification of a nonphysician such as a pharmacist for inquiring about the woman's reasons for wanting contraception, because engaging in such inquiry requires a fund of knowledge and clinical skills about reproductive medicine that a nonphysician does not possess.

5.5.5 Conscientious Objection to Referral for Induced Abortion and Feticide

5.5.5.1 Invoking Individual Conscience Bears the Burden of Proof

Some physicians invoke conscientious objection to referral for induced abortion and feticide. These objections often originate in the physician's religious convictions about the moral status of the fetus. While this is no doubt a matter that the physician must take seriously, patients are not in a relationship of any kind with the physician's individual conscience but in a professional relationship. The ethical concept of medicine as a profession is a secular idea in that it can be understood without reference to any religious beliefs or moral theologies about the moral status of the fetus. Invoking conscientious objection therefore bears the burden of proof.

5.5.5.2 Beneficence-Based and Autonomy-Based Indications

In the language of professional medical ethics referral has *both* beneficence-based and autonomy-based indications.[25] (See Chapter 9.) The ethical principle of beneficence in professional ethics in obstetrics creates a prima facie ethical obligation to provide clinical management that in deliberative clinical judgment is reliably predicted to result in net clinical benefit for the pregnant patient. This ethical principle requires *direct* referral of patients for medically indicated intervention. The ethical principle of respect for autonomy in professional ethics in obstetrics creates the prima facie ethical obligation to empower the pregnant woman to make informed and voluntary decisions about the clinical management of her pregnancy. Respect for autonomy requires only *indirect* referral of patients for intervention that has only autonomy-based indications.[26]

5.5.5.3 Beneficence-Based Direct Referral

Beneficence-based ethical obligations are implemented in one of two ways. The obstetrician is competent and willing to perform the service in question and offers or recommends it to the patient. The alternative is that the obstetrician is not competent or willing to perform the service in question and makes a referral to another physician. Fulfilling the beneficence-based ethical obligation to see to it that the patient receives medical care for which there is a beneficence-based indication is accomplished by direct communication to the referral physician. Such direct referral is required because simply providing patients with referral information (which is the definition of indirect referral) does not ensure that the referral will be accomplished and the patient's clinical needs met in a timely and effective fashion. For example, an obstetrician suspects appendicitis in a pregnant patient. The obstetrician has a prima facie beneficence-based ethical obligation to see to it that the patient receives prompt surgical attention, an obligation that is fulfilled by ensuring that a general surgeon does indeed see the patient promptly.

5.5.5.4 Autonomy-Based Indirect Referral

Sometimes patients request medical intervention that is not beneficence based but is clinically safe and effective in achieving the patient's goal. These procedures have only autonomy-based indications. This is by definition the case for cosmetic procedures to improve appearance. The indications for termination of pregnancy in a healthy woman are also autonomy based, because beneficence-based clinical judgment provides physicians with no professional competence either to make decisions about remaining pregnant or about continuing a pregnancy in which a fetal anomaly, of whatever severity, has been diagnosed; these are, instead, the personal decisions of each individual pregnant woman. Pregnant women appeal to a wide range of cultural, familial, religious, and personal beliefs that physicians are not professionally competent in beneficence-based clinical judgment to evaluate. This underscores an important difference from cosmetic procedures: the values and beliefs on which pregnant women base their requests for termination of pregnancy involve more fundamental concerns than improving one's appearance. ACOG is therefore correct to emphasize that respect for autonomy requires every physician to acknowledge and respect such values and beliefs and not discriminate against patients based on differences of these values and beliefs from those of the physician.[27]

The crucial question becomes: What is the ethical obligation in professional ethics in obstetrics regarding referral for medical intervention that has *only* autonomy-based indications? Because the reason for the patient's referral is based on the patient's personal reasons and goals and not on medical indications, there is no beneficence-based ethical obligation to ensure that the referral occurs. The physician's ethical obligation is only to empower the exercise of autonomy by the patient, by giving the patient referral information, without taking any additional steps to ensure the referral actually occurs. Because the indications for referral are exclusively autonomy-based, direct referral is not ethically obligatory, but is permissible.

There is an inescapable beneficence-based obligation, however, that shapes the physician's response. Given the sorry history of incompetently performed abortions, which unfortunately is not altogether past, the physician has a prima facie beneficence-based ethical obligation to protect the patient from loss of future fertility, health, or even her life. It is not realistic to expect a physician to know all of the physicians or nonphysicians who incompetently perform abortions. However, it is realistic to expect a physician to know that there are healthcare organizations, such as Planned Parenthood,[28] in which the physician can have confidence that an abortion, should it be elected by the pregnant woman, would be done competently. It is not necessary to provide names of particular physicians, but it is necessary to inform the patient about responsible healthcare organizations such as Planned Parenthood. It is a violation of the obstetrician-gynecologist's prima facie beneficence-based ethical obligation to the patient not to provide such information on the basis of the physician's individual or private conscience-based objection to induced abortion or feticide. In our view, simply informing the patient that she is free to seek a second opinion,[29] without providing information about responsible healthcare organizations, is not consistent with beneficence-based obligations to pregnant women.

By definition, the exercise of autonomy in response to indirect referral for abortion is solely the pregnant woman's freedom and responsibility. It is therefore a mistake for the physician to think that the physician is somehow a party to, or complicit in, the patient's subsequent exercise of autonomy to seek termination of pregnancy. This marks yet another important difference between direct and indirect referral, because in direct referral the physician is indeed a direct party to the referral and the performance of the procedure.

5.5.5.5 Polarized Positions Are Unnecessary

Our ethical analysis of direct and indirect referral has important implications for the current, politicized polarization between advocates for conscience-based exceptions to make referrals for termination of pregnancy and advocates for an obligation to make unconditional referrals for termination of pregnancy.[27,29] This polarization becomes unnecessary when one acknowledges the ethical distinction between direct and indirect referral and the fact that ethical analysis of indirect referral does not and need not include reference to the individual conscience of the physician. There is no intrinsic ethical conflict between the prima facie beneficence-based ethical obligation to make an *indirect* referral, which is all that is ethically required with regard to termination of pregnancy, and the physician's individual or private conscience.

Individual conscience regarding termination of pregnancy is consistent with indirect referral to responsible healthcare organizations that will provide professional counseling and competently performed termination of pregnancy. To repeat, the physician cannot reasonably be understood to be a party to, or complicit in, a subsequent decision that is the sole province of the patient's subsequent exercise of autonomy in consultation with a referral physician. Physicians without conscience-based objections to termination of pregnancy are free to make a direct referral.

References

1. Chervenak FA, McCullough LB, Hale RW. Guild interests: an insidious threat to professionalism in obstetrics and gynecology. Am J Obstet Gynecol 2018; 219: 581–584.
2. Porter D, Porter R. Patient's Progress: Doctors and Doctoring in Eighteenth Century England. Cambridge: Cambridge University Press, 1989.
3. Gregory J. Lectures on the Duties and Qualifications of a Physician. London: W. Strahan and T. Cadell, 1772. In McCullough LB, ed. John Gregory's Writings on Medical Ethics and the Philosophy of Medicine. Dordrecht, the Netherlands: Kluwer Academic, 1998: 161–248.
4. McCullough LB. John Gregory and the Invention of Professional Medical Ethics and the Profession of Medicine. Dordrecht, the Netherlands: Springer, 1998.
5. Percival T. Medical Ethics; or, A Code of Institutes and Precepts, Adapted to the Professional Conduct of Physicians and Surgeons. London: Johnson & Bickerstaff, 1803.
6. American College of Obstetricians and Gynecologists. Committee Opinion No. 390. Ethical decision making in obstetrics and gynecology. Obstet Gynecol 2007; 110: 1479–1487.
7. National Academy of Medicine. Conflicts of Interest in Medical Research, Education, and Practice. Washington, DC: National Academies Press, 2009.
8. Hillman BJ, Joseph CA, Mabry MR, et al. Frequency and costs of diagnostic imaging in office practice: a comparison of self-referring and radiologist-referring physicians. N Engl J Med 1990; 323: 1604–1608.
9. International Association for Medial Ultrasound. Practice parameters. Available at www.aium.org/resources/guidelines.aspx (accessed March 1, 2019).
10. Jain C. ACOG Committee Opinion No. 723. Guidelines for diagnostic imaging during pregnancy and lactation. Obstet Gynecol 2019; 133: 186.
11. Choo EK, Byington CL, Johnson NL, Jagsi R. From #MeToo to #TimesUp in health care: can a culture of accountability end inequity and harassment? *Lancet* 2019; 393: 499–502.
12. Holroyd-Leduc JM, Straus SE. #MeToo and the medical profession. CMAJ 2018; 190: E972–E973.
13. Bayer T, Coverdale J, Chiang E. A national survey of physicians' behaviors regarding sexual contact with patients. South Med J 1996; 89: 977–982.
14. McCullough LB, Chervenak FA, Coverdale J. Ethically justified guidelines for defining sexual boundaries between obstetrician-gynecologists and their patients. Am J Obstet Gynecol 1996; 175: 496–500.
15. Johns Hopkins Hospital. Hospital agrees to pay $190 million over recording of pelvic exams. Available at www.nytimes.com/2014/07/22/us/johns-hopkins-settlement-190-million.html (accessed March 1, 2019).
16. 'Just the grossest thing': Women recall interactions with U.S. C. doctor. Available at www.nytimes.com/2018/05/17/us/USC-gynecologist-young-women.html. Accessed March 1, 2019.
17. Anonymous. Our family secrets. Ann Intern Med 2015; 163: 321.
18. von Staden H. "In a pure and holy way:" personal and professional conduct in the Hippocratic Oath. J Hist Med Allied Sci 1996; 51: 404–437.
19. Pernick MS. Bioethics and history. In Baker RB, McCullough LB, eds. The Cambridge World History of Medical Ethics. New York: Cambridge University Press, 2009: 16–20.
20. Hoffmann F. Medicus politicus; sive, regulae prudentiae secundum quas medicus juvenis studia sua & vitae rationem dirigere debet. (The Politic Doctor, or Rules of Prudence according to which a Young Physician Should Direct his Studies and Reason of Life). Leiden: Philip Bonk, 1738.
21. Tong R. Feminine and Feminist Ethics. Belmont, CA: Wadsworth, 1993.
22. American Psychiatric Association. Principles of Medical Ethics with Annotations Especially Applicable to Psychiatry. 2013. Available at https://www.psychiatry.org/psychiatrists/practice/ethics (accessed March 1, 2019).
23. American College of Obstetricians and Gynecologists. ACOG Committee Opinion No. 723. Sexual misconduct. Obstet Gynecol 2007; 110: 441–444.
24. Selective Service System. Conscientious objection and alternative service. Available at www.sss.gov/consobj (accessed March 1, 2019).
25. Chervenak FA, McCullough LB. Obstetric ethics and the abortion controversy. Am J Ethics Med 1994; 3: 3–6. https://www.psychiatry.org/psychiatrists/practice/ethics (accessed March 1, 2019).
26. Chervenak FA, McCullough LB. Reply (re: The ethics of direct and indirect referral for termination of pregnancy). Am J Obstet Gynecol 2008; 199: 232e1–3.26.
27. American College of Obstetricians and Gynecologists. Committee on Ethics. Committee Opinion Number 385. The limits of conscientious refusal in reproductive medicine. Obstet Gynecol 2007; 110: 1203–1208.
28. Planned Parenthood. Available at www.plannedparenthood.org/ (accessed March 1, 2019).
29. American Association of Pro-Life Obstetricians and Gynecologists. AAPLOG response to the ACOG Ethics Committee Opinion #385, titled "The limits of conscientious refusal in reproductive medicine." February 6, 2008. Available at www.consciencelaws.org/ethics/ethics079-004.aspx3. Accessed March 1, 2019.

Section 2 Pedagogy of Professional Ethics in Obstetrics and Gynecology

Chapter 6

Teaching Professional Ethics in Obstetrics and Gynecology

GOAL
This chapter provides guidance on teaching professional ethics in obstetrics and gynecology.

OBJECTIVES
On completing study of this chapter, the reader will:

Describe how to teach the discipline of ethical reasoning

Identify pedagogical tools for teaching professional ethics in obstetrics and gynecology

Identify pedagogical methods for teaching professional ethics in obstetrics and gynecology

Demonstrate how a preventive ethics approach to drift away from professionalism should be used in graduate medical education

Apply guidance on teaching professional ethics in obstetrics and gynecology to learners, including medical students, residents in obstetrics and gynecology, fellows in subspecialties of obstetrics and gynecology, and clinical colleagues

TOPICS

6.1 Teaching the Basics of Professional Ethics in Obstetrics and Gynecology	94
6.2 Teaching the Discipline of Ethical Reasoning	95
6.2.1 Precision of Thought and Speech	95
6.2.2 Going Where Arguments Take One and Nowhere Else	95
6.3 Pedagogical Tools	96
6.3.1 Formal Assessment Tool for the Normative Ethics Literature	96
6.3.1.1 Does the Article Address a Focused Ethics Question?	96
6.3.1.2 Are the Results of the Article Valid?	97
6.3.1.3 What Are the Results?	98
6.3.1.4 Will the Results Help Me in Clinical Practice? In Innovation and Research? In Organizational Culture? In Health Policy and Advocacy?	98
6.3.2 Structured Reviews of the Normative Ethics Literature	98
6.4 Pedagogical Methods	98
6.4.1 Case-Based Teaching Using an Ethics Workup	98
6.4.2 "Fast Ethics": Teaching Ethics on Rounds	99
6.4.3 Preparing a Grand Rounds Presentation on Professional Ethics in Obstetrics and Gynecology	99
6.4.4 What Makes a Great Teacher of Professional Ethics in Obstetrics and Gynecology?	100
6.5 A Distinctive Challenge in Graduate Medical Education: Preventing Drift Away from Professionalism	101
6.5.1 The Commitment to the Ethical Concept of Medicine as a Profession	101

6.5.2 Drift Away from an Organizational Culture of Professionalism   102
    6.5.2.1 Restricted Duty Hours   102
    6.5.2.2 Supervision by Attending Physicians   103
    6.5.2.3 Compounding Factors   103
6.6 A Preventive Ethics Response to Reduced Accountability   103
  6.6.1 Performing a Critical Appraisal of the Organizational Culture of the Residency   104
  6.6.2 Defining Components of Professional Accountability in Milestones   104
  6.6.3 Mastering the Skillset of Patient Safety and Quality   104
  6.6.4 Enhancing the Role of ACGME   105

Key Concepts

Argument-based ethical reasoning
Descriptive ethics
Discipline of ethical reasoning
Ethical concept of medicine as a profession
Ethical principles
Normative ethics
Patient
Virtues

6.1 Teaching the Basics of Professional Ethics in Obstetrics and Gynecology

Medical educators know well one of the fundamental tasks of medical education: teaching the basics again and again to learners at all levels: undergraduate, graduate, postgraduate, and continuing medical education. Teaching professional ethics in obstetrics and gynecology is no exception. The basics of professional ethics in obstetrics and gynecology include

1. The three commitments that define the ethical concept of medicine as a profession: to scientific and clinical competence, the necessary and sufficient condition for patient safety and quality; to the primacy of the patient's health-related interests and to keeping individual self-interest systematically secondary; and to the primacy of the patient's health-related interests to keeping guild interests systematically secondary. The existence of medicine as a profession is not guaranteed; whether we have a profession of medicine is a function of obstetrician-gynecologists making the commitment to the ethical concept of medicine as a profession as medical students and then strengthening and sustaining that commitment as residents, fellows, and practicing physicians. See Chapters 1 and 2.

2. Becoming a patient, a living human being under the protection of the evidence-based clinical judgment and argument-based ethical judgment of a physician who sustains these three commitments. A living human being becomes a patient when she is presented to a physician and there exist clinical interventions reliably expected to benefit that human being clinically. Becoming a patient is a beneficence-based concept. See Chapters 1 and 2.

3. Specifying the prima facie ethical principles of beneficence, nonmaleficence, respect for autonomy, and healthcare justice, so that they become clinically applicable, practical guides to clinical ethical judgment, decision making, patient care, clinical innovation and research, organizational culture, and health policy advocacy for women and children. Professional ethics in obstetrics and gynecology does not countenance absolute ethical principles, including respect for autonomy as an absolute ethical principle. See Chapters 2 and 18.

4. Empowering patients, or their surrogate decision makers, in the simple consent, informed consent, assisted consent, assent, and surrogate decision-making processes. See Chapter 3.

5. Confidentiality, a prima facie beneficence-based and autonomy-based ethical obligation to protect health-related information from those without authorized access to it, especially those who are not bound by the professional ethical obligation of confidentiality. Confidentiality is consistent

with routine sharing of information about a patient by all healthcare professionals responsible for her clinical care. See Chapter 4.
6. Professionally responsible management of conflicts of interest and conflicts of commitment. See Chapter 5.

The first long-term goal of teaching professional ethics in obstetrics and gynecology is that, by the conclusion of residency training, these basics have become guides to the obstetrician-gynecologist in all aspects of patient care, in clinical innovation and research, organizational culture, and in advocating for women's and children's health policy. The second long-term goal of teaching professional ethics in obstetrics and gynecology is to sustain the professionalism of medical students, residents, fellows, practicing physicians, and clinical innovators and researchers.

6.2 Teaching the Discipline of Ethical Reasoning

6.2.1 Precision of Thought and Speech

Clarity in clinical discourse is essential for patient safety and quality. Clarity is required because, in the absence of clarity and precision, the risks of miscommunication with clinical colleagues and with female and pregnant patients increase. Precision of thought and speech is essential for clarity in clinical discourse. There is a direct parallel to the first component of ethical reasoning, ethical analysis or gaining clarity about clinically relevant ethical concepts. Precision of thought and speech is essential for clarity in the discourse of professional ethics in obstetrics and gynecology. The discipline of ethical reasoning is therefore expressed in precision and clarity of thought. (See Chapter 1.)

To support teaching the discipline of ethical reasoning about the material in each chapter of this book, we include for each chapter a statement of goals and objectives, topics covered, and a list of the key concepts that each chapter invokes. Teaching the material in each chapter can usefully begin with a review of these concepts, so that learners aim for clear and precise mastery of the technical vocabulary of professional ethics in obstetrics and gynecology, just as they aim for precise mastery of the technical vocabulary of anatomy, physiology, diagnosis, treatment planning, and prognosis. As a pedagogical aide memoire we have gathered all of the Glossary of Key Concepts into a single, alphabetical listing, with definitions, that appears after Chapter 18.

6.2.2 Going Where Arguments Take One and Nowhere Else

As we explained in Chapter 1, the second component of ethical reasoning is ethical argument: identifying the implications of clearly expressed clinically relevant ethical concepts for clinical practice, organizational culture, innovation and research, and health policy. One is intellectually required to accept these implications, which become the conclusions of ethical reasoning. This is directly analogous to the discipline of evidence-based clinical reasoning: one is required to improve clinical practice, innovation and research, and health policy on the basis of the best available evidence. Intellectual integrity requires that one accept the conclusions of ethical reasoning, unless, as explained in Chapter 1, one can find an error in ethical analysis or argument, correct the error, and develop a superior line of ethical reasoning. This is known as argument-based ethical reasoning.[1]

We have developed a tool for critical appraisal of ethical reasoning, i.e., for the normative ethics literature of professional ethics in obstetrics and gynecology, which asks what professional ethics in obstetrics and gynecology ought to be.[1] This tool can be used in teaching, for example in lectures, small groups, and journal clubs, to assess an article and in creating a structured review of the literature on a clinical topic, such as covert placement of psychiatric medications in patients' food.[2] We created this tool because none exists for the normative ethics literature in medicine. The components of the tool are adapted from tools for the critical appraisal of the clinical literature,[3] including critical appraisal of reviews,[3] randomized clinical trials,[4,5] practice guidelines,[6,7] qualitative studies,[8,9] and economic analyses.[10,11]

Deploying this tool requires attention to an important distinction: descriptive ethics in obstetrics and gynecology and normative ethics in obstetrics and gynecology.[1,12] The literature of descriptive medical ethics uses empirical methods of the social sciences to obtain data that describe the actual ethical judgments, practices, and policies of physicians and healthcare organizations, of patients and their families, and of the larger society. In addition, these articles report the results of ethically justified interventions for their clinical effects. Descriptive ethics articles use accepted methods of empirical research, such as interviews analyzed with qualitative methods and questionnaire research analyzed with quantitative methods.[12] Such empirical studies are common in the medical literature and should be critically appraised using appropriate methodology that has already been well described.[3-11]

By contrast, the literature of normative medical ethics is argument based and uses the tools of ethical analysis and argument to explore the implications of ethical concepts for what clinical practice and organizational and healthcare policy ought to be. Normative ethics scholarship offers reasoned conclusions about what clinical judgment, decision making, and behavior *ought to be* the case, rather than descriptions of what *is* the case.

Scholarship in normative medical ethics appears as review articles, clinical opinions, editorials, and statements from professional associations of physicians. Books, both authored and edited, are a major component of the normative ethics literature. Unlike the practice with textbooks in medicine, which are expected to synthesize current knowledge, edited volumes in normative ethics often make original and even innovative contributions to the literature.

Normative ethics articles and books should not be judged solely on the basis of their source – an individual physician, a research group, or a professional association – no matter how prominent and accomplished.[12-14] Instead, these works should be held to standards of intellectual rigor that are in their own way as demanding as those of evidence-based medicine and other standards for evaluating the medical and scientific literature.

A basic distinction for the normative ethics literature needs to be made between reasoned argument, i.e., conclusions that meet the standards of argument-based ethics because they are supported by ethical analysis and argument, and mere opinions, offered without such support. Plato (ca .427–ca. 338 BCE) in dialogues such as *Republic* has Socrates teach again and again that reasoned argument must be distinguished from "mere" opinion and that the latter commands no intellectual respect, even if it comes from the most renowned authorities.[15] Common errors of ethical reasoning are identified in Chapter 1.

It is often said that there is no right or wrong answer in ethics. This is a disservice to physicians turning to the normative medical ethics literature.

There are well argued and poorly argued positions and they can be reliably distinguished. The latter appeal to "gut feeling," free-floating intuition, and unsystematic clinical ethical judgment and decision making, rather than judgment and decision making that meet standards of careful reflection and argument that are the hallmarks of argument-based medical ethics.

6.3 Pedagogical Tools

6.3.1 Formal Assessment Tool for the Normative Ethics Literature

The appraisal tool for the normative ethics literature is summarized in Table 6.1.[1] We have adapted this tool from recent work on critical appraisal of the medical literature reporting the results of qualitative research.[8,9]

6.3.1.1 Does the Article Address a Focused Ethics Question?

As in the literature of basic and clinical science, normative ethics articles should have a clear, well-defined focus. This focus should be reflected in the title and made explicit in the introductory section of the article in a clearly stated focused question or purpose. There are a number of possible domains for the focus of normative ethics literature, including theoretical issues, clinical issues for a specific patient population, research issues for a specific population, organizational culture, and health policy and advocacy issues.

The importance of the issue should be explained. Importance can be theoretical as well as clinical. The issue may be important for clinical care, organizational culture, clinical innovation and research, or for advocacy and public policy.

The importance of the issue should be justified. The justification for addressing the issue may be descriptive, e.g., data concerning its prominence in surveys of physicians' attitudes, or normative, e.g., ethical analysis and argument. Finally, the article should identify the perspective from which the importance of the issue is claimed, including that of physicians, clinical innovators and investigators, patients, patients' families and other support networks, payers, healthcare organization leadership, and experts and public officials concerned with health policy and advocacy. The relevance of this consideration is that the target audience for the article should be clear.

Chapter 6: Teaching Professional Ethics in Obstetrics and Gynecology

Table 6.1 An argument-based, comprehensive assessment tool for critical appraisal of the normative ethics literature in medicine.[1]

1. Does the article address a focused ethics question?
   a. Does the article address a clearly stated and focused ethical issue or problem?
   b. Is the issue important and why?
   c. Is justification for the importance presented?
   d. From whose perspective is importance claimed?
2. Are the results of the article valid?
   a. Was the literature search complete?
   b. Are the analysis and argument of cited articles reported clearly and accurately?
   c. What is the quality of the article's ethical analysis and argument?
3. What are the results?
   a. What are the conclusions of the articles ethical analysis and argument?
4. Will the results help me in clinical practice? Innovation and research? In health policy?
   a. Will the help be practical?
   b. Will the help be theoretical?
   c. How should the reader change his or her thinking, attitudes, practices, or policies?

6.3.1.2 Are the Results of the Article Valid?

The validity of the results in a normative ethics article rest primarily on the quality of its ethical analysis and argument and whether the article meets the standards of argument-based ethics. The literature of normative ethics in medicine is now very large, making it highly unlikely that there is no prior relevant literature that needs to be considered. As in basic and clinical science literature, it is crucial to elucidate the search strategies, including key words, databases, bibliographies, and other sources used. The first question to ask, therefore, is, How adequate was the article's search strategy? Inasmuch as both are major forms of scholarship in bioethics, are both articles and books cited? An additional, though not necessarily obligatory, level of thoroughness would be references to the "gray" literature, which includes abstracts and presentations from professional meetings and articles in languages other than English. A final, crucial, consideration is whether the article identifies and addresses different viewpoints.

The next question is, What was the completeness of the background and literature review? Major positions on the issue should be presented in a clear and unbiased fashion. How these positions have developed and their critical interaction should be explained, so that the reader is provided with an as-comprehensive-as-possible account of the best thinking on the subject. These major positions should be critically appraised for their strengths and weaknesses and how well they responded to criticisms that have been advanced against them or how they are capable of responding to criticisms that could be advanced against them.

The third question brings us to the heart of the critical appraisal of normative ethics work: What is the quality of the article's analysis and argument? Quality turns on both validity and soundness. Validity concerns the formal qualities of ethical analysis and argument. (See Chapter 1.) Are relevant clinical and other facts clearly identified and supported? Are key concepts clearly stated and reasonably related to clinical information? Are these concepts used with consistent meaning throughout the argument? Do the reasons given for the position, the premises of the argument, fit together into a coherent whole? Is the conclusion that follows from those premises clearly stated? Normative ethics in medicine is not an "ivory tower" enterprise; it concerns issues of vital importance in clinical practice and research and in organizational management and health policy. Physician readers are therefore entitled to expect authors of normative medical ethics scholarship to take a clinically relevant and applicable stand.

Soundness concerns the substance of the ethical analysis and argument, including especially whether the conclusion should be regarded as reliable, i.e., one on which the physician can act with confidence that patient care, clinical innovation and research, organizational culture, and health policy and advocacy will be improved as a result. Reliable arguments are those in which a clear warrant or defense is given for each premise or reason offered in support of the conclusion. Unsupported premises or reasons are not acceptable. In most cases at the current time, the reliability of the conclusions of normative ethics articles is conceptually and theoretically based. There is an emerging literature that goes one step further and studies whether, using accepted tools of health services research, implementing the conclusions of well-argued positions can be documented as improving the outcomes of patient care.[12]

In preventing readers' bias,[13,14] it is helpful to identify the disciplines represented among the authors. The normative medical ethics literature is distinctive in that work of high quality by nonclinicians should influence the clinical judgment and decision making of physicians, just as work on infectious disease by microbiologists or on pharmacokinetics by pharmacologists rightly influences clinical judgment and practice. Normative ethics work therefore should not be dismissed simply because none of the authors are physicians or accepted simply because all of the authors are physicians.

At the same time, the reader should beware of positive or negative bias toward an article, based on the reputation of the author(s) or of the journal. Just as in the basic and clinical sciences, the standing of authors and journals is no guarantee of quality.

6.3.1.3 What Are the Results?

The results of normative ethics work are the conclusions of ethical analysis and argument. As emphasized, there should be clearly stated and easy to find in the article.

6.3.1.4 Will the Results Help Me in Clinical Practice? In Innovation and Research? In Organizational Culture? In Health Policy and Advocacy?

The results of normative ethics articles and books can be helpful in three ways. First, they may have important practical implications, especially if the article incorporates evidence to support the clinical utility of acting on the conclusions of the article. The quality of the empirical evidence cited should be assessed in the same way as evidence should be assessed in any medical or scientific article.[3-11] The results for clinical practice, clinical innovation and research, organizational culture and leadership, or health policy and advocacy should be assessed as well. Second, they may have important theoretical implications, which

do not depend on whether an intervention was performed and evaluated. Finally, readers of the normative ethics literature should ask themselves how they should change their thinking (clinical judgment and reasoning), attitudes (toward patients, their families, and legal institutions), clinical practice, or organizational policies and practices. This is a crucial step in the literature on evidence-based medicine and is similarly crucial here.

6.3.2 Structured Reviews of the Normative Ethics Literature

This critical appraisal tool can be readily adapted to become the basis for creating a structured review of the normative ethics literature on a selected topic.[2] Articles from the normative ethics literature can be scored in domains relevant to a successful article. First, the patient population should be identified. Second, a clinically useful article in the normative ethics literature should address a focused question, a standard that is not uniformly met unfortunately. Third, the article should include a statement of the search strategy that identifies the topic, the search terms used to search databases, and the databases searched. PubMed will play a prominent role, inasmuch as it captures virtually all of the clinically pertinent normative ethics literature. Fourth, the article should include ethical analysis (clearly stated relevant concepts) and argument (clearly identified implications of these concepts). Fourth, the conclusion(s) of the article should be clearly stated. Fifth, the clinical (or research or policy) implications should be clearly identified and follow from the conclusion(s). We have found useful in our teaching for the reviewer to assign a score to each of the five domains: 0 = unsatisfied; 0.5 = partially satisfied; and 1 = satisfied. The range scores when the five domains are summed will be 0 to 5. Articles can then be ranked by their overall score, with this result used to determine which articles should be considered the most relevant to answering the focused question.

6.4 Pedagogical Methods

6.4.1 Case-Based Teaching Using an Ethics Workup

The discipline of ethical reasoning, like the discipline of clinical reasoning, requires an orderly process, following iterative steps of an Ethics Work-Up. (See Table 6.2.)

Table 6.2 Ethics work-up.

1. Identify the clinical facts.
2. A question or questions about the ethical challenges of the case should be clearly stated, using normative language.
3. For each question, classify the ethical challenge using the categories in this book.
4. Identify the medically reasonable alternatives (evidence-based, beneficence-based; see Chapter 1) for the management of the patient's condition and their benefits and risks.
5. The medically reasonable alternatives should be presented to the patient or the patient's surrogate in the informed decision-making process.
6. If the patient or the patient's surrogate authorizes one of the medically reasonable alternatives, it should be implemented.
7. If the patient or the patient's surrogate refuses to authorize any medically reasonable alternative, implement the process of informed refusal.

1. Identify the clinical facts. The account of the patient's history, current condition, treatment plan, and prognosis should be concisely stated.
2. A question or questions about the ethical challenges of the case should be clearly stated, using normative language, e.g., Is it ethically permissible to offer nonaggressive obstetric management when the fetus has been diagnosed with a serious anomaly?
3. For each question, classify the ethical challenge using the categories in this book, e.g., the diagnosis and management of fetal anomalies.
4. Identify the medically reasonable alternatives (evidence-based, beneficence-based; see Chapter 1) for the management of the patient's condition and their benefits and risks.
5. The medically reasonable alternatives should be presented to the patient or the patient's surrogate in the informed decision-making process.
6. If the patient or the patient's surrogate authorizes one of the medically reasonable alternatives, it should be implemented.
7. If the patient or the patient's surrogate refuses to authorize any medically reasonable alternative, implement the process of informed refusal, as described in Chapter 3.

6.4.2 "Fast Ethics": Teaching Ethics on Rounds

On clinical rounds – "fast ethics,"[16] if you will – teachers should be alert to ethical challenges in a clinical case, especially those that have the potential to develop into ethical conflicts. The following approach has proven useful to the authors:

1. It strikes me that there is an ethical challenge in this case. Then state it as one would in Step 3 in Section 6.4.1.
2. Identify and clearly state clinically relevant concepts.
3. Ask learners to identify the implications of those concepts for the care plan.
4. Identify what should be done, who should be responsible for doing it, and a follow-up plan.

Learners should be alerted to an important limitation: the well-known time constraints on teaching on clinical rounds. Step 4 is designed to address this limitation, making follow-up especially important.

6.4.3 Preparing a Grand Rounds Presentation on Professional Ethics in Obstetrics and Gynecology

A grand rounds presentation in ethics should always begin with a focused question and objectives, followed by a concise review of the components of ethical reasoning: ethical analysis and argument. The discipline of ethical reasoning – going where the conclusions of ethical reasoning take us and nowhere else – and its analogy to the discipline of clinical reasoning – going where the evidence takes us and nowhere else – should be emphasized. This emphasis prepares learners to be open to reasoned challenges to their own clinical ethical judgments. This openness sets the stage for reasoned debate and dispassionate exploration of differences in reasoned ethical judgments. Such differences should be expected when there is ethical controversy about a topic.

If the presentation is broad in scope, the topic area should be clearly stated. The question to be addressed should be clearly stated in normative terms and well embedded in the chapters of this book and the peer-reviewed literature, e.g., When is it ethically permissible to refer one's patient to a clinical trial?

The first step in addressing the question is to present the results of one's structured review, using the critical appraisal tool described in Section 6.3.1. The search methods for papers should be described and the scoring of articles based on the steps of the critical appraisal.[2] The reasoning in the highest-scored papers should be presented, followed by the presenter's judgment of how the question should be answered. This becomes the basis for giving the appropriate weight to the highest quality papers in answering the focused question.

If the presentation is about a current or recent case, then the case should be presented and discussed following the steps of the Ethics Work-Up in Section 6.4.1. The implications for how similar cases from the past were managed should be identified, to improve patient safety and quality. These become implications for how similar cases in the future should be managed.

6.4.4 What Makes a Great Teacher of Professional Ethics in Obstetrics and Gynecology?

Gary Sutkin and colleagues describe the qualities of the excellent clinical educator and these apply to teaching professional ethics in obstetrics and gynecology.[17] The excellent teacher creates a positive learning environment. The importance of professional ethics in obstetrics and gynecology for maintaining patients' trust should be emphasized and the excellent teacher does not hesitate to express enthusiasm for this subject matter. The excellent teacher also wants all learners to succeed in mastering the basics of professional ethics in obstetrics and gynecology and signals strong approval when learners exhibit progress toward mastery of these basics.

The excellent teacher pays close attention to the pedagogical process. Successful ethical reasoning is a direct function of asking clinically pertinent questions and in the proper order. Once a clinical case has been classified, e.g., a request for nonindicated hysterectomy or refusal of cesarean delivery in a birth plan, learners should be asked: What are the clinically pertinent questions to ask? The teacher should know what the clinically pertinent questions are but remain silent. The goal is to have learners work together to formulate the clinically pertinent questions. These questions should be based on the content of chapters in this book as well as current peer-reviewed literature.

There is a tendency among learners to move quickly to answers to questions and criticism of those answers. Allowing this tendency to be actualized disrupts the discipline of ethical reasoning and therefore a sustained focus on what is important. When a learner formulates a question, the teacher should ask: Is it possible to formulate this question more precisely and clearly? Posing this question allows other learners to join in. There are often learners who are quiet and who often have a great deal to contribute. They should be asked, once a question has been formulated: What do you think? Sutkin and colleagues identify questioning skills, especially the Socratic method of building on learners' responses so that they own the intellectual and clinical results.

John Goldie and colleagues also identify the importance of the interpersonal skills of promoting participation by learners.[18] The great teachers also know that, when they ask a question, they wait for learners' answers and do not immediately jump in, a very bad pedagogical habit that discourages learner participation and therefore their progress toward mastery of the key concepts and their use in ethical reasoning in obstetrics and gynecology.

The next step is to put the clinically pertinent questions in order: Which questions need to be asked first, because the answers to the other depend on these questions being asked first? For example, if concern is raised about the patient's decision-making capacity, the first clinically pertinent question to ask becomes: Is there any clinically sound reason to question the patient's capacity to make decisions for herself? Putting questions in a proper order prevents overwhelming learners by staying focused on what is most important and also manages practical considerations of time and resources. If not all clinically pertinent questions can be addressed at the moment, the teacher should guide learners strategically by keeping the focus on the question or questions that need to be answered first and then following up in clinical case conferences.

In the course of a student clerkship or residency rotation there is time to pursue higher-order concerns, especially integrating and synthesizing key concepts and their relationship to the ethical concept of medicine as a profession, which is the basis of professional ethics in obstetrics and gynecology. One way to do this is to ask learners toward the end of a clerkship or rotation how the various ethical topics that have been addressed relate to each other, so that learners are encouraged to make meaningful connections, a crucial skill when dealing with a fresh ethical challenge in patient care. Another important skill to promote is that of argument-based critical appraisal of the normative ethics literature in obstetrics and gynecology. Learners can be assigned in teams to complete such an appraisal for a topic that has arisen repeatedly on rounds. Journal clubs can and should be used to develop the skill of argument-based critical appraisal. Themes of recurring importance in clinical teaching should be worked up for lectures and grand rounds presentations.

Excellent teachers should be role models of professional integrity and support learners when they set ethically justified limits based on professional integrity. For example, there is now strong consensus that the once common practice of conducting a pelvic examination on an anesthetized female patient without her consent is ethically impermissible.[19] This is because every female patient has an autonomy-based right to decline to allow students and residents to learn the skills of pelvic examination by examining her. Respecting this right to refuse will not adversely affect the learning experience, because paid, nonpatient volunteers, who teach and assess learners, have now become the pedagogical norm. A learner who objects to participating in pelvic examination of an anesthetized female patient on the basis of professional integrity is ethically justified in doing so and should not be penalized in any way. Indeed, maintenance of an organizational culture based on professional integrity requires review and possible sanction of faculty supervisors in such cases.

6.5 A Distinctive Challenge in Graduate Medical Education: Preventing Drift Away from Professionalism

Professionalism is one of the core competences required of all graduate medical education programs accredited by the Accreditation Council for Graduate Medical Education (ACGME)[20] and is emphasized by the American Medical Association[21] and in the Physician Charter.[22] Here we identity an unintended risk to professionalism in residency training, reduced accountability, and propose a preventive ethics approach (see Chapter 3) to the pedagogically responsible management of this risk.[23] We base our approach on the three commitments that define the ethical concept of medicine as a profession. (See Chapters 1 and 2.) We then explain how recent, positive changes in graduate medical education inadvertently can result in the risk of drift away from an organizational culture of professionalism in residency education. We then propose practical proposals for a preventive ethics response to pedagogically responsible management of this risk.[24]

6.5.1 The Commitment to the Ethical Concept of Medicine as a Profession

As explained in Chapters 1 and 2, professionalism is based on the ethical concept of medicine as a profession. Many believe that this concept originates in the Hippocratic oath and ethics texts in the Hippocratic Corpus. However, scholarship in the history of medical ethics has shown that this concept originates in the medical ethics of two eighteenth-century physician-ethicists, John Gregory (1724–1773) of Scotland and Thomas Percival (1740–1804) of England.[25-27] (See Chapter 1.) Their ethical concept of medicine as a profession requires physicians to make three commitments: to scientifically and clinically competent patient care; to the protection and promotion of the patient's health-related interests while keeping individual self-interest systematically secondary; and to the protection and promotion of the patient's health-related interests while keeping group or guild self-interest systematically secondary. Making these commitments grounds the characteristics of medical professionalism that appear in such sources as the American Medical Association Code of Medical Ethics[21] and the Physician Charter.[22]

Both Gregory and Percival presciently emphasized accountability, i.e., physicians being open to the routine critical appraisal and improvement of the processes and outcomes of patient care. Gregory called for accountability of physicians for these commitments to a panel of scientifically sophisticated laypersons.[26] Percival called for accountability of physicians and surgeons to their peers who would constitute a hospital committee charged with reviewing the processes of patient care and their outcomes and reporting these results, which were then to be used by the physicians and surgeons to improve processes and outcomes.[27] Both proposals were radical for their time and it was only in the early twentieth century that Percival's proposal for peer review was widely adopted, but separately for medical and surgical specialties in case conferences such as tumor boards. Gregory's proposal was adopted by the contemporary patient safety and quality movement that has insisted on physicians' accountability to other healthcare professionals, nurses especially, and to scientifically sophisticated non-healthcare professionals such as biostatisticians, epidemiologists, and ethicists. The resulting multidisciplinary approach to accountability for patient safety and quality, in effect, blends Gregory's and Percival's proposals. The historical origins of this approach were not appreciated by the early advocates of the patient safety and quality movement.

6.5.2 Drift Away from an Organizational Culture of Professionalism

A major legacy of Gregory and Percival is the current recognition that creating an organizational culture of accountability is essential for patient safety and quality, to which professionalism commits all physicians. An organizational culture can be defined as the mission and values of the organization, its policies and practices, its priorities (especially as implicitly expressed in operating and capital budgets), what leaders reward and discourage, what leaders tolerate, and, crucially, what leaders tolerate that should not be tolerated. An organizational culture of professionalism promotes accountability for patient safety and quality, based on the ethical concept of medicine as a profession, at every level of the organization. Failure to sustain an organizational culture of professionalism constitutes a risk to professionalism itself and therefore should not be tolerated by organizational leaders.[28]

An organizational culture of professionalism in residency training should promote accountability for patient safety and quality as an essential component of the professionalism requirement of the ACGME. The emergence of an organizational culture of reduced accountability would be antithetical to the professionalism requirement. No academic leader intends to produce such an organizational culture. However, organizational culture can incrementally drift away from professionalism when academic leaders tolerate learners' responses to changes that have been well intentioned but incentivize development of the attitudes and behaviors of reduced accountability among residents. If not appreciated for what they are, these attitudes and behaviors can be inadvertently tolerated by academic leaders and become risks to professionalism.

We conducted a literature search to determine whether this drift, which should be understood as an unintended risk to professionalism in residency education, has been previously described. Our PubMED search combined the following search items: "residents" with "decreased accountability," "accepting responsibility," "decreasing responsibility," and "accepting accountability." These same terms were then combined with "graduate medical education." One citation directly addressed the accountability of graduate medical educations for its processes and outcomes but not of residents themselves.[29] We also performed two Google searches using the combined search of "reduced accountability of residents" + "postgraduate medical education" and the sole search of "organizational culture of reduced accountability." Both searches produced no relevant results.

We concluded that a drift toward reduced accountability of individual residents or residents as a group and a concomitant unprofessional organizational culture of reduced accountability in graduate medical education has not been previously appreciated. We believe that the origins of this drift can be found in two important and positive changes in residency education and how residents might respond to them: restricted duty hours and increased residency supervision. These changes have been directed to sustaining an organizational culture of patient safety and quality. We therefore want to be clear that we support these improvements. At the same time there is an unappreciated risk in the form of attitudes and behaviors that residents adopt as they respond to these changes in ways that promote an incremental drift away from professionalism. Because it is often incremental, this drift can be difficult to detect.

6.5.2.1 Restricted Duty Hours

Restricted duty hours constitute a welcome change from unrestricted duty hours, because they aim at reducing fatigue-related errors of judgment and practice.[30] How a program interprets and implements this requirement can incentivize sustained professionalism or a drift away from it. ACGME intends for this requirement to be a "living document" and not rigid.[30] For example, a program might adopt a flexible approach that allows residents to continue the management of a patient's condition for a short period of time beyond the daily limit on hours, when this is required for the resident's learning experience. By contrast, a program might adopt a less flexible or even inflexible approach or be perceived by residents to create disincentives for a focused learning opportunity. Such perceptions can be fostered when an attending upbraids a resident for wanting to remain involved in a patient's care for a short time for educational purposes but is told to leave and not jeopardize the program's accreditation.

Left unchecked, these practices risk incremental drift away from a professional organizational culture to a bureaucratic organizational culture, in which adherence to rules and therefore "looking good" for reaccreditation become detached from the educational mission. The result is that individual and group self-interest in not getting into trouble over adherence to restricted duty hours becomes dominant, undermining the second and third commitments of the ethical concept of medicine as a profession. The commitment to scientific and clinical competence then begins to erode, as important educational opportunities are lost when residents leave at the precise end of their shift rather than continue the management of an educationally important case for a short time.

The word "shift" is crucial because this attitude is characteristic of a "shift mentality."[31] In the context of the ethical concept of medicine as a profession, a shift mentality is through-and-through self-interested. In a bureaucratic organizational culture, becoming self-interested is correctly perceived by residents, individually and as a group, as survival positive. Thus does the drift away from an organizational culture of professionalism begin in a way that is invisible to program leaders for the simple reason that incremental changes in attitudes are invisible. The behavior that manifests changed attitudes, however, is visible. A key aspect of a preventive ethics response to the drift away from a professional organizational culture is to be alert to the development of such behavior, as outlined in Section 6.6.

6.5.2.2 Supervision by Attending Physicians

Increased attending supervision is another important change, inasmuch as it is meant to enhance both patient safety and opportunities for teaching and learning. The risk of supervision is that it may impede the progressive assumption of responsibility, which is a core goal of residency education. The most troubling risk of increased supervision is that it may incentivize infantilization of residents. Because human beings do not welcome stress and because residency is already stressful, it is easier for residents to take the path of least resistance by embracing infantilization as stress reductive and survival positive while often at the same time resenting infantilization. The result is to create an organizational culture in which the individual and group self-interest in avoiding the burdens of accountability becomes a driving force that undermines the second and third commitments of the ethical concept of medicine as a profession.

6.5.2.3 Compounding Factors

The risk of slowing residents' assumption of accountability may be compounded by two factors. The first is the positive experience in some academic medical centers of reducing professional liability by increasing safety and quality through such measures as assigning a laborist to oversee all peripartum management and increasing attending involvement in patient care.[32] The effect of such a change is to diminish the role of senior-level residents in safety and quality, for which they were directly responsible in the past. This change can delay or impair residents in becoming scientifically and clinically competent to function independently, thus undermining the first component of the ethical concept of medicine as a profession.

The second factor is the effect on professional formation of a less challenging clinical and academic schedule for medical students in many medical schools. To be sure, this can make undergraduate medical education less stressful and more humane and thus more conducive to learning than it was in the past. However, there is a risk: in its worst forms, this otherwise positive change has become, in the judgment of the authors, coddling of medical students that has created a sense of entitlement rather than a sense of increasing responsibility for patient care and the increasing accountability that goes hand in hand with increasing responsibility.

6.6 A Preventive Ethics Response to Reduced Accountability

No one intends to create an organizational culture of reduced accountability in graduate medical education any more than physicians and physician leaders intend to create an unsafe and low-quality clinical environment. Intent is not the issue; impact on the organizational culture of a residency program's practices is. We have described how a residency program can drift into such a culture by tolerating risks to professionalism, which should never occur. This is because tolerating risks to professionalism in effect normalizes deviance: its most insidious form occurs when the risks of positive changes go unrecognized and therefore unmanaged. Preventive ethics comprises the skill set of recognizing the risk of incremental drift away from an organizational culture of professionalism and adopting policies and practices to prevent this risk.

6.6.1 Performing a Critical Appraisal of the Organizational Culture of the Residency

To prevent diminished accountability and its risks to successful professional formation, program directors and department chairs should first critically appraise the organizational culture of the residency from the perspective of the ethical concept of medicine as a profession. This includes, especially, identifying residents' behaviors that are not compatible with professionalism and incentives to such behaviors created by faculty behaviors. Prime among these is a rigid enforcement of restricted duty hours, especially informal enforcement, because this is the strongest incentive to residents to develop bureaucratic and shift mentalities.

The preventive ethics response to the incremental development of these attitudes is to promote a professionally responsible adherence to duty hour requirements, for example, by faculty encouraging residents to continue care of a complicated case by taking the time to educate both the current and new teams about the case and reaching an agreed upon plan for its continued management by the new team. This can be accomplished efficiently if the residency is structured to emphasize thorough, rather than perfunctory, educational hand-offs based on patient safety and quality. Program policy should emphasize professional responsibility and accountability by requiring that the original resident or resident team follow up on patients they had previously taken care of when they return to duty. For example, residents should follow all patients postpartum whom they delivered, do postoperative rounds on patients on whom they performed surgery, and care for their patients if they are readmitted with complications. These are all observable and therefore measurable pedagogical activities, permitting the faculty and program director to monitor them. The monitoring should include a judgment by the educational team about the progressive assumption of accountability for patient safety and quality and these judgments should be reviewed periodically with each resident to identify progress and areas for improvement. The medical school office of graduate medical education should support this approach to restricted duty hours. There is some evidence that some programs have implemented a flexible approach[33] and that residents adapt well to a flexible approach[34]

6.6.2 Defining Components of Professional Accountability in Milestones

It has become commonplace for the evaluation of residents to be based on milestones that, in turn, are based on the core competencies. For the professionalism core competency, the academic association for each specialty and subspecialty should define new professionalism milestones that reflect mastery of professional ethics in obstetrics and gynecology: the observable and therefore measurable intellectual and behavioral components of assumption of professional accountability for each year, culminating in demonstrable, independent assumption of professional accountability in the final year. For example, milestones related to professional attitudes should have both intellectual and behavioral components. This information should be disseminated to the residents and to all faculty and fellows with responsibility for graduate medical education. Residents should self-evaluate their progress or regress and faculty should do the same on a form designed in a pedagogically meaningful way. The review with each resident of progress in milestone achievement should incorporate these evaluations. The medical school office of graduate medical education should support this approach to the evaluation of residents.

6.6.3 Mastering the Skillset of Patient Safety and Quality

Mastering the skillset of patient safety and quality is an essential component of residency education and therefore the supervision of residents by faculty. Experienced faculty may know these components so well that they have become implicit. Some faculty supervisors then make the mistaken pedagogical assumption that residents learn this skillset by observation and osmosis. This assumption is false. To prevent this assumption from shaping the learning experience, supervisory faculty should define the components of the skillset and how they function together to produce patient safety and quality. They will then be in a position to teach the components of the skillset didactically, by demonstration and by observing and evaluating residents in their progressive development and deployment of the skillset. The goal is to inculcate the enduring, self-critical habits of professional accountability for patient safety and quality required of an independent, professional physician.

6.6.4 Enhancing the Role of ACGME

The policies and practices of ACGME have a profound effect on the organizational culture of residency training, because the accreditation process creates powerful incentives for compliance by residency program directors, faculty, and departmental chairs.[35] The accreditation process should require programs to include in their self-study a section on preventive ethics approaches to drift away from an organizational culture of professionalism, obstacles to implementing preventive ethics approaches, and progress in removing such obstacles.

References

1. McCullough LB, Coverdale JH, Chervenak FA. Argument-based ethics: a formal tool for critically appraising the normative medical ethics literature. Am J Obstet Gynecol 2004; 191: 1097–1102.
2. McCullough LB, Coverdale JH, Chervenak FA. Constructing a systematic review for argument-based clinical ethics literature: the example of concealed medications. J Med Philos 2007; 32: 65–76.
3. Oxman AD, Cook DJ, Guyatt GH. Users' guide to the medical literature. VI. How to use an overview. JAMA 1994; 272: 1367–1371.
4. Guyatt GH, Sackett DL, Cook DJ. Users' guide to the medical literature. II. How to use an article about therapy or prevention. A. Are the results of the study valid? JAMA 1993; 270: 2598–2601.
5. Guyatt GH, Sackett DL, Cook DJ. Users' guide to the medical literature. II. How to use an article about therapy or prevention. B. What were the results and will they help me in caring for my patients? JAMA 1994; 271: 59–63.
6. Wilson MC, Hayward RS, Tunis SR, Bass EB. Users' guides to the medical literature. VIII. How to use clinical practice guidelines. A. Are the recommendations valid? JAMA 1995; 274: 570–574.
7. Wilson MC, Hayward RS, Tunis SR, Bass EB. Users' guides to the medical literature. VIII. How to use clinical practice guidelines. B. What are the recommendations and will they help you in caring for your patients? JAMA 1995; 274: 1630–1632.
8. Giacomini MK, Cook DJ. Users' guides to the medical literature: XXIII. Qualitative research in health care A. Are the results of the study valid? Evidence-Based Medicine Working Group. JAMA 2000; 284: 357–362.
9. Giacomini MK, Cook DJ. Users' guides to the medical literature: XXIII. Qualitative research in health care B. What are the results and how do they help me care for my patients? Evidence-Based Medicine Working Group. JAMA 2000; 284: 478–482.
10. Drummond MF, Richardson WS, O'Brien BJ, Levine M, Heyland D. Users' guides to the medical literature. XIII. How to use an article on economic analysis of clinical practice. A. Are the results of the study valid? Evidence-Based Medicine Working Group. JAMA 1997; 277: 1552–1557.
11. O'Brien BJ, Heyland D, Richardson WS, Levine M, Drummond MF. Users' guides to the medical literature. XIII. How to use an article on economic analysis of clinical practice. B. What are the results and will they help me in caring for my patients? Evidence-Based Medicine Working Group. JAMA 1997; 277: 1802–1806.
12. Sugarman J, Sulmasy DP, eds. Methods in Medical Ethics, 2nd ed. Washington, DC: Georgetown University Press, 2010.
13. Chervenak FA, McCullough LB. What is obstetric ethics? J Perinat Med 1995; 23: 331–341.
14. Owen R. Reader bias. JAMA 1982; 247: 2533–2534.
15. Plato. Republic. In Hamilton E, Cairns H, eds. The Collected Dialogues of Plato. Princeton, NJ: Princeton University Press, 1969: 575–844.
16. Wear S. Teaching bioethics at or near the bedside. J Med Philos 2002; 27: 433–445.
17. Sutkin G, Wagner E, Harris I, Schiffer R. What makes a good clinical teacher in medicine? A review of the literature. Acad Med 2008; 83: 452–466.
18. Goldie J, Dowie A, Goldie A, Cotton P, Morrison J. What makes a good clinical student and teacher? An exploratory study. BMC Med Ed 2015; 15: 40. DOI 10.1186/s12909-015-0314-5.
19. Adashi EY. Teaching pelvic examination under anesthesia without patient consent. JAMA 2019; 321: 732–733.
20. NEJM Knowledge+ Team. Exploring the ACGME core competencies: professionalism (Part 7 of 7). Available at https://knowledgeplus.nejm.org/blog/exploring-acgme-core-competencies/ (accessed March 1, 2019).
21. American Medical Association. AMA Code of Medical Ethics. Available at www.ama-assn.org/delivering-care/ama-code-medical-ethics (accessed March 1, 2019).
22. Project of the ABIM Foundation, ACP-ASIM Foundation, European Federation of Internal Medicine. Medical professionalism in the new millennium: a physician charter. Ann Intern Med 2002; 136: 243–246.
23. Doukas DJ, McCullough LB, Wear S, Lehmann LL, Nixon LL, et al. for the Project to Rebalance and Integrate Medical Education (PRIME) Investigators. The challenge of promoting professionalism through medical ethics and humanities education. Acad Med 2013; 88: 1624–1629.
24. Chervenak FA, McCullough LB, Grünebaum A. Preventing incremental drift away from professionalism in graduate

medical education. Am J Obstet Gynecol 2018; 219: 589.e1-589.e3.

25. Chervenak FA, McCullough LB, Brent RL. The professional responsibility model of obstetrical ethics: avoiding the perils of clashing rights. Am J Obstet Gynecol. 2011; 205: 315.e1–5.

26. McCullough LB. John Gregory and the Invention of Professional Medical Ethics and the Profession of Medicine. Dordrecht, the Netherlands: Springer, 1998.

27. Percival T. Medical Ethics; or, A Code of Institutes and Precepts, adapted to the Professional Conduct of Physicians and Surgeons. London: Johnson & Bickerstaff, 1803.

28. Chervenak FA, McCullough LB. The diagnosis and management of progressive dysfunction of health care organizations. Obstet Gynecol 2005; 105: 882–887.

29. Weinstein DF. The elusive goal of accountability in graduate medical education. Acad med 2015; 90: 1188–1190.

30. Burchiel KJ, Zetterman RK, Ludmerer KM, Philibert I, Brigham TP, et al. The 2017 ACGME common work hour standards: promoting physician learning and professional development in a safe, humane environment. J Grad Med Ed 2017; 9: 692–696.

31. Van Eaton EG, Horvath KD, Pellegrini CA. Professionalism and the shift mentality: how to reconcile patient ownership with limited work hours. Arch Surg 2005; 104: 230–235.

32. Grünebaum A, Dudenhausen J, Chervenak FA, Skupski D. Reduction of cesarean delivery rates after implementation of a comprehensive patient safety program. J Perinat Med 2013; 41: 51–55.

33. Szymczak JE, Brooks JV, Volpp KG, Bosk CL. To leave or to lie? Are concerns about a shift-work mentality and eroding professionalism as a result of duty-hour rules justified? Milbank Q 2010; 88: 350–381.

34. Stroud L, Oulanova O, Szecket N, Ginsburg S. "The benefits make up for whatever is lost": altruism and accountability in a new call system. Acad Med 2012; 87: 1421–1427.

35. Accreditation Council on Graduate Medical Education. Milestones. Available at www.acgme.org/What-We-Do/Accreditation/Milestones/Overview (accessed March 1, 2019).

Section 3 Professionally Responsible Clinical Practice

Chapter 7

Prevention of Pregnancy

GOAL
This chapter provides guidance on deliberative clinical judgment and decision making about preventing pregnancy in professional ethics in gynecology.

OBJECTIVES
On completing study of this chapter, the reader will:
  Identify the biopsychosocial concept of fertility
  Describe the role of deliberative clinical judgment in decision making about prevention of pregnancy
  Describe the role of directive counseling in decision making about prevention of pregnancy
  Describe the role of assisted decision making in decision making about prevention of pregnancy
  Describe the role of pediatric assent in decision making about prevention of pregnancy
  Describe the role of surrogate decision making in decision making about prevention of pregnancy
  Identify clinical implications of the ethical principle of healthcare justice for prevention of pregnancy
  Apply guidance on deliberative clinical judgment and decision making about preventing pregnancy in professional ethics in gynecology in clinical practice

TOPICS

7.1	The Biopsychosocial Concept of Fertility	108
	7.1.1 The Role of the Biologic Concept of Sex in the Biopsychosocial Concept of Fertility	108
	7.1.2 The Biologic Concept of Fertility: A Clinical Condition with Two Meanings	108
	7.1.3 The Biopsychosocial Concept of Fertility	108
7.2	Medically Reasonable Alternatives for the Prevention of Pregnancy	109
	7.2.1 Four Groups of Methods to Prevent Pregnancy	109
7.3	Decision Making about the Management of Fertility	109
	7.3.1 Beneficence-Based Deliberative Clinical Judgment	109
	7.3.2 Autonomy-Based Clinical Judgment	109
	7.3.3 The Role of Directive Counseling	109
	7.3.4 The Role of Shared Decision Making	110
	7.3.5 Impermissible Scope of Beneficence-Based Deliberative Clinical Judgment	110
7.4	Assisted Decision Making	111
	7.4.1 Assisted Decision Making with Patients with Major Mental Disorders	111
7.5	Pediatric Assent	112
7.6	Surrogate Decision Making	112
7.7	Organizational Policy	113

Section 3: Professionally Responsible Clinical Practice

7.8 Healthcare-Justice–Based Deliberative Clinical Judgment and Advocacy — 113
   7.8.1 Access to Clinical Management of Fertility — 113
   7.8.2 Court-Ordered Clinical Management of Fertility — 113

Key Concepts

Assisted decision making
Biopsychosocial concept of health and disease
Coercion
Directive counseling
Ethical principle of beneficence in professional ethics in gynecology
Ethical principle of respect for autonomy in professional ethics in gynecology
Ethical principle of healthcare justice in professional ethics in gynecology
Fertility
Force
Manipulation
Medically reasonable alternative
Pediatric assent
Professional autonomy
Shared decision making
Surrogate decision making
Undue influence

7.1 The Biopsychosocial Concept of Fertility

7.1.1 The Role of the Biologic Concept of Sex in the Biopsychosocial Concept of Fertility

The biologic concept of sex is an essential component of the biologic concept of fertility. It is used to categorize human beings according to reproductive role: only the capacity to produce gametes, or the capacity to produce gametes and initiate a pregnancy. Sex was once thought to be dimorphic, but modern genomics of chromosomes has abandoned dimorphism for a concept of biologic sex as ranging along a continuum between these two productive roles. In other words, like all other human traits, biologic sex displays variation.

7.1.2 The Biologic Concept of Fertility: A Clinical Condition with Two Meanings

Fertility is a clinical condition, not a disease and not a disability. The biologic concept of fertility has at least two biologic meanings. One meaning of "fertility" applies to both males and females of the human species: the capacity to produce gametes capable of fusing with gametes from the other sex to become zygotes. Another meaning of "fertility" applies to females of the human species: the capacity to produce ova that can fuse with spermatozoa to become zygotes that can embed in the uterine wall and initiate pregnancy.

Gender is the psychosocial construction of biologic sex. Like biologic sex and all other human traits, gender displays variation. There is variation in gender identity as well as in sexual orientation. Given these two levels of variation, multiple relationships between biologic sex and gender occur in the human species.

7.1.3 The Biopsychosocial Concept of Fertility

The foregoing biologic meaning of "fertility" is not a clinically or ethically adequate account of the concept of fertility, because, like all human traits, the condition of fertility should also be understood as a biopsychosocial trait.[1] The biopsychosocial concept of health and disease was developed by George Engel (1913–1999) as an antidote to biomedical reductionism or the belief that attention only to the biomedical component of health and disease is scientifically and clinically adequate. This is certainly not the case for psychiatry, Engel's specialty. His remarkable contribution to the history of medicine was to show that biologic reductionism is scientifically and clinically inadequate to the concept of health and disease in all medical specialties. The psychological and social dimensions of health and disease must always be included, in order to make deliberative clinical judgments that are scientifically and clinically comprehensive and therefore scientifically and clinically adequate.

The biologic concept of fertility in its two meanings described in Section 7.1.2 requires expansion on the basis of the biopsychosocial concept of health and

Chapter 7: Prevention of Pregnancy

disease: clinical conditions such as fertility that are not diseases but have clinically significant biomedical, psychological, and social dimensions. Consider, for example, the desire, even expectation, in many extended families that one's children will have children, expressed in the frequently heard question: "When will you be giving me a grandchild?" This expectation can become very strong in faith communities that understand themselves to be commanded by God to populate the earth with his people.[2] Consider also the well-known and potentially adverse psychosocial dimensions of teenage pregnancy,[3,4] especially when it is followed by childbirth and becoming a teenage mother, the potentially serious psychosocial consequences of an unwanted pregnancy, or the very grave psychosocial consequences of pregnancy resulting from rape.

7.2 Medically Reasonable Alternatives for the Prevention of Pregnancy

As explained in Chapter 2, the first step in the decision-making process with regard to the female patient is to deploy beneficence-based deliberative clinical judgment to identify the medically reasonable alternatives for prevention of pregnancy, for a female patient who is heterosexually active or might become heterosexually active. The clinical benefits and harms that shape deliberative beneficence-based clinical judgment should be understood in terms of the biopsychosocial benefits and harms of preventing pregnancy and the probability of these outcomes.

7.2.1 Four Groups of Methods to Prevent Pregnancy

The American College of Obstetricians and Gynecologists (ACOG) has made available on its public website educational materials for patients about managing fertility, "Your Birth Control Choices."[5] ACOG identifies four groups of methods:

1. "Permanent and highly effective:" vasectomy to achieve male sterilization (>99% effectiveness) and female sterilization methods: tubal ligation and Essure® (97%–99% effectiveness)
2. "Works best," with effectiveness ranging from 94% to 99%: implantable contraception or long-acting reversible contraception (LARC), hormone intrauterine device, copper intrauterine device, and injection of Depo-Provera
3. "Works well," with effectiveness ranging from 91% to 99%: ring, patch, pill, and mini-pill
4. "Works less well," with effectiveness ranging from 58% to 98%, with variation among methods: male condom, diaphragm, female condom, withdrawal, fertility awareness, and emergency contraceptive pill

7.3 Decision Making about the Management of Fertility

7.3.1 Beneficence-Based Deliberative Clinical Judgment

The ethical principle of beneficence in professional ethics in gynecology creates the prima facie ethical obligation of the physician to provide clinical management that in deliberative clinical judgment is predicted to result in net clinical benefit for the female patient and therefore protect and promote the female patient's health-related interests. The biologic goal of the four groups of methods is to prevent pregnancy. In deliberative clinical judgment, methods that have the highest rates of effectiveness should be considered clinically superior to options that are progressively less effective in preventing pregnancy.

7.3.2 Autonomy-Based Clinical Judgment

The ethical principle of respect for autonomy in professional ethics in gynecology creates the prima facie ethical obligation of the gynecologist to empower the female patient to make informed and voluntary decisions about the management of her fertility by providing her with information about the medically reasonable alternatives for its clinical management.

7.3.3 The Role of Directive Counseling

Sometimes the biomedical component of the biopsychosocial concept of fertility becomes justifiably prominent in deliberative clinical judgment about the prevention of pregnancy. There are two such clinical circumstances.

When deliberative clinical judgment supports a reliable prediction that pregnancy will pose a high probability of pregnancy-related death of the female patient, preventing pregnancy becomes a medically reasonable alternative. This is an extremely rare

109

clinical circumstance. Unmanaged fertility in such clinical circumstances is no longer a medically reasonable alternative. When there is more than one medically reasonable form of clinical management for the female patient's condition and one is clinically superior, the gynecologist should recommend it. This means that, to minimize the risk of death from contraindicated pregnancy, the gynecologist should recommend permanent prevention of pregnancy. The options in the "permanent and highly effective" group are clinically superior to options in the second and third groups. The gynecologist should therefore recommend that the female patient consider the options in this first group.

When pregnancy is reliably predicted to create a high probability of the risk of serious, far-reaching, and irreversible pregnancy-related harm to the health of the female patient, the gynecologist should recommend a choice from among the options in the first three groups of methods. The gynecologist should recommend against the fourth group of methods because of their higher failure rates.

7.3.4 The Role of Shared Decision Making

When pregnancy is not contraindicated, the biomedical component of the biopsychosocial concept of fertility becomes co-equal with the psychosocial dimensions of preventing pregnancy. All three components – the biomedical, the psychological, and the social – must be considered. Whether to become pregnant is not a medical decision, although it has a medical component, as just described. The decision to become pregnant in such clinical circumstances is biopsychosocial. The gynecologist therefore should initiate shared decision making with the female patient: eliciting her values and beliefs related to becoming pregnant as the starting point for decision making. The goal should be to provide the female patient with the opportunity to develop a clinically comprehensive cognitive and evaluative understanding of the four groups of methods and the options within each group. (See Chapter 3.)

If the female patient expresses an interest in preventing pregnancy, subsequent decision making should be guided by the ethical principle of respect for autonomy, which creates the prima facie ethical obligation of the gynecologist to empower the patient with information about each of the four groups of methods, as just described. Effectiveness and reversibility should be explained. The "permanent" methods are most effective and potentially reversible, Essure more so than tubal ligation. The next two groups are highly effective and reversible. The fourth group is the least effective and also reversible.

Autonomy-based clinical judgment should give priority to reversible means of preventing pregnancy, to keep open the option of initiating pregnancy. This is an especially compelling consideration regarding permanent methods, because their potential for reversibility is limited.

In the deliberative clinical judgment of the gynecologist, claims about the psychosocial benefit of preventing pregnancy for a female patient with no clinical contraindications to pregnancy should have a solid evidence base. Such evidence exists for preventing the psychosocial sequelae of teenage pregnancy in straitened economic or socially chaotic circumstances[2,3] and preventing pregnancy in a female patient with major depression or other serious mental illness or disorder that has been refractory to treatment.[6-9] These potential biopsychosocial outcomes of pregnancy should be explained to patients reliably considered in deliberative clinical judgment to be at risk for them.

Sometimes claims about the psychosocial benefit to a female patient with no clinical contraindications to pregnancy lack a reliable evidence base, e.g., a clinical impression that pregnancy or parenting may go badly for a patient with mild depression. To prevent bias, the gynecologist should offer consideration of preventing pregnancy when there is reliable evidence of predicted biopsychosocial harm of unmanaged fertility but make no recommendation when the evidence is unreliable. Counseling should therefore be nondirective, with exploration of methods guided by the patient's values and beliefs.

7.3.5 Impermissible Scope of Beneficence-Based Deliberative Clinical Judgment

The scope of deliberative beneficence-based clinical judgment pertains to the patient's health-related interest and the critical appraisal of the reliability in deliberative clinical judgment of the evidence for net clinical benefit. The scope of deliberative beneficence-based clinical judgment therefore does not include reference to other interests of the female patient, for example the judgment that a female patient should not become pregnant for psychosocial reasons that lack an evidence base and are therefore at risk of bias. To make such judgments is to claim intellectual and moral authority over a patient that lacks a foundation in beneficence-based and professional-integrity–based clinical judgment and is therefore ethically impermissible.

7.4 Assisted Decision Making

Female patients with mental illnesses and disorders may exhibit impairment in the components of decision-making capacity. The gynecologist should evaluate the female patient's decision-making capacity and implement clinical management designed to reverse these impairments. This is known as assisted decision making, which is described in detail in Chapter 3. These patients can exhibit what we have characterized as chronically and variably impaired autonomy.[6–9]

An important aspect of assisted decision making for patients who exhibit chronically and variably impaired autonomy is to prevent paternalism, which is the interference with the autonomy of the female patient justified by appeal to beneficence-based clinical judgment about what the patient ought to value and authorize.[10] The gynecologist has a prima facie autonomy-based ethical obligation not to engage in paternalism for an additional reason: the claim of the gynecologist to determine for the female patient what she ought to value is not compatible with the professional virtue of integrity in professional ethics in gynecology.

7.4.1 Assisted Decision Making with Patients with Major Mental Disorders

The need for assisted decision making becomes greater when the female patient has a major mental disorder, such as bipolar disorder, a psychotic disorder, or major depression. Patients with major mental disorders are at risk of unwanted, or even forced pregnancy, maternal complications of pregnancy, and loss of children to others to raise. Patients with major mental disorders may have impairments of decision-making capacity that call into question whether assisted decision making will be challenging. This clinical reality may evoke a strong sense of frustration or even foreboding that may discourage the gynecologist from undertaking assisted decision making. A psychiatric consult could be invaluable in assessing the impairments and identifying ways to manage them. (See Chapter 3.)

This collaborative approach will help the keep the clinical focus where it belongs: maximizing the opportunity for the patient to achieve assisted decision making about prevention of pregnancy. This approach becomes a powerful antidote to two clinical ethical errors. The first is managing the challenges of assisted decision by flying a false flag of autonomy, i.e., assuming that a patient with patent impairments of decision making would not benefit from psychiatric consultation aimed at improving her decision-making capacity. The second is to assume the opposite and that the patient should be protected from herself and decision making turned over to a surrogate decision maker, a form of paternalistic thinking that thwarts assisted decision making.

Assisted decision making aims at respect for the female patient's autonomy. When assisted decision making is successful, the patient with a major mental disorder becomes able to make decisions for herself. The informed consent process should be followed. (See Chapter 3.) Given the ease of use for the female patient, LARC should be emphasized as a medically reasonable alternative. Like any other patient making decisions for herself, there is a risk that she will make decisions that increase her psychosocial risks. In beneficence-based and nonmaleficence-based deliberative clinical judgment, such risks should be considered serious but their probability cannot be reliably predicted. The maternal complications of pregnancy can be managed with reasonable safety. Raising her child herself should not be ruled out in advance, especially when psychosocial supports can be arranged before she delivers and are ready to support her when she returns home with her newborn child.

The professional virtue of self-effacement creates the prima facie ethical obligation to prevent bias in clinical judgment about the needs of patients whose mental health is compromised and whose social circumstances are challenging in ways that few gynecologists directly experience. The professional virtue of self-sacrifice complements this ethical obligation with the prima facie ethical obligation not to be influenced by one's personal responses to female patients with major mental disorders, especially the quite natural sense of foreboding that occurs when one contemplates the future of patients in fragile or chaotic social circumstances.

The long history of neglect of patients with major mental disorders includes invoking the social costs of such patients and their children and eugenics.[6–9] Both concerns lack an evidence base and therefore should not be permitted to influence clinical judgment. Gynecologists should advocate for preventing these concerns from shaping health policy. Sustained adherence to respect for autonomy in the assisted decision-making process should be deployed as an antidote to these insidious and powerful, but always unacceptable, sources of bias.

There is a distinct advantage of assisted decision making for patients who have been forced (use of psychological or physical pressure to control the patient's decision-making process) or coerced (the use of force accompanied by a threat[10]) into decisions about preventing pregnancy by family members, partners, sexual predators, or traffickers. The assisted decision-making process has the untapped potential to empower these women to gain increased control over their reproductive capacity and also to link with social service agencies that can help them escape from those who would disrespect their autonomy and degrade them as human beings.

Implementing assisted decision making for female patients with major mental disorders is undeniably time consuming. Shortage of staff and other resources, combined with the time demands, can result in patients not receiving medically reasonable clinical management of fertility. The ethical principle of healthcare justice makes this outcome ethically impermissible. Leaders of healthcare organizations and private and public payers have the healthcare-justice–based prima facie ethical obligation to see to it that compensation is based on documented time and other resource requirements and that assessment of productivity takes account of the special needs of this patient population.

7.5 Pediatric Assent

Female patients who are adolescents are sometimes functional equivalents of adults under federal and some state laws with respect to the prevention of pregnancy. Hospital policy should be explicitly based on such law and provide clear guidance to the gynecologist for how to proceed, especially when surgical sterilization is being considered. Questions about such organizational policy should be directed to organizational legal counsel.

Chapter 3 provides an account, based on ethics statements from the American Academy of Pediatrics, of the concept of pediatric assent.[11,12] This concept recognizes that, absent legal status as an adult, some adolescent female patients may not exhibit adult-like decision-making capacity. Nonetheless, they should be engaged in a developmentally appropriate way in decision making about the management of fertility. The more adult-like the adolescent female patient's developmental status, the more weight that should be given to her values, judgments, and preferences by the gynecologist and her parent(s) or guardian.

The biopsychosocial risks of teenage pregnancy and teenage motherhood, as noted in Section 7.1.3, can be serious, far-reaching, and potentially irreversible. This is especially the case when the adolescent is in an abusive relationship or a relationship with an older male, because the greater the age difference, the greater the potential for undue influence (the use of psychological pressure to reduce perception of other options as available to direct the patient to elect the preferred option of the inducer), force, or coercion to have sexual intercourse, including especially unprotected sexual intercourse. This is also especially the case for women who have been trafficked. Prevention of pregnancy and of sexually transmitted infections become urgent beneficence-based concerns in such a social context. Given the ease of use for the female patient, LARC should be emphasized as a medically reasonable alternative. The gynecologist should be especially alert to attempts by a male partner to exert undue influence, force, or coercion on her decision-making process, which can substantially reduce or eliminate voluntary decision making.

7.6 Surrogate Decision Making

As explained in Chapter 3, efforts of assisted decision making to reverse impaired components of decision-making capacity may fail. These patients need a surrogate decision maker, as designated in applicable law. Adolescents who have not been granted by law adult status will have decisions made about the clinical management of infertility made for them by their parents or guardians, acting as the child's surrogate decision makers.

As explained in Chapter 3, two standards guide surrogate decision making. The first is the substituted judgment standard: making a decision based on a reliable account of the patient's values and beliefs. Female patients with mental illnesses and disorders may retain an intact capacity to express what is important to them. Adolescent female patients may have a mature capacity to express what is important to them. To support the legally designated surrogate decision maker to meet the substituted judgment standard, the gynecologist should support effective communication of the female patient's values and beliefs to her surrogate decision maker.

Some female patients have cognitive disabilities that make them unable to engage in any of the components of decision making. For these patients the surrogate decision maker should follow the best interests standard, understood biopsychosocially. It will be very difficult for family caregivers who are legally designated surrogate decision makers not to take into account the biopsychosocial caregiving burdens on them of unmanaged fertility, especially because these female patients are vulnerable to sexual exploitation by predatory males. Setting limits on these caregiving burdens is ethically justified because doing so protects the biopsychosocial health and well-being of female patients. Surrogates should be supported in expressing limits on their caregiving capacity, reflecting on how they might be reduced with social and other supports. Making a judgment about limits is consistent with their ethical obligation to protect and promote the female patient's biopsychosocial health and well-being.

7.7 Organizational Policy

There should be a legally based and ethically justified comprehensive organizational policy to guide the gynecologist in the informed-consent, assisted-decision-making, assent, and surrogate-decision-making processes. Guidance should be as clear and detailed as possible. The policy should state clearly when legal counsel should be consulted and when a clinical ethics consultation is advisable.

7.8 Healthcare-Justice–Based Deliberative Clinical Judgment and Advocacy

As explained in Chapters 1 and 2, the ethical principle of healthcare justice in professional ethics in medicine generally and in professional ethics in obstetrics and gynecology specifically creates a prima facie ethical obligation to see to it that each patient receives medically reasonable clinical management of her condition or diagnosis. In resource-rich settings such as the United States, healthcare justice creates a prima facie ethical obligation to ensure that every woman with childbearing potential has access to contraception. Financial, religious, or other sociocultural barriers should not be permitted in health policy, because they are incompatible with professional ethics in gynecology. In resource-limited settings in which it is not possible to fulfill this ethical obligation in every case, the ethical principle of healthcare justice in professional ethics in medicine generally and in professional ethics in obstetrics and gynecology specifically creates an ethical ideal. The goal of providing access to contraception for every woman with childbearing potential should be clearly stated and pursued in incremental steps. Failure to make steady progress toward this goal should not be permitted in health policy.

7.8.1 Access to Clinical Management of Fertility

The ethical principle of healthcare justice in professional ethics in obstetrics and gynecology creates a prima facie ethical obligation to educate all women with intact fertility about techniques to manage it. In resource-limited settings, self-administered management of fertility is always a possibility. The goal of health policy and advocacy for women's health should be identifying and mitigating social, cultural, and political barriers to educating women and supporting them in self-administered management of fertility.

7.8.2 Court-Ordered Clinical Management of Fertility

Court-ordered prevention of pregnancy has occurred in response to judgments of courts that the risks to the life, health, and well-being of current children create a reliable basis to predict recurrence of such risk for future possible children.[13] Protecting the welfare of children, who are vulnerable to social circumstances over which they have no control, is one of the core responsibilities of society, acting through the instruments of self-government.

Thomas Percival (1740–1804), one of the coinventors of professional ethics in medicine (see Chapter 1), was perhaps the first to argue for the autonomy of the profession of medicine from state power.[14] For example, while Percival accepted the authority of the state to restrict abortion (at that time, before the invention of aseptic procedures, induced abortion was very dangerous and often fatal), he criticized the harsh legal penalties meted out to women. He argued that, given the very high risk of morbidity and mortality of induced abortion, no woman would be acting in her right mind to attempt or procure an induced abortion. It follows, he pointed out, that a condition for committing a crime, *mens rea* (intention to engage in wrongdoing), was not intact. Penalties therefore should be reduced.

Percival's line of reasoning applies directly to court-ordered prevention of pregnancy. Court-ordered prevention of pregnancy is biopsychosocially highly invasive. In deliberative clinical judgment and following Percival's line of reasoning, this use of state power is unnecessary in cases in which less invasive alternatives have been not used thoroughly. They have not yet been shown to fail to protect vulnerable children. Given this evidence, Percival would, justifiably, assert professional autonomy in the form of opposition to court orders of implantable, long-acting contraception. Only after all other options in the four groups of methods identified by ACOG have been tried and failed would such an invasive use of state power become worthy of consideration for compatibility with professional ethics in gynecology.

In the rare instance in which court-ordered prevention of pregnancy is not compatible with the professional ethics in gynecology, especially the professional virtue of integrity, it becomes ethically impermissible to accept the judgment of the state about what is in the health-related interests of a patient. For example, a court order issued in the absence of evidence of systematic failure of other alternatives, including LARC, should be considered an ethically impermissible violation of the autonomy of the female patient. It follows that gynecologists should refuse to implement such a court order and work with organizational leadership and legal counsel to appeal such orders. Organizational leaders should commit the organization's resources to sustained support of colleagues who take this ethically justified position.

References

1. Engel GL. The need for a new medical model: a challenge for biomedicine. Science 1977; 196: 129–136.
2. Engelhardt, H.T. Jr. The discourses of Orthodox Christian medical ethics. In Baker RB, McCullough LB, eds. Cambridge World History of Medical Ethics. New York: Cambridge University Press, 2009: 211–217.
3. American College of Obstetricians and Gynecologists. ACOG committee opinion. Condom availability for adolescents. Int J Obstet Gynecol 1995; 49: 347–351.
4. American College of Obstetricians and Gynecologists. ACOG Committee Opinion No. 392. Intrauterine device and adolescents. Obstet Gynecol 2007; 110: 1493–1495.
5. American College of Obstetricians and Gynecologists Store. Available at https://sales.acog.org/Default/aspx. (Accessed March 1, 2019)
6. Coverdale J, Chervenak FA, McCullough LB, Bayer T. Ethically justified clinically comprehensive guidelines for the management of the depressed pregnant patient. Am J Obstet Gynecol 1996; 174: 169–173.
7. Coverdale J, McCullough LB, Chervenak FA, Bayer T, Weeks S. Clinical implications of respect for autonomy in the psychiatric treatment of pregnant patients with depression. *Psychiatr Serv* 1997; 48: 209–212.
8. McCullough LB, Coverdale J, Chervenak FA. Ethical challenges of decision making with pregnant patients who have schizophrenia. Am J Obstet Gynecol 2002; 187: 696–702.
9. Coverdale J, McCullough LB, Chervenak FA. Assisted and surrogate decision making for pregnant patients who have schizophrenia. *Schizophr Bull* 2004; 30: 659–664.
10. Beauchamp TL, Childress JF. Principles of Biomedical Ethics, 7th ed. New York: Oxford University Press, 2013.
11. American Academy of Pediatrics. Committee on Bioethics. Informed consent, parental permission, and assent in pediatric practice. Pediatrics 1995; 95: 314–317.
12. Katz AL, Webb SA. Committee on Bioethics. American Academy of Pediatrics. Informed consent in decision-making in pediatric practice. Pediatrics 2016; 138: pii: e20161485.
13. Board of Trustees. American Medical Association. Requirements or incentives for the use of long-acting contraceptives. JAMA 1992; 267: 1818–1821.
14. Percival T. Medical Ethics; or, A Code of Institutes and Precepts, adapted to the Professional Conduct of Physicians and Surgeons. London: Johnson & Bickerstaff, 1803.

Chapter 8

Initiation of Pregnancy

GOAL
This chapter provides an ethical framework for decision making about initiation of pregnancy.

OBJECTIVES
On completing study of this chapter, the reader will:

Identify the meanings of "in vitro embryo" and "in vivo embryo" in reproductive medicine

Identify the ethical concept of the moral status of the embryo

Describe implications for the concept of the moral status of the embryo for embryo transfer

Describe the concept of the moral status of the embryo for preimplantation analysis

Describe implications for the concept of the moral status of the embryo for responding to requests for a high number of embryos for transfer

Describe ethically justified innovation and research in reproductive medicine

Describe ethically justified preconception counseling

Apply the ethical framework for decision making about initiation of pregnancy in clinical practice

TOPICS

8.1 Two Roles of the Obstetrician-Gynecologist in the Initiation of Pregnancy	116
8.1.1 Assisted Reproduction	116
8.1.2 Preconception Counseling	116
8.2 Precision of Thought and Speech	117
8.2.1 The In Vitro Meaning of "Embryo" in Reproductive Medicine	117
8.2.2 The In Vivo Meaning of "Embryo" in Reproductive Medicine	117
8.3 In Vitro Assisted Reproduction	117
8.3.1 The Ethical Concept of Moral Status	117
8.3.1.1 Does an Embryo Have Independent Moral Status?	117
8.3.1.2 Does an Embryo Have Dependent Moral Status?	118
8.3.1.3 How Many Embryos Should Be Transferred?	118
The Indispensable Role of Self-Regulation	118
One Embryo Should Be Transferred	119
Exceptions	119
8.3.1.4 Preimplantation Analysis of the In Vitro Embryo	119
8.3.1.5 Responding to Requests for a High Number of Embryos to Be Transferred	120
8.3.1.6 Seamless Patient Care	120
8.4 Manipulation of the In Vitro Embryo: Clinical Innovation and Research	120

8.5 Preconception Counseling 120
    8.5.1 Anticipating Moral Risk 121
    8.5.2 Counseling about Obstetric Management 121

Key Concepts

- Dependent moral status
- Ethical concept of the fetus as a patient
- Ethical principle of beneficence in professional ethics in gynecology
- Ethical principle of beneficence in professional ethics in obstetrics
- Ethical principle of respect for autonomy in professional ethics in gynecology
- Ethical principle of respect for autonomy in professional ethics in obstetrics
- Fetus as a patient
- Independent moral status
- Informed consent process
- In vitro embryo
- In vivo embryo
- Moral risk
- Moral status
- Patient
- Preventive ethics
- Privacy
- Right
- Right to privacy
- Right to reproductive privacy

8.1 Two Roles of the Obstetrician-Gynecologist in the Initiation of Pregnancy

Obstetrician-gynecologists play two important roles in the initiation of pregnancy. The first is the medically assisted initiation of pregnancy, usually to manage infertility in the female patient or her partner or both. The second is preconception counseling to anticipate and prevent ethical challenges in assisted initiation of pregnancy.

8.1.1 Assisted Reproduction

Modern assisted reproductive technology now takes many forms to assist a female patient – with her partner or alone – to become pregnant. These include the spectrum of infertility treatments, such as artificial insemination, in vitro fertilization in its various forms, and gestational carriers. These and other reproductive technologies do not aim to cure infertility but to manage its sequelae, just as other incurable, chronic conditions and diagnoses are managed in other medical specialties, such as congestive heart failure or progressive dementia. Infertility can be understood as a disease when its etiology has been reliably identified. When its etiology cannot be reliably identified, infertility can be understood as a biomedical condition that can result in the psychosocial disability of not being able to have children. By using assisted reproductive technology, the obstetrician-gynecologist provides clinical management of infertility by technologically assisting the initiation of pregnancy, hence the phrase "assisted reproductive medicine."

With the use of assisted reproductive technologies in the reproductive endocrinology and infertility (REI) laboratory embryos are created by fertilization of ova with sperm. The result is to make the human embryo directly accessible to the REI team. The in vitro embryo's general morphological condition, genetics, and genomics can be analyzed. The embryo can also be manipulated using techniques to alter its genome. The ethical concept of the moral status of embryo is an essential component of this first aspect professional ethics in reproductive medicine, a subfield of professional ethics in obstetrics and gynecology.

8.1.2 Preconception Counseling

In addition to assisting in the initiation of pregnancy directly, obstetrician-gynecologists also engage in the clinical management of fertility by providing preconception counseling for at risk and other women and their partners, including genetic and genomic analysis to reach a deliberative clinical judgment about risk assessment that the woman and her partner can incorporate into their decision-making processes. The informed consent process, especially its deployment in preventive ethics (see Chapter 3), is an essential component of this second aspect of professional ethics in reproductive medicine, a subfield of professional ethics in obstetrics and gynecology.

8.2 Precision of Thought and Speech

8.2.1 The In Vitro Meaning of "Embryo" in Reproductive Medicine

The word "embryo" has two distinct meanings in reproductive medicine. The first meaning is: "the fertilized ovum after it has begun the process of cell division"[1] in a petri dish or other vessel in a reproductive endocrinology and infertility or other laboratory. This first meaning is the in vitro definition of "embryo" and is the meaning used in in vitro fertilization.

8.2.2 The In Vivo Meaning of "Embryo" in Reproductive Medicine

The second meaning is: the biologic entity that comes into existence when the blastocyst implants in the uterine wall until the eighth week of development, after which it becomes a fetus.[2] This is the in vivo definition of "embryo" and is the meaning used in obstetrics and gynecology.

8.3 In Vitro Assisted Reproduction

Ethical challenges arise concerning in vitro assisted reproduction because technologies such as in vitro fertilization create embryos. The resulting embryos are analyzed for suitability for transfer. When this analysis is invasive of the embryo to obtain a single cell, it should be described as preimplantation analysis. (See Chapter 10.) This nomenclature should replace "preimplantation diagnosis" because genomic analysis yields more than diagnostic information, as discussed in Section 8.3.1.4. "Preimplantation diagnosis" is therefore a nomenclature that fails to prepare the female patient and her partner for the range of information that can be produced by genomic analysis. The ethical challenges of in vitro assisted reproduction arise because of the contested moral status of the embryo.

8.3.1 The Ethical Concept of Moral Status

The attribution of moral status to an entity means that others have the ethical obligation to recognize the existence of that entity and to protect its interests, i.e., its stakes in its present and future. As explained in Chapter 2, there are two kinds of moral status, independent moral status and dependent moral status.

8.3.1.1 Does an Embryo Have Independent Moral Status?

Independent moral status means that some property or properties constitutive of the entity that it has independently of all other entities originate moral status. (See Chapter 2.) In philosophical ethics a paradigm of independent moral status is known as a "person." In the history of Western metaphysics, a branch of philosophy, the ethical concept of independent moral status and therefore the ethical concept of being a person, applies only to individuals.

In Western metaphysics an entity becomes an individual if and only if it satisfies two criteria (which can be thought of as joint inclusion criteria for being an individual).[3] The first criterion is that the entity is distinct from other entities: we can pick it out separately from other entities. An in vitro embryo is distinct because it can be picked out from other embryos using microscopy, thus satisfying the first criterion for being an individual. The second criterion is indivisibility: the entity cannot divide into two entities of the same species. In embryological development this division is known as twinning. Twinning, a phenomenon with which obstetricians are already familiar, has important metaphysical implications, which we now briefly explore.

As long as the embryo retains the potential to twin, it is divisible, not indivisible, into two human beings. It follows necessarily that an embryo that can twin is not an individual and therefore cannot have independent moral status. It also follows necessarily that the ethical concept of being a person cannot apply to the embryo with the potential to twin. No in vitro embryo has independent moral status. It follows that no in vitro embryo is a person. No in vivo embryo is a person as long as that embryo has the potential to twin.

The embryo that no longer has the potential to twin is indeed an individual, because it has become indivisible. However, while it is metaphysically necessary for being a person that one is an individual, it is metaphysically insufficient for being a person, by itself, that one is an individual. One must also be an entity that self-generates the constitutive property that is the basis for independent moral status as an individual. In Western metaphysics, it is generally accepted that an entity with the constitutive property of rational self-consciousness, which is a function of highly developed sensory and nervous systems, has become a person.[4,5] Neither the in vitro embryo nor the in vivo embryo has such sensory and nervous systems. It necessarily follows that neither the in vitro embryo nor the in vivo embryo is a person.

Some Western philosophers hold that the capacity for awareness of pain establishes the basis for the independent moral status of an individual as a person. Awareness of pain is a function of highly developed sensory and nervous systems. Neither the in vitro embryo nor the in vivo embryo has such sensory and nervous systems. It necessarily follows that neither the in vitro embryo nor the in vivo embryo can be in pain. It also follows that neither has independent moral status and that neither, therefore, can be a person.

In professional ethics of obstetrics and gynecology the ethical concept of independent moral status, or being a person, has no clinical application to the in vitro embryo or in vivo embryo. This has an important implication: the ethical justification of creating and manipulating in vitro embryos does not require further engagement with the metaphysics of being an individual and being a person. There is a further advantage. The metaphysics of being an individual and being a person is distinctively Western, calling into serious question whether the ethical concept of the embryo having independent moral status is a transnational, transcultural, and transreligious concept. The ethical concept of the in vitro embryo as a person should be expunged from professional ethics in in vitro assisted reproduction in the professional ethics of obstetrics and gynecology.

8.3.1.2 Does an Embryo Have Dependent Moral Status?

The second kind of moral status is known as "dependent" moral status: an entity occupies a social role that has been created to protect all entities in that role. In Chapter 2, we explain that the fetus, when it is a patient, has dependent moral status. The obstetrician-gynecologist therefore has prima facie beneficence-based ethical obligations to protect the life and health of the fetal patient, obligations that in all cases must be balanced against prima facie beneficence-based and prima facie autonomy-based ethical obligations to the pregnant patient. The question "Does an embryo have dependent moral status?" thus becomes: "Should the in vitro embryo be considered a patient?"

As explained in Chapters 1 and 2, an individual human being becomes a patient when he or she is presented to a physician and there exist forms of clinical management that are reliably expected to protect and promote that individual's health-related interests. The in vitro embryo, as explained just above, is not an individual, although biologically it is surely human. The in vitro embryo can become a fetal patient, provided that the woman into whose uterus it will be transferred authorizes transfer, pregnancy ensues, and she confers moral status of being a patient on the previable fetus. This authorization is solely a function of the woman's informed and voluntary decision. (See Chapter 3.) It follows that the in vitro embryo therefore becomes a patient solely as a function of the pregnant woman's autonomous decision to transfer that embryo in the attempt to initiate a pregnancy. Remaining in vitro embryos that are not transferred are not patients. It is therefore permissible in professional ethics in obstetrics and gynecology to destroy unused embryos. In bioethics generally, the moral status of stored unused embryos is controversial.

8.3.1.3 How Many Embryos Should Be Transferred?
The Indispensable Role of Self-Regulation

The law of reproductive medicine in the United States is governed by a landmark US Supreme Court ruling, *Griswold v. Connecticut*, from 1965.[6] The state of Connecticut had prohibited the use of birth control by persons, including married couples. Assisting others to use birth control was also prohibited. The Court ruled that this restriction was not permissible under the Constitutional concept of privacy. Privacy means that individuals, alone or in concert with others, have a zone of protected decision making and action into which the state is not permitted to intrude in the absence of a compelling state's interest. While "compelling state's interest" is not precisely defined in the common law, it generally means that the state may exercise its police power to protect the life, health, and property of others and that privacy may give way for this police power to be exercised. The Court held that reproductive decisions made by a married couple with their physician creates no risk of such harm to others. The Connecticut law was struck down, because the state has no compelling interest in interfering with the zone of privacy between a married couple and their physician in making and implementing reproductive decisions. Subsequent rulings expanded the right to reproductive privacy to unmarried women and men in their relationship with their physician.

Griswold has had an enduring, unexpected implication: the state may not intrude into the privacy of the REI laboratory because that would be an impermissible exercise of its police powers to interfere with the right to reproductive privacy of the relationship of the female patient and her partner with their REI physician. The result is that reproductive medicine is not directly legally regulated in the United States. This means that professional self-regulation becomes a paramount ethical obligation in professional ethics in obstetrics and gynecology, in order to create and sustain efficacy and safety of embryo transfer after in vitro fertilization.

One Embryo Should Be Transferred

The in vitro embryo can become an in vivo embryo and fetal patient only with the informed consent of the woman into whose uterus it is to be transferred and who confers this dependent moral status. The ethical justification of transfer is beneficence based. Transfer should occur only when it is a medically reasonable alternative: transfer is technically possible and there exist forms of clinical management that in deliberative clinical judgment are reliably predicted to result in net clinical benefit for the pregnant, fetal, and neonatal patient. When transfer is technically possible, its efficacy is established. When transfer in deliberative clinical judgment is reliably predicted to result in net clinical benefit for the pregnant, fetal, and neonatal patient, its safety is established.

This means that it is ethically permissible to transfer an embryo or embryos if and only if there is an evidence base for the efficacy and safety of transfer. The number of embryos to be transferred should therefore be consistent with the safety of the ensuing pregnancy for the pregnant, fetal, and neonatal patient. Safety is jeopardized when three or more embryos are transferred because of the risks of mortality and morbidity for pregnant, fetal, and neonatal patients from a higher-order pregnancy. Safety is marginally decreased when two embryos are transferred. To minimize these risks, one embryo should be transferred. There are justified exceptions when the woman's condition requires more than one embryo to be transferred to achieve efficacy balanced against safety.[7–9] Whenever two or more embryos are justifiably transferred, the woman should be informed about what is known as moral risk to her: having to confront a morally challenging or unwelcome decision about feticide to reduce the risks of a multifetal pregnancy.[10] Some women may elect to avoid this risk and accept only one embryo for transfer, aware that efficacy may be reduced.

Exceptions

There may be clinical conditions that warrant the transfer of two embryos, to increase its efficacy. The relative risk to the life and health of fetal and neonatal patients in a twin pregnancy when compared to a singleton pregnancy is very small and clinically manageable. This means that, when deliberative clinical judgment supports the prediction of increased efficacy for well-defined clinical circumstances, transferring two embryos may be considered medically reasonable. Existing guidelines from such organizations as the American Society for Reproductive Medicine (ASRM),[7] the American College of Obstetricians and Gynecologists (ACOG),[8] or the European Society of Human Reproduction and Embryology[9] (ESHRE) should be followed. The informed consent process should include information about the in vitro fertilization group's outcomes, including both percent of pregnancies initiated and percent of livebirths.

8.3.1.4 Preimplantation Analysis of the In Vitro Embryo

The removal of a single cell for genetic and genomic analysis displays efficacy and safety. Such analysis can produce a range of results about the embryo: a genetic or genomic diagnosis of an embryo; risk assessment, i.e., the increased likelihood of disease in a future child; pharmacogenomic information about medication of the future child; alleles of uncertain clinical significance, i.e., not previously reported alleles in genes known or suspected to be pathogenic; and previously unreported alleles in healthy genes, the clinical significance of which is unknown.[11] These categories of results can also apply by implication to the individuals whose gametes have been used to create the embryo. These categories apply directly in "trio" testing, because tissue is obtained from analysis of genomic material from patients who have contributed the gametes used to create the embryo.

Counseling the female patient and her partner about the interpretation of results should take account of the fact that reports from genome laboratories can be cognitively demanding for the obstetrician-gynecologist and will be even more cognitively demanding for the female patient and her partner. The results should be organized into the foregoing five categories and presented in order of clinical significance for which embryo(s) are considered appropriate for transfer. The likelihood of there being no results in any of the five categories is very low, given the inherent errors of human reproduction. This should be explained, so that the woman and her partner are disabused of the search for the "perfect baby."[12] (See Chapter 13.) It should be made very clear from the outset that the decision about which embryos she considers appropriate to transfer is the woman's decision and that the gynecologist's professional judgment may differ, in which case the differences will need to be mediated. The REI laboratory should have a policy to guide such mediation that expressly states the laboratory's exclusion criteria, which should be consistent with guidance from ASRM,[7] ACOG,[8] or ESHRE.[9]

8.3.1.5 Responding to Requests for a High Number of Embryos to Be Transferred

A request from a female patient to depart from these guidelines establishes only that she has made such a request. The goal should be to transform her request into an informed decision. (See Chapter 3.) The obstetrician-gynecologist should pursue this goal by informing the female patient of the risks of high-order pregnancy and recommending that the guidelines be followed for her benefit and for the benefit of future fetal and neonatal patients. If this attempt to transform her request into an informed decision in the informed consent process fails to persuade her to withdraw her request, then the REI team should, as a matter of professional integrity, refuse the request. The REI team leader should document this process in detail.

8.3.1.6 Seamless Patient Care

The referring obstetrician has a prima facie beneficence-based ethical obligation to send a complete medical history and the results of the infertility work-up. REI teams should not be put in a position in which their plan of care is not based on sufficient clinical information about the patient. The obstetrician-gynecologist leader of the REI team has a prima facie beneficence-based and professional-integrity–based ethical obligation to the patient to ensure seamless transfer of care to the patient's obstetrician after transfer of the embryo(s). The referring obstetrician should receive a clinical report, especially detailing any complications or poor prognosis, so that her obstetrician has the clinical information that he or she needs to create an appropriate care plan with the pregnant woman.

8.4 Manipulation of the In Vitro Embryo: Clinical Innovation and Research

Because of the privacy protections of US common law explained in Section 8.3.1.3, private REI laboratories have been able to develop reproductive medicine technologies with limited accountability to governmental regulatory agencies. A major clinical ethical challenge is emerging: performing experiments that genomically manipulate the embryo in the absence of a reliable prediction about short-term and long-term outcomes in deliberative clinical judgment. This challenge will occur in the context of a history that sometimes has put advances in reproductive medicine for development on the basis of enthusiasm: the belief in clinical benefit of an advance in the absence of evidence needed to make a reliable prediction about outcomes.[13] When an experiment is performed to benefit a patient, in this case a woman who wants to initiate pregnancy, it is clinical innovation. (See Chapter 17.) When an experiment is performed to create generalizable knowledge it is clinical research. (See Chapter 17.)

As explained in Chapter 17, it is ethically impermissible to engage in clinical innovation or research without prospective review and approval. This change creates the ethical obligation of obstetrician-gynecologists specialized in REI to support and implement a system of peer-reviewed accountability for clinical innovation and research in in vitro assisted reproduction as an essential component of self-regulation. This accountability includes documented adherence to the ethically justified criteria for innovation and early-phase clinical research and for randomized clinical trials that are presented in Chapter 17. REI physicians should be alert to and implement ethics statements from ASRM and other relevant professional associations intended to promote integrity-based clinical innovation and research.

8.5 Preconception Counseling

The obstetrician-gynecologist also assists reproduction by means of preconception counseling. This counseling should be understood and undertaken as using the informed consent process as a preventive ethics tool, to prepare the female patient for consideration of initiating a pregnancy using assisted reproductive technology. The female patient and her partner should be provided with information about the medically reasonable alternatives for the management of infertility and the clinical benefits and risks of each medically reasonable alternative for the pregnant, fetal, and neonatal patient.

8.5.1 Anticipating Moral Risk

In Chapter 13 we describe the information that should be provided to every woman who becomes pregnant. The same information should be provided to a woman contemplating clinical use of assisted reproductive technology. Following accepted guidelines, should more than one embryo be transferred, the obstetrician-gynecologist should explain that the option of feticide to achieve a singleton pregnancy may be offered. For women who have a conscience-based moral objection to feticide, this may be experienced as unwelcome or worse. This is known as taking moral risk for the patient in decision making.[10] The obstetrician-gynecologist should reach agreement with the woman in advance on the parameters of clinical management of a multifetal pregnancy that are acceptable to the woman. If she becomes pregnant with multiple fetuses, this agreement should be reviewed early in her pregnancy, revised per the pregnant patient's preferences, and implemented.

Subsequent decision making about the disposition of her pregnancy should focus on empowering the woman with clinical information that is salient to her decision-making process. This information should be presented free of bias. It is ethically impermissible to limit information based on the obstetrician's personal beliefs or applicable law. It is also ethically impermissible to make any recommendation of any kind, especially one based on the obstetrician's personal beliefs. Counseling therefore should be strictly nondirective. A shared decision-making process should be adopted and driven by the patient's informational needs, values, and beliefs. She should be encouraged to draw on her social supports as she deems valuable. She should be supported in her decision about whom to involve and assured that the professional virtue of confidentiality will be adhered to and as required by law.

8.5.2 Counseling about Obstetric Management

Every pregnant patient should also be informed that a normal, low-risk pregnancy can become high-risk quickly and without warning, especially during the intrapartum period. A pregnant woman with a multifetal pregnancy should be informed about the risks of prematurity in counseling that should involve a neonatologist. During such perinatal counseling, as explained in Chapter 2, the obstetrician-gynecologist should think like a pediatrician when counseling about neonatal outcomes. This means basing deliberative clinical judgment about resuscitation and admission to the neonatal intensive care unit on the best interests of the child standard in professional ethics in pediatrics. Chapter 11 provides guidance about the professionally responsible management of periviability. Chapter 12 provides guidance about intrapartum management. Chapter 15 provides guidance on setting professionally responsible limits on life-sustaining treatment.

References

1. Society for Assisted Reproductive Technology. Embryo. In "Topics." Available at www.sart.org/topics/topics-index/embryo/ (accessed March 1, 2019).
2. American College of Obstetrics and Gynecology. How your fetus grows during pregnancy. Frequently Asked Questions. 156 Pregnancy. Available at www.acog.org/-/media/For-Patients/faq156.pdf?dmc=1&ts=20180615T1523286650 (accessed March 1, 2019).
3. Gracia JE. Introduction to the Problem of Individuation in the Early Middle Ages, 2nd ed. Munich: Philosophia Verlag, 1988.
4. Engelhardt HT, Jr. The Foundations of Bioethics, 2nd ed. New York: Oxford University Press, 1995.
5. Beauchamp TL, Childress JF. Principles of Biomedical Ethics, 7th ed. New York: Oxford University Press, 2013.
6. *Griswold v. Connecticut* 381 U.S. 479 (1965).
7. Practice Committee of the American Society for Reproductive Medicine. Performing the embryo transfer: a guideline. Fertil Steril 2017; 107: 882–896.
8. American College of Obstetricians and Gynecologists, Society for Maternal-Fetal Medicine. ACOG Practice Bulletin No. 144: Multifetal gestation: twin, triplet, and higher-order multifetal pregnancies. Obstet Gynecol 2014; 123: 1118–1132.
9. European Society of Human Reproduction and Embryology. ESHRE Revised Guidelines for Good Practice in IVF Laboratories. Available at file:///C:/Users/mccullou/Documents/Downloads/ESHRE_IVF_labs_guideline_15122015_FINAL.pdf (accessed March 1, 2019).

10. Faden RR, Becker C, Lewis C, Freeman J, et al. Disclosure of information to patients in medical care. Med Care 1981; 19: 718–733.
11. McCullough LB, Brothers KB, Chung WK, Joffe S, Koenig BA, Wilfond B, Yu JH. Clinical Sequencing Exploratory Research (CSER) Consortium Pediatrics Working Group. Professionally responsible disclosure of genome sequencing results in pediatric practice. Pediatrics 2015; 136: e974–982.
12. Chervenak FA, McCullough LB, Brent RL. The perils of the imperfect expectation of the perfect baby. Am J Obstet Gynecol 2010; 203: 101.e1–5.
13. Chervenak FA, McCullough LB. Preventing enthusiasm in response to clinical advances. BJOG 2019; 126: 890.

Chapter 9

Induced Abortion and Feticide

GOAL
This chapter provides an ethical framework for offering, recommending, performing, and referring for induced abortion and feticide.

OBJECTIVES
On completing study of this chapter, the reader will:
    Identify an ethical framework for offering induced abortion and feticide
    Identify an ethical framework for recommending induced abortion and feticide
    Identify an ethical framework for performing induced abortion and feticide
    Identify an ethical framework for referring induced abortion and feticide
    Describe ethically justified decision making with, by, and for patients with depression and psychoses
    Describe an ethically justified role of conscientious objection to induced abortion and feticide
    Apply the ethical framework for offering, recommending, performing, and referring for induced abortion and feticide in clinical practice

TOPICS

9.1 Ethical Challenges of Counseling Pregnant Women about Induced Abortion and Feticide	124
9.2 Precision of Thought and Speech	124
9.3 Induced Abortion and Feticide before Viability in Professional Ethics of Obstetrics	125
9.4 Offering Induced Abortion and Feticide	125
9.4.1 After Viability	125
9.4.2 Before Viability: Beneficence-Based Justifications	126
9.4.2.1 When Pregnancy Poses a Threat to the Health or Life of the Pregnant Patient	126
9.4.2.2 When Pregnancy Poses a Threat to the Life or Health of the Coexistent Fetus(es)	126
9.4.3 Before Viability: Autonomy-Based Justifications	126
9.5 Recommending Induced Abortion or Feticide	127
9.5.1 Risk to the Health or Life of the Pregnant Woman	127
9.5.2 Increased Risk to the Health or Life of the Fetus(es)	127
9.5.3 Diagnosis of a Serious Fetal Anomaly	128
9.5.4 Complications that Threaten the Health or Life of the Pregnant Woman and Fetal Salvage Is Hopeless	128
9.5.5 Ethical Justifications	128
9.6 Decision Making With, By, and For Patients with Depression and Psychoses	128
9.7 Conscientious Objection to Offering or Recommending Induced Abortion or Feticide	129
9.8 Performing Induced Abortion and Feticide	129

Section 3: Professionally Responsible Clinical Practice

9.9 Invoking Conscientious Objection to Performing Induced Abortion or Feticide	130
9.10 Confidentiality	131
9.11 Referring for Induced Abortion and Feticide	131
9.11.1 Direct Referral	131
9.11.2 Indirect Referral	131

Key Concepts

Assisted decision making
Best interests standard of surrogate decision making
Chronically and variably impaired autonomy
Confidentiality
Conscientious objection
Direct referral
Ethical principle of beneficence in professional ethics in gynecology
Ethical principle of beneficence in professional ethics in obstetrics
Ethical principle of nonmaleficence in professional ethics in obstetrics and gynecology
Ethical principle of respect for autonomy in professional ethics in gynecology
Ethical principle of respect for autonomy in professional ethics in obstetrics
Feticide
Indirect referral
Induced abortion
Severe fetal anomaly
Substituted judgment standard of surrogate decision making
Surrogate decision making
Termination of pregnancy

9.1 Ethical Challenges of Counseling Pregnant Women about Induced Abortion and Feticide

Counseling pregnant women about induced abortion and feticide presents the obstetrician with a distinct set of challenges.[1,2] The American Medical Association[3] and the American College of Obstetricians and Gynecologists[4] have provided general guidance. Based on the ethical principles of beneficence and respect for autonomy in professional ethics in obstetrics and gynecology (see Chapter 2), this chapter provides practical, clinically comprehensive ethical guidance on when to offer, recommend, perform, and refer for abortion and feticide.

9.2 Precision of Thought and Speech

"Abortion" and "feticide" are often used without precision. Failure to be clear about their precise meanings violates the requirement of clarity in ethical analysis, the first step in ethical reasoning. (See Chapter 1.) "Abortion" and "feticide" have precise, descriptive, medical meanings that are independent of their ethical significance.

According to Stedman's Medical Dictionary, abortion is the "[e]xpulsion from the uterus of an embryo or fetus before viability."[5] Abortion can occur spontaneously or be induced. Induced abortion, because it occurs before viability, will result in the death of the embryo(s) or fetus(es). Feticide is defined as the "[d]estruction of the embryo or fetus in the uterus"[5] independently of gestational age and is not dependent on whether the uterus is emptied. Feticide can be performed by such means as intracardiac injection of potassium chloride or ligation of the umbilical cord.[5]

"Multifetal pregnancy reduction" is the use of feticide to cause the death of fetus(es), which typically remains in the ongoing pregnancy.[6] The more precise terminology is "selective feticide," because of the vagueness of the word "reduction," especially for pregnant patients and those involved with them in their decision making. (See Chapter 3.) Termination of pregnancy is the "[i]nduced ending of a pregnancy"[3] or ending of gestation, independently of gestational age, and is not dependent on whether survival occurs. In light of this definition, "selective termination" can be confusing and should not be used, because selective feticide does not end the pregnancy of the surviving fetus(es). In this book, we use "induced abortion" rather than simply "abortion" to be precise that spontaneous abortion is not included. We use "feticide" with the foregoing descriptive meaning. We emphasize that "induced abortion" and "feticide" are value-neutral, medical terms. The use of these terms therefore does not entail ethical judgments about their ethical permissibility or impermissibility.

9.3 Induced Abortion and Feticide before Viability in Professional Ethics of Obstetrics

As explained in Chapter 2, in professional ethics in obstetrics the previable fetus is a patient if and only if the pregnant woman confers this moral status on her fetus. Whether the fetus has properties that generate independent moral status (moral status originating in intrinsic properties of the fetus) or has dependent moral status from another source (moral status conferred on the fetus, e.g., in a faith community) is an ethical controversy with a millennia-long history. It is plain from this history that this controversy has persisted – and will continue to do so – because there is no single philosophical or theological methodology or authority that all must accept as the basis for its resolution. It follows that the pregnant woman is free to confer, withhold, or having once conferred withdraw the dependent moral status of being a patient on the basis of her values and beliefs. There is no single authoritative perspective that all must accept as an ethically justified constraint on this exercise of her autonomy. The pregnant woman is therefore free to decide for herself whether a particular perspective on the morality of induced abortion and feticide before viability has moral authority for her. Her obstetrician, partner, family, society, and the state have an autonomy-based ethical obligation to respect her decision making in this matter by not interfering with it.

Induced abortion and feticide before viability cause the death of the fetus. Induced abortion and feticide before viability are ethically permissible in professional ethics in obstetrics when the pregnant woman does not confer the moral status of being a patient on her fetus, because induced abortion and feticide before viability do not cause the death of a fetal patient. Induced abortion and feticide before viability are therefore ethically permissible in professional ethics in obstetrics.

9.4 Offering Induced Abortion and Feticide

There is no general beneficence-based or autonomy-based ethical obligation to offer every pregnant patient an induced abortion. Instead, there are specific clinical circumstances in which offering an induced abortion or feticide becomes ethically obligatory, with distinct beneficence-based autonomy-based justifications.

9.4.1 After Viability

After viability, there is a beneficence-based prohibition against feticide of viable fetuses grounded in the prima facie beneficence-based ethical obligation to protect the life and health of the fetal patient. (See Chapters 9 and 11.) As a consequence, both the obstetrician and the pregnant woman have beneficence-based obligations to protect the health and life of the viable fetal patient. It follows that it is ethically impermissible to offer feticide for viable fetuses, including fetuses with either severe anomalies or less-than-severe anomalies, such as Down syndrome or achondroplasia. Less-than-severe anomalies do not involve a high probability of death or a high probability of the absence or virtual absence of cognitive developmental capacity.[7,8]

When a serious fetal anomaly has been diagnosed in a viable fetus, induction of labor and nonaggressive obstetric management (no fetal monitoring, all indications for intervention are maternal) are ethically permissible. "Serious fetal anomaly" means that there is a certain or near certain diagnosis of an anomaly that is reliably expected either to result in death, even with aggressive obstetric and neonatal intervention, or short-term survival with severe and irreversible deficit of cognitive developmental capacity.[7,8]

Live-born infants with a certain or near certain diagnosis of an anomaly that is reliably expected to result in death, even with aggressive obstetric and neonatal intervention, are born with a terminal condition as defined in applicable advance directive law. The concepts of physiologic futility or imminent demise futility also apply. (See Chapter 15.) Live-born infants with a certain or near certain diagnosis of an anomaly that is reliably expected to result in short-term survival with severe and irreversible deficit of cognitive developmental capacity are born with an irreversible condition as defined in applicable advance directive law. The concepts of imminent demise futility or interactive capacity also apply. (See Chapter 15.) In both clinical circumstances, the limits of the prima facie beneficence-based ethical obligation to provide aggressive obstetric and neonatal management have therefore been reached, making it ethically permissible to allow such fetal and neonatal patients to die. Induction of labor does not introduce risk of mortality; the severe anomaly has already done so. Feticide followed by induction of labor for viable fetuses is not clinically necessary. It is ethically permissible in such cases to forego aggressive obstetric and neonatal clinical management and to provide palliative and hospice care for live-born infants.

9.4.2 Before Viability: Beneficence-Based Justifications

There are two beneficence-based justifications that make offering induced abortion or feticide before viability ethically obligatory.

9.4.2.1 When Pregnancy Poses a Threat to the Health or Life of the Pregnant Patient

The first is based on a deliberative clinical judgment that continued pregnancy poses a threat to the health or life of the pregnant patient. Preexisting conditions, such as severe cardiac disease or some forms of cancer, can pose such threats.[9] (See Chapter 14.) When the best available evidence supports the clinical judgment that continued pregnancy poses a risk to the pregnant woman's health or life, she should be informed about this clinical reality and offered the alternative of induced abortion.

It is important to appreciate that this beneficence-based justification will evolve over time as new evidence accumulates about the risks of pregnancy from preexisting conditions or the complications of pregnancy. Some women, because of moral convictions about the general moral status of the fetus, will refuse this offer. They should be informed that their refusal increases the risk that their health could be severely compromised and that they could die. The final decision to remain pregnant or to elect induced abortion is ultimately a function of the pregnant woman's autonomy because the obstetrician's clinical expertise does not extend to the question of whether one should remain pregnant in such clinical circumstances. The importance of her pregnancy and how to weigh this value against the value of reducing her risks of morbidity and mortality are personal judgments that each pregnant patient must make for herself. Her decision should therefore be respected by her obstetrician.

9.4.2.2 When Pregnancy Poses a Threat to the Life or Health of the Coexistent Fetus(es)

The second beneficence-based justification for offering feticide before viability is based on deliberative clinical judgment that continued pregnancy poses a threat to the life or health of the coexistent fetus(es), such as in the case of a higher-order pregnancy or twin pregnancy in which the continued existence of an anomalous fetus poses a threat to the health or life of the co-twin. Current evidence supports the deliberative clinical judgment that these risks can be reduced by selective feticide.[6] When the best available evidence supports the clinical judgment that continued multifetal, previable pregnancy poses a risk to the health or life of the other fetus(es), the pregnant woman should be informed about this clinical reality and offered the alternatives of selective feticide and induced abortion. Some women, because of moral convictions about the general moral status of the fetus, will refuse this offer. They should be informed that their refusal increases the risk that the pregnancy could end before viability without any surviving fetuses or end prematurely after viability, with increased risk of infant mortality and morbidity from premature delivery. The final decision to remain pregnant, to elect induced abortion, or to elect selective feticide is ultimately a function of the pregnant woman's autonomy and should be respected by her obstetrician.

9.4.3 Before Viability: Autonomy-Based Justifications

When the best available evidence supports the deliberative clinical judgment that a continued previable pregnancy does not pose an increased risk to the health or life of the pregnant woman or fetuses, the only remaining justification for offering induced abortion or feticide is autonomy based. There are six clinical circumstances in which induced abortion should be offered to empower the pregnant woman's decision making about the disposition of her pregnancy. First, in all cases of rape and incest induced abortion should be offered so that the pregnant patient becomes aware that she has the right to decide whether to end her pregnancy. Second, some pregnant women will request an induced abortion. Third, a previable pregnancy will be diagnosed with an anomaly, e.g., by ultrasound. Fourth, a complication occurs that threatens the successful continuation of a previable pregnancy, such as preterm premature rupture of membranes. Fifth, a complication may be present during pregnancy that jeopardizes maternal health or life, such as cancer or severe eclampsia. Sixth, some pregnant women will directly, and sometimes indirectly, express concern about remaining pregnant or will be concerned about multiple births and prefer for economic or other personal reasons to have a singleton pregnancy. Obstetricians should respond to women in the first five groups by discussing the option of induced abortion and, when appropriate, explaining time limitations. Obstetricians should respond to women in the sixth group by discussing the options of induced abortion or selective feticide for multiple pregnancies and, when appropriate, explaining time limitations.

In response to the offer of induced abortion, obstetricians should expect pregnant women to sort themselves into three subgroups.[10] Some will want to continue the pregnancy because they decide to accept any child who results, regardless of health status. Some will not want to remain pregnant and will elect induced abortion. Some will be uncertain about whether to continue the pregnancy. Respecting the autonomy of pregnant women means that obstetricians should respect this self-sorting, by limiting their role to providing information in a nondirective fashion (offering but not recommending induced abortion) that these women can use to resolve their uncertainty. Nondirective counseling, or shared decision making, is required because the decision to remain pregnant, although it has a medical component, is a psychosocial decision to be made on the basis of the values and beliefs of each individual woman. Attempting to bias a woman's decision assumes, falsely, that physicians have the professional competence to decide for a woman with a previable pregnancy that she should or should not remain pregnant. Commitment to the ethical concept of medicine as a profession does not create such competence, which only the pregnant woman therefore possesses.

Nondirective counseling should guide obstetricians in discussing induced abortion with women with previable pregnancies who remain uncertain. "Nondirective counseling" means that obstetricians should refrain from making, suggesting, or implying a recommendation about continuation or termination of a previable pregnancy, which is a defining feature of shared decision making. (See Chapter 3.) Directive counseling toward continuation of a previable pregnancy based on the alleged benefit to the pregnant woman of providing information about fetal development or showing images of fetal development, or to prevent remorse or regret, lacks an evidence base. Such directive counseling, even when required by law, is inconsistent with respect for the pregnant woman's autonomy. Such directive counseling is therefore an ethically impermissible distortion of the obstetrician's professional role in the informed consent process. All women should be informed that their decision making about termination is time limited, given the legal availability of induced abortion in the applicable jurisdiction. In addition, to respect autonomy, the obstetrician should provide frank, evidence-based information about maternal or fetal conditions, even if doing so is emotionally distressing. Obstetricians need to make the time available for the sometimes extensive and iterative discussions required to disclose the medical facts and assist the woman to assimilate those medical facts into her decision-making process.

9.5 Recommending Induced Abortion or Feticide

There are four clinical circumstances in which recommendations of induced abortion or feticide might be considered.

9.5.1 Risk to the Health or Life of the Pregnant Woman

The first is in a situation in which a maternal condition, or treatment of such a condition, results in increased risk to the pregnant woman's health or life should she continue her pregnancy.

9.5.2 Increased Risk to the Health or Life of the Fetus(es)

The second is in a situation in which continued pregnancy without induced abortion or feticide substantially increases the risk to the health or life of the other fetus(es).

9.5.3 Diagnosis of a Serious Fetal Anomaly

The third is for feticide as a component of termination of pregnancy when a serious fetal anomaly has been diagnosed.

9.5.4 Complications that Threaten the Health or Life of the Pregnant Woman and Fetal Salvage Is Hopeless

The fourth occurs in complications that threaten the woman's health or life and salvage of the fetus is clinically hopeless. Recommendations are not ethically justified for the first three, which are paradigm clinical circumstances for which shared decision making should be used. For the fourth, a recommendation for induced abortion or feticide followed by induction of labor should be made.

9.5.5 Ethical Justifications

The first and second categories can be addressed together. The first requires balancing the life and health of the pregnant woman against the health and life of the fetal patient in rare cases, such as some forms of cancer[9] or mirror syndrome. The second category requires balancing the life and health of multiple fetal patients. These judgments, at first, appear to be purely beneficence based, and therefore within the scope of the obstetrician's professional competence to make recommendations, but on closer examination they are not. This is because these judgments involve deciding which health or life is more important. This judgment is ultimately not beneficence based but autonomy based, appealing to the cultural, religious, and other individual beliefs of the pregnant woman. Respecting the pregnant woman's autonomy means that the physician should be nondirective and not seek to bias the woman's decision-making process, e.g., by "soft pedaling" the benefits or overemphasizing the risks of continued pregnancy. No recommendation of induced abortion or feticide is permitted when the woman is undecided about how to balance her and the fetal patient's interests. Individual conscience is not implicated because physicians are not responsible for or complicit in the ultimate balancing judgments that pregnant women will make in these tragic circumstances after they been informed about them by their physician. Conscientious objection is therefore ethically impermissible. (See Chapter 5.)

Third, given the nature of severe fetal anomalies, one might think that recommendation of induced abortion or feticide would be justified, e.g., for anencephaly or trisomy 13. Women with serious moral convictions about the moral status of the fetus, especially women with religious convictions about the sanctity of fetal life, may experience a recommendation of induced abortion or feticide as profoundly disrespectful of their autonomy. They may also experience moral distress when offered this alternative. However, offering an alternative, although distressful, is not profoundly disrespectful of the conscience and convictions of such pregnant women and is, therefore, ethically permissible.

The fourth category is straightforward in beneficence-based clinical judgment. For complications such as preterm premature rupture of membranes with chorioamnionitis, the fetal condition is hopeless clinically and the woman's health, and perhaps life, is in danger. There is, therefore, no beneficence-based obligation to the fetus, and there is a strong beneficence-based obligation to the pregnant woman to protect her health or life, which makes a recommendation for induced abortion ethically obligatory.

9.6 Decision Making With, By, and For Patients with Depression and Psychoses

In Chapter 3 we explained the concept of assisted decision making and its clinical application, especially with regard to patients with mental illnesses and disorders. The clinical application of assisted decision making during pregnancy must take account of the maternal risks of untreated depression and psychosis. Over time, depression may result in chronically and variably impaired autonomy that can in different ways influence all of the steps of decision making described in Chapter 3.[11-14] In particular, a sense of worthlessness or hopelessness resulting from depression may impair the patient's evaluative understanding. Psychosis can impair cognitive understanding as well. These impairments may adversely influence the patient to want termination of pregnancy. Instead of acceding to this request, the obstetrician should implement assisted decision making, with psychiatric consultation as necessary. The goal should be to mitigate the effects of depression, so that the patient can achieve the minimum threshold for each step of decision making and so that a paternalistic response can be prevented. The obstetrician should not assume that depression automatically means that the patient is irreversibly impaired in her decision-making capacity, because in almost all cases patients with depression can succeed at assisted decision making. When they do, the nondirective approach described earlier should be used. To set the stage for assisted decision, one of us (JHC) in his practice asks the patient what her thoughts might have been, absent her depression.

Patients with psychoses present more complex challenges. They may be able to succeed at assisted decision making, in which case nondirective counseling should proceed. A major difference from depression is that patients with psychoses will fail to do so more often. For example, a pregnant patient who denied the very existence of her pregnancy is not able to participate in decision making. When this is the case, the legally designated surrogate should become involved. To achieve the substituted judgment of surrogate decision making, the patient should be asked what is important for her about her pregnancy and about becoming a mother. The obstetrician and surrogate decision maker should aim to elicit the patient's long-standing values and beliefs, so that the surrogate decision maker should base his or her decision making on them. This approach should aim for a decision made *with* and *for* the patient *by* the surrogate decision maker.

Sometimes, this effort to meet the substituted judgment standard will not be successful. The best interests standard should then be implemented by the obstetrician. We emphasize that the best interests standard does not automatically support termination of pregnancy, because the outcomes of pregnancy for pregnant, fetal, and neonatal patients when the pregnant patient has psychosis are not uniformly or predictably adverse. Decision making based on the best interests standard can be dauntingly complex. The antidote is a thorough decision making process by a multidisciplinary team, including social work, chaplaincy, nursing, and ethics consultation. The professional virtues of self-effacement and self-sacrifice create a prima facie ethical obligation of the team to manage their understandable sense of foreboding when working with the surrogate to reach a considered judgment about the implications of the best interests standard for the continuation of pregnancy.

A comprehensive biopsychosocial assessment of the patient and her social circumstances and supports is essential. When these can be effectively organized to support her throughout the remainder of her pregnancy, continuation of her pregnancy may be in her best interests. The judgment that continuation of her pregnancy may not be in her best interests should be approached with great caution, to prevent bias. In all such cases, the obstetrician and psychiatrist should follow organizational policy about termination of pregnancy for this patient population. Such policy should place the burden of proof on the clinical ethical judgment that termination of pregnancy is in the patient's interest.

9.7 Conscientious Objection to Offering or Recommending Induced Abortion or Feticide

Conscientious objection to offering induced abortion or feticide when justified in professional ethics in obstetrics and gynecology is not ethically permissible. (See Chapter 5.) Individual conscience, i.e., the values and beliefs of an obstetrician that arise from sources outside the ethical concept of medicine as a profession, such as upbringing or religion, does not justifiably place limits on the ethics of offering induced abortion or feticide when the aforementioned ethical justifications apply. There are two reasons why this is the case.

The first is that every obstetrician's autonomy-based prima facie ethical obligation to provide information in the informed consent process to empower a pregnant woman's decision making is a matter of professional ethics in obstetrics, not individual conscience. (See Chapter 3.) Second, one cannot predict how women will sort themselves in response to offering induced abortion or feticide. Subsequent decisions are a function ultimately of the pregnant woman's autonomy. It is, therefore, a mistake to think that offering induced abortion or feticide makes the obstetrician somehow responsible for or complicit in the informed, deliberative, and voluntary decisions of a pregnant patient that may not be consistent with the obstetrician's individual conscience. The obstetrician does not control the pregnant woman's decision-making process; she controls it.[15]

9.8 Performing Induced Abortion and Feticide

There are two ethical issues concerning performing induced abortion or feticide. The first concerns the method of terminating the pregnancy. The second concerns whether conscientious objection places ethically justified barriers on an individual obstetrician's performing induced abortion or feticide.

Before viability, it is ethically permissible in the professional ethics of obstetrics and gynecology, and therefore in professional conscience, to perform an induced abortion. As explained in Chapter 2, the pregnant woman is free to withhold or withdraw the moral status of being a patient from the previable fetus at her discretion. Induced abortion of the previable fetus in such circumstances, therefore, does not involve the killing of a patient and is permissible in professional ethics of obstetrics. For the same reason, performing feticide in a previable pregnancy is ethically permissible in professional ethics in obstetrics.

Pregnant women should not be presumed to understand that expelling the near-viable fetus with a severe anomaly from the uterus could result in a live birth and that feticide can prevent this outcome. In such circumstances, live birth creates an increased risk of preventable neonatal morbidity with no offsetting benefit. There is therefore a beneficence-based obligation of the obstetrician and the pregnant woman to prevent this risk. Refusal of feticide can also be seen as contradictory because election of termination of pregnancy means that the pregnant woman does not wish to have a child from her current pregnancy. Such contradictory thinking may be evidence of confusion on the woman's part or significant impairment of her capacity for autonomous decision making. In such a setting, it is reasonable for the obstetrician to require that the pregnant woman accept feticide as a condition for performing termination of her pregnancy. Performing feticide in this setting also exonerates the physician from being accused of performing a so-called "partial-birth abortion." This is a phrase with no clinical meaning and therefore should not be used by obstetricians. The correct account is that the physician is evacuating the uterus after ethically justified iatrogenic fetal demise.

9.9 Invoking Conscientious Objection to Performing Induced Abortion or Feticide

Some obstetricians may invoke conscientious objection, based on judgments of individual conscience, that prohibit participation in induced abortion or feticide. Respecting individual conscience means that such obstetricians should be free to refuse to perform induced abortion or feticide. This has the important implication that a requirement of residents or fellows to participate in induced abortion or feticide is ethically impermissible.[16] However, as explained in Section 9.7, there is no ethically justified conscience-based objection to participation in the decision-making processes described earlier. Residency programs are therefore ethically justified to require that trainees have an appropriate fund of knowledge about these procedures and an appropriate fund of knowledge and clinical skills in managing their complications. (See Chapter 5.)

Obstetricians with individual-conscience-based objections to induced abortion or feticide must keep in mind, when they refuse to perform the procedure, that individual conscience does *not* govern the obstetrician's professional role. It is, therefore, impermissible for the obstetrician, on the basis of individual conscience, to express judgments about the morality of a woman's election of induced abortion or feticide, or of colleagues who perform these procedures, because doing so is inconsistent with nondirective counseling regarding induced abortion before viability.

The obligation of a community to ensure access to termination of pregnancy services involves complex and controversial appeals to healthcare justice as the basis for health policy. While it could be argued that every community has such a social-justice–based obligation, healthcare justice creates prima facie ethical obligations that, because they are prima facie and not absolute, can be justifiably limited by the individual conscience of the obstetrician but only when the result of doing so is that no pregnant women loses access to termination of pregnancy services. Respect for individual conscience, therefore, creates a controlling ethical obligation not to mandate violations of individual conscience as a matter of heath policy. An important exception is termination of pregnancy for maternal indications in a medical emergency, such as obstetric hemorrhage or severe intrauterine infection, conditions for which there is no time to transfer the care of the pregnant woman to another physician or facility. It is ethically impermissible to invoke conscientious objection in such circumstances, because protecting the life and health of patients in medical emergencies is a paramount beneficence-based and nonmaleficence-based ethical obligation in professional ethics in obstetrics and gynecology.

9.10 Confidentiality

Pregnant patients who elect induced abortion or feticide should be assured that ethical and legal obligations of confidentiality will be fulfilled: Others will be informed about the patient's decision only with her explicit permission or, in the case of minors, as required by applicable law. (See Chapter 4.) In particular, should she elect absolute confidentiality, her husband or partner should not be informed. Obstetricians have no professional competence to make judgments about the appropriateness of the pregnant woman's decision in this matter and therefore should respect her autonomous decisions about whom she wants to be informed by the physician.

9.11 Referring for Induced Abortion and Feticide

9.11.1 Direct Referral

Referral for induced abortion and feticide is straightforward in professional ethics in obstetrics for obstetricians who do not have conscience-based objections to induced abortion. They can make direct referrals, and the referring obstetrician sees to it that the patient will be seen by a colleague competent and willing to perform the procedure.[15]

9.11.2 Indirect Referral

Direct referral appears not to be an option for obstetricians with a conscience-based objection to induced abortion or feticide, because of the explicit involvement of the obstetrician in the subsequent termination of a pregnancy. To concomitantly respect the pregnant patient's autonomy and the individual conscience of obstetricians opposed to induced abortion or feticide, an indirect referral for termination of pregnancy should be made. Indirect referral is both autonomy based and beneficence based. When it is obligatory to offer induced abortion or feticide, respect for the pregnant woman's autonomy in previable pregnancies requires the obstetrician to inform her that induced abortion or feticide is an option. Beneficence requires the obstetrician to protect the life and health of the pregnant patient. The ethical principle of beneficence in professional ethics in obstetrics therefore creates a prima facie ethical obligation to provide information about clinics or agencies, such as Planned Parenthood in the United States, that provide competent and safe induced abortion or feticide. The obstetrician's individual conscience is not violated, because whether an induced abortion or feticide subsequently occurs is solely a function of the pregnant woman's autonomy after she visits the clinic or agency of her own accord. The referring obstetrician is, therefore, not responsible for or complicit in a subsequent induced abortion or feticide. Conscientious objection thus cannot be invoked. There are therefore no conscientious-objection-based constraints on the beneficence-based ethical obligation to protect the pregnant patient's life and health.

In summary, direct referral for induced abortion or induced abortion and feticide is not ethically required but is ethically permissible. Conscientious objection to direct referral for induced abortion or feticide has merit; conscientious objection to indirect referral does not have merit in professional ethics in obstetrics.[15]

References

1. Chervenak FA, McCullough LB, Brent RL. The professional responsibility model of obstetric ethics: avoiding the perils of clashing rights. Am J Obstet Gynecol 2011; 205: 515.e1–5.
2. Chervenak FA, McCullough LB. An ethically justified practical approach to offering, recommending, performing, and referring for induced abortion and feticide. Am J Obstet Gynecol. 2009; 201: 560.e1–6.
3. American Medical Association. Code of Medical Ethics Opinion 4.2.7. Abortion. Available at www.ama-assn.org/delivering-care/ethics/abortion (accessed March 1, 2019).
4. American College of Obstetricians and Gynecologists. Committee on Ethics. Ethics in Obstetrics and Gynecology. Available at www.acog.org/-/media/Committee-Opinions/Committee-on-Ethics/co390.pdf?dmc=1&ts=20181231T2040174286 (accessed March 1, 2019).
5. Stedman's Medical Dictionary. Available at online.statref.com/DictionaryHelp/DictionaryHelp (accessed March 1, 2019).
6. American College of Obstetricians and Gynecologists. Committee on Ethics. Multifetal Pregnancy Reduction. ACOG Committee Opinion Number 369. Obstet Gynecol 2007; 109: 1511–1515.
7. Chervenak FA, McCullough LB, Campbell S. Is third trimester abortion justified? Brit J Obstet Gynaecol 1995; 102: 434–435.
8. Chervenak FA, McCullough LB, Campbell S. Third trimester abortion: is compassion enough? Brit J Obstet Gynæcol 1999; 106: 293–296.
9. Chervenak FA, McCullough LB, Knapp RC, Caputo TA, Barber HR. A clinically comprehensive ethical framework for offering and recommending cancer treatment before and during pregnancy. Cancer 2004; 100(2): 215–222.

10. Chervenak FA, McCullough LB, Sharma G, Davis J, Gross S. Enhancing patient autonomy with risk assessment and invasive diagnosis: an ethical solution to a clinical challenge. Am J Obstet Gynecol 2008; 199: 19.e1–4.

11. Coverdale J, Chervenak FA, McCullough LB, Bayer T. Ethically justified clinically comprehensive guidelines for the management of the depressed pregnant patient. Am J Obstet Gynecol 1996; 174: 169–173.

12. Coverdale J, McCullough LB, Chervenak FA, Bayer T, Weeks S. Clinical implications of respect for autonomy in the psychiatric treatment of pregnant patients with depression. Psychiatr Serv 1997; 48: 209–212.

13. McCullough LB, Coverdale J, Chervenak FA. Ethical challenges of decision making with pregnant patients who have schizophrenia. Am J Obstet Gynecol 2002; 187: 696–702.

14. Coverdale J, McCullough LB, Chervenak FA. Assisted and surrogate decision making for pregnant patients who have schizophrenia. Schizophr Bull 2004; 30: 659–664.

15. Chervenak FA, McCullough LB. The ethics of direct and indirect referral for termination of pregnancy. Am J Obstet Gynecol 2008; 199: 232.e1–232.e3.

16. Chervenak FA, McCullough LB. Does obstetric ethics have any role to place in the obstetrician's response to the abortion controversy? Am J Obstet Gynecol 1990; 163: 1425–1429.

Chapter 10: Fetal Analysis

GOAL
This chapter provides an ethical framework to guide decision making about fetal analysis.

OBJECTIVES
On completing study of this chapter, the reader will:
- Identify precise nomenclature for fetal analysis
- Describe role for nondirective counseling or shared decision making
- Describe how pregnant women will respond to the offer of fetal analysis
- Describe ethically justified use of results of fetal analysis
- Apply the ethical framework to guide decision making about fetal analysis in clinical practice

TOPICS

10.1 Fetal Analysis and Decision Making about Obstetric Management	134
10.2 Providing Clinical Information about Options for Fetal Analysis Using Precise Nomenclature	134
10.2.1 Deceptively Imprecise Current Nomenclature	134
10.2.2 Replacement Nomenclature: Noninvasive Fetal Analysis or Invasive Fetal Analysis	135
10.2.2.1 Fetal Analysis	135
10.2.2.2 Noninvasive or Invasive Method	135
10.2.2.3 New Nomenclature	135
10.2.3 Communication among Obstetricians	135
10.2.4 Communication with Patients	135
10.3 Nondirective Counseling or Shared Decision Making	136
10.4 How Pregnant Women Will Respond to an Offer of Fetal Analysis	136
10.4.1 Refusal of All Forms of Fetal Analysis	137
10.4.2 Election of Invasive Fetal Analysis	137
10.4.3 Election of Noninvasive Fetal Analysis	137
10.4.3.1 Free Fetal DNA Analysis	137
10.4.4 Uncertainty about What to Do	138
10.5 Use of Results from Fetal Analysis	138

Section 3: Professionally Responsible Clinical Practice

> **Key Concepts**
>
> Directive counseling
> Ethical principle of beneficence in professional ethics in obstetrics
> Ethical principle of respect for autonomy in professional ethics in obstetrics
> Fetal analysis
> Informed consent process
> Invasive fetal analysis
> Moral risk
> Nondirective counseling
> Noninvasive fetal analysis
> Shared decision making

10.1 Fetal Analysis and Decision Making about Obstetric Management

The ethical principle of respect for autonomy in professional ethics in obstetrics creates the obstetrician's prima facie ethical obligation to empower the pregnant patient to make informed and voluntary decisions about obstetric management. This ethical obligation has two components. The first is providing her with clinical information about options for fetal analysis using nomenclature that is precise.[1] The second is supporting the pregnant woman's understanding and use of this information.[2]

10.2 Providing Clinical Information about Options for Fetal Analysis Using Precise Nomenclature

Precision of thought and speech by physicians is essential for excellent patient care and an effective informed consent process.[3,4] The need for precision increases as the gravity of the clinical stakes increase. In prenatal evaluation and counseling the stakes are especially high because termination of a pregnancy might be considered. The current nomenclature of "prenatal testing," "prenatal screening," and "prenatal diagnosis" – along with their subsets of "ultrasound testing," "ultrasound screening," "ultrasound diagnosis," "noninvasive prenatal testing," "noninvasive prenatal screening," and "noninvasive prenatal diagnosis" – has become so imprecise that clinical misinterpretation and distortion of the informed consent process are increasingly difficult to prevent. Obstetricians and their patients are at chronic risk of confusion and miscommunication that can impair the pregnant patient's informed decision making about the evaluation of the fetus' condition. Further compounding this problem is the fact that there is no agreement on a standard nomenclature.

10.2.1 Deceptively Imprecise Current Nomenclature

"Testing" has two components: information gathering and analysis of that information or results. It is commonly assumed that all testing is diagnostic and that a binomial answer will be given: presence or absence of a diagnosis. It is true that testing is diagnostic but the range of results is not so clear-cut. Laboratory and imaging analysis often produces nondiagnostic results. These include findings of uncertain clinical significance, e.g., echogenic fetal bowel on ultrasound examination or previously unreported chromosome variation.

"Screening" can mean assessing risk of disease in an individual patient, such as Pap smear screening. But "screening" can also mean performing diagnostic testing in a population to measure the prevalence of a specific condition, such as anonymous serology to measure the prevalence of HIV infection, to plan for allocation of public health resources in a community. The use of "screening test" compounds this ambiguity, because it suggests that the screening test will provide a definitive diagnostic answer.

The use of "diagnosis" suggests that imaging or laboratory analysis always produces a diagnosis. However, this is not always the case. Sometimes such analysis produces results that may trend toward a diagnosis but do not confirm it or may be uncertain in their clinical significance.

The use of "invasive" and "noninvasive" describe the *method* by which information is gathered. They do not describe testing or screening, because these terms pertain to *analysis* of information.

When these terms are combined, e.g., "noninvasive prenatal screening," the potential for confusion among obstetricians and their patients increases. This confusion is likely to infect the informed consent process, putting it at risk of becoming misleading. Phrases formed by combining the terms sound precise but they are not; they are unintentionally deceptively imprecise.

10.2.2 Replacement Nomenclature: Noninvasive Fetal Analysis or Invasive Fetal Analysis

To prevent this completely unintended deceptive imprecision we propose a clinically precise, comprehensive replacement nomenclature to be used among obstetricians and other physicians and by obstetricians with their patients in the informed consent process.

10.2.2.1 Fetal Analysis

The phrase "fetal analysis" should be used and "testing" or "screening" should not be used. We make this proposal because "analysis" is a very well understood, precise clinical term: interpreting information about the fetus' condition. In addition, it is also very well understood that the results of laboratory or imaging analysis of the fetus are not limited to the presence or absence of a diagnosis. Positive and negative diagnoses are surely categories of results of analysis but not the only category. Understood in a clinically comprehensive fashion, the results of laboratory and imaging analysis sort into the following well known clinical categories:

> Positive Diagnosis: Presence of pathology that requires a plan of clinical management.
> Negative Diagnosis: Absence of pathology that enables reassurance but does not guaranty a "normal" fetus, much less a "perfect baby."[5] *(See Chapter 13.)*
> Risk Assessment: Gradations of probability of the presence of a fetal anomaly or of future occurrence of disease or disability that require further analysis to make a specific diagnosis.
> Results of Uncertain Clinical Significance: Anatomy or physiology that is related to known pathology, for which there is no known treatment plan and that therefore should be prospectively observed for evolution into pathology.
> Pharmacogenomics (when genomic analysis is performed): Increased precision of drug selection and drug dosing).

10.2.2.2 Noninvasive or Invasive Method

"Noninvasive" and "invasive" describe the method by which information is gathered for fetal analysis. A noninvasive method does not penetrate the maternal abdomen, uterus, or amniotic cavity. An invasive method penetrates the maternal abdomen, uterus, or amniotic cavity. Even though the skin and vein are penetrated, a maternal blood draw is characterized as noninvasive, because it poses no risk of clinical harm to the fetus.

The techniques used in noninvasive or invasive method function as modifiers:

Noninvasive fetal analysis using ultrasound or magnetic resonance imaging

Noninvasive fetal analysis using maternal blood draw

Invasive fetal analysis using amniocentesis

Invasive fetal analysis using chorionic villus sampling

Invasive fetal analysis using fetal blood or tissue sampling

10.2.2.3 New Nomenclature

The new nomenclature should convey the distinction between fetal analysis with a noninvasive method and fetal analysis with an invasive method, using various techniques. The techniques need not be part of the new nomenclature. This new nomenclature is designed to be precise and therefore facilitate effective communication among physicians and with pregnant women. For ease of use the new nomenclature:

Noninvasive Fetal Analysis (fetal analysis with various noninvasive methods)

Invasive Fetal Analysis (fetal analysis with various invasive methods)

10.2.3 Communication among Obstetricians

Communication among obstetricians about fetal analysis has two components. When obstetricians communicate about the method of fetal analysis to each other they should first identify the technique of either noninvasive or invasive method from among the above five conceptually clear, clinically precise categories. When obstetricians report the results of fetal analysis to another physician, the results should be labeled and described in the conceptually clear, clinically precise category or categories of results listed in Section 10.2.2.1.

10.2.4 Communication with Patients

Communication with the pregnant patient about fetal analysis has six components. We propose the

Table 10.1 Guide to information to be provided the informed consent for fetal analysis.

1. The concept of fetal analysis
2. The purpose of fetal analysis
3. The distinction between noninvasive fetal analysis and invasive fetal analysis
4. The techniques of noninvasive and invasive method
5. The range of results of each technique of fetal analysis
6. Categories of results of genome sequencing

following guide to the informed process as a tool for maintaining its quality. (See Table 10.1.) The pregnant woman should be informed about

1. The concept of fetal analysis: interpreting information about the condition of the fetus(es).
2. The purpose of fetal analysis: To support the woman's exercise of her autonomy in making an informed and voluntary decision about the management of her pregnancy.
3. The distinction between noninvasive fetal analysis and invasive fetal analysis. Invasive fetal analysis penetrates the maternal abdomen, uterus, or amniotic cavity and thereby creates some degree of risk of fetal loss, whereas noninvasive fetal analysis does not penetrate these structures and therefore creates no risk of fetal loss or other clinical harms to the fetus.
4. The two techniques of a noninvasive method and the three techniques of an invasive method, with a description of each, the range of results that can be expected, and their clinical risks.
5. Information about the range of results from each technique:
   a. The results of noninvasive ultrasound may include positive diagnosis, negative diagnosis with no guaranty of a "normal" fetus, results of uncertain clinical significance, and risk assessment.
   b. The results of noninvasive maternal blood draw are currently limited to risk assessment and therefore should *not* be expected to be diagnostic with no guaranty of a "normal" fetus. The purpose of this risk assessment is to inform decision making about the use of an invasive method.
   c. The results of the three techniques of an invasive method may include positive diagnosis, negative diagnosis with no guaranty of a "normal" fetus, results of uncertain clinical significance, and risk assessment.
6. When genome sequencing (whole exome sequencing or whole genome sequencing) is a component of analysis, the results may include positive diagnosis, negative diagnosis with no guaranty of a "normal" fetus, results of uncertain clinical significance, risk assessment, and increased precision in drug selection and dosing (pharmacogenomics).

10.3 Nondirective Counseling or Shared Decision Making

The decision to remain pregnant has a medical component: the health status of the fetus. This medical component, however, is only one component of the biopsychosocial clinical reality of pregnancy.[6] Judgments about the psychosocial dimensions are the exclusive province of the pregnant woman. The exercise of her capacity for autonomous decision making is decisive.

Respect for the pregnant patient's autonomy in presenting fetal analysis to her requires that the presentation be nondirective. Fetal analysis should be performed as described in Section 10.2.2.2. The pregnant woman should be supported to understand this information. The obstetrician should not make a recommendation about whether to accept fetal analysis or of a specific form of fetal analysis. The obstetrician should also refrain from introducing conscious and, to the extent possible, nonconscious bias into the communication process. This means that the options should only be offered. This is also known as shared decision making: the patient's values and beliefs should guide the evaluation of her options by the pregnant woman.[7] (See Chapter 3.) She is free to draw on her social resources in doing so. For the pregnant woman who is without social resources, the obstetrician should ask if she would welcome support and provide it if asked. The obstetrician may need to deploy assisted decision making to help the patient make her own decisions. (See Chapter 2.)

10.4 How Pregnant Women Will Respond to an Offer of Fetal Analysis

In response to this routine offer of options for the evaluation of pregnancy, patients will exercise their autonomy along one of four pathways.[8] The ethical principle of respect for autonomy in professional ethics in obstetrics creates the prima facie ethical obligation of the obstetrician to respect the pregnant woman's response.

10.4.1 Refusal of All Forms of Fetal Analysis

Some women will refuse all forms of fetal analysis. The concept of moral risk is important to appreciate in these circumstances.[9] Moral risk occurs when a patient obtains information that opens an option that is, for that patient, morally unacceptable to elect. The concept of moral risk in the setting of fetal analysis means that some women will not want to confront the moral risk of making a decision about termination or continuation of pregnancy based on the results of any form of fetal analysis. On the basis of their religious or other moral beliefs they will be ethically justified to refuse all forms of fetal analysis. This is why their decisions in all cases should be treated with respect.

Respect for the patient's autonomy requires physicians to recognize that some women will not consider termination of pregnancy as morally acceptable under any circumstances and therefore will find risk-assessment and diagnostic information irrelevant to their decision to continue the pregnancy. Religious and other moral beliefs will play a central role in such decisions and must command respect from physicians.

10.4.2 Election of Invasive Fetal Analysis

Some women will elect invasive fetal analysis prior to noninvasive fetal analysis for risk assessment for a variety of reasons, such as unwillingness to accept the birth of a child with any detectable abnormality, including trisomy 21. Such women should be informed that opting for noninvasive fetal analysis for risk assessment first could provide information relevant to opting for invasive fetal analysis but will take some time. Some women will nonetheless elect invasive fetal analysis, because it can rule out trisomy 21 and other detectable anomalies promptly, and consequently accept the risks of invasive fetal analysis. Their reasons for making such a decision are their own and should therefore command respect from their obstetrician. Once such women have made an informed decision for invasive fetal analysis, it should be performed or an appropriate referral made. For these women and for those in the first pathway, once they have made an informed decision, recommending risk assessment should be regarded as potential paternalism, i.e., an attempt to interfere with the exercise of the woman's autonomy,[10] based on the physician's judgment that she has made a bad choice.

10.4.3 Election of Noninvasive Fetal Analysis

Some women will elect noninvasive fetal analysis for risk assessment. They should understand that risk assessment is not diagnostic and that it may provide a revised risk assessment for fetal Down syndrome or other fetal anomalies. In response to the results of noninvasive fetal analysis for risk assessment, pregnant women will sort themselves along three branching routes.

One route will be taken by women who judge the estimation of risk to be acceptable and will elect to continue their pregnancy without further fetal analysis, including invasive fetal analysis. At the other end of the spectrum, a second route will be taken by women who judge the estimation of risk to be unacceptable to them and will elect invasive fetal analysis. The obstetrician should either perform, or refer the patient for, invasive fetal analysis, with the patient's informed consent for the procedure.

The third route will be taken by women who are uncertain about whether the estimation of risk is acceptable. These women should be provided with information about available additional, noninvasive fetal analysis that could be performed during the first and second trimesters to better define their risk. The American College of Obstetricians and Gynecologists (ACOG) Practice Bulletin provides information on these alternatives.[11] The pregnant woman should be offered support to think through her options. If she accepts support it should be provided, drawing on colleagues in other disciplines such as social work and chaplaincy as appropriate.

10.4.3.1 Free Fetal DNA Analysis

Free fetal DNA analysis is a form of noninvasive fetal analysis for risk assessment. The obstetrician should be clear with the pregnant woman that this fetal analysis is *not* diagnostic for fetal aneuploidy at this time. The obstetrician therefore should not describe free fetal DNA analysis as a diagnostic test. In addition, it is not currently endorsed as a medically reasonable alternative for risk assessment for all pregnant women. ACOG states that pregnant women "at increased risk of aneuploidy can be offered testing with free fetal DNA."[12] Norton and colleagues state that the role for free DNA testing in routine noninvasive risk assessment remains to be determined.[13] Norton and colleagues go beyond the ACOG statement and state that this new technology may be used as a "second-tier test for those patients who screen positive by conventional aneuploidy screening."[13] If free fetal DNA analysis becomes accepted as appropriate for all pregnant women, it will become a medically reasonable alternative for noninvasive fetal analysis for routine prenatal risk assessment.

10.4.4 Uncertainty about What to Do

Some women will be uncertain about what to do. The obstetrician should explore the reasons for their uncertainty with them and be especially attentive to incomplete understanding of information that has been provided and confusion about the distinction between a risk assessment and diagnosis. If, as a result of a thorough informed consent process, the patient wishes to postpone her decision, she should be informed about the time-limited nature of such postponement. The obstetrician should be sure to point out that, if she postpones her decision too long for first-trimester noninvasive fetal analysis for risk assessment to be performed, her only options will become second-trimester noninvasive fetal analysis for risk assessment, invasive fetal analysis, or neither.

10.5 Use of Results from Fetal Analysis

Sometimes the results of fetal analysis are used by the pregnant woman in decision making about the disposition of her pregnancy. There is evidence that pregnant women are capable of making informed decisions using the results of fetal analysis.[14] When a fetal anomaly is diagnosed, the obstetrician has an autonomy-based prima facie ethical obligation to offer induced abortion or feticide. Chapter 13 provides a detailed account of this ethical obligation and its implications for performing and referring for induced abortion and feticide.

References

1. Chervenak FA, McCullough LB, Dudenhausen J. Fetal analysis with invasive method (FA-I) and fetal analysis with non-invasive method (FA-NI): replacing current, deceptively imprecise clinical nomenclature. J Perinal Med 2017; 45: 985–987.
2. Chervenak FA, McCullough LB. Ethical dimensions of first-trimester aneuploidy screening. Clin Obstet Gynecol 2014; 57: 226–231.
3. Chervenak J, McCullough LB, Chervenak FA. Surgery without consent or miscommunication? A new look at a landmark case. Am J Obstet Gynecol 2015; 212: 586–590.
4. Wielgos M, Chervenak FA, McCullough LB, Dudenhausen JW. Deliberative clinical ethical judgment: an essential component of contemporary obstetrics. J Perinat Med 2013; 41: 627–630.
5. Chervenak FA, McCullough LB, Brent RL. The perils of the imperfect expectation of the perfect baby. Am J Obstet Gynecol 2010; 203: 101.e1–5.
6. Engel G. A unified concept of health and disease. IRE Trans Med Electron 2009; 10.1109/IRET-ME.1960.5008004. Originally appeared in Perspect Biol Med 1960; 13: 48–57.
7. Kon AA. The shared decision-making continuum. JAMA 2010; 304: 903–904.
8. Chervenak FA, McCullough LB, Sharma G, Davis J. Gross G. Enhancing patient autonomy with risk assessment and invasive diagnosis: an ethical solution to a clinical challenge. Am J Obstet Gynecol 2008; 199: 19.e1–19.e4.
9. Faden RR, Becker C, Lewis C, Freeman J, et al. Disclosure of information to patients in medical care. Med Care 1981; 19: 718–733.
10. Beauchamp TL, Childress JF. Principles of Biomedical Ethics, 7th ed. New York: Oxford University Press, 2012.
11. American College of Obstetricians and Gynecologists. Committee on Practice Bulletins. Screening for fetal chromosomal abnormalities. Obstet Gynecol 2007; 109: 217–227.
12. American College of Obstetricians and Gynecologists. Committee on Genetics. The Society for Maternal-Fetal Medicine. Publications Committee. Noninvasive prenatal testing for aneuploidy. Obstet Gynecol 2012; 120: 1532–1534.
13. Norton ME, Rose NC, Benn P. Noninvasive prenatal testing for fetal aneuploidy: clinical assessment and a plea for restraint. Obstet Gynecol 2013; 121; 847–850.
14. Nicolaides KH, Chervenak FA, McCullough LB, Avgidou K, Papageorghiou A. Evidence-based obstetrics ethics and informed decision-making by pregnant woman about invasive diagnosis after first-trimester assessment of risk for trisomy 21. Am J Obstet Gynecol 2005; 193: 322–326.

Chapter 11 Periviability

GOAL
This chapter provides an ethical framework to guide decision making about periviable birth.

OBJECTIVES
On completing study of this chapter, the reader will:

Identify professional ethics in perinatal medicine as having an obstetric component and a pediatric component
Describe the continuum of deliberative clinical judgment about the clinical management of periviability
Describe a multidisciplinary team approach to counseling about delivery
Describe ethically justified responses to requests to "do everything"
Apply the ethical framework to guide decision making about periviable birth in clinical practice

TOPICS

11.1 Viability	140
11.2 Periviable Birth	140
11.3 Professional Ethics in Perinatal Medicine	140
11.3.1 The Obstetric Component of Professional Ethics in Perinatal Medicine	141
11.3.2 The Pediatric Component of Professional Ethics in Perinatal Medicine	141
11.4 The Continuum of Deliberative Clinical Judgment about the Clinical Management of Periviability	142
11.4.1 Intrapartum Management	142
11.4.1.1 Consensus Statement from the American College of Obstetricians and Gynecologists and the Society for Maternal–Fetal Medicine	142
11.4.1.2 Limits of Deliberative Clinical Obstetric Judgment	143
11.4.2 Evaluation of the Neonatal Patient for Clinical Application of Specified Concepts of Futility	143
11.4.3 Resuscitation as a Trial of Intervention	143
11.4.4 Neonatal Critical Care as a Trial of Intervention	143
11.5 A Multidisciplinary Team Approach to Counseling before Delivery	143
11.5.1 Clarifying Who Is the Decision Maker with the Perinatal Team	143
11.5.2 A Multidisciplinary Approach	144
11.6 Responding to Requests to "Do Everything"	144
11.6.1 A Preventive Ethics Approach	144
11.6.2 Addressing Incomplete or Inaccurate Information	144
11.6.3 Moral Theological Considerations	145
11.6.4 Hope and Coping with Loss	145

Key Concepts

Anatomic futility
Best interests of the child standard in professional ethics in pediatrics
Critical care as a trial of intervention
Ethical concept of the fetus as a patient
Ethical principle of beneficence in professional ethics in obstetrics
Ethical principle of nonmaleficence in professional ethics in obstetrics and gynecology
Ethical principle of respect for autonomy in professional ethics in obstetrics
Futility
Hope
Imminent demise futility
Interactive capacity futility
Medically reasonable alternative
Physiologic futility
Preventive ethics
Professional ethics in perinatal medicine
Resuscitation as a trial of intervention
Trial of intervention

11.1 Viability

Viability in professional ethics in obstetrics and gynecology is a function of both fetal physiology and available resuscitation and life-sustaining treatment. Viability is therefore the biological capacity of a liveborn infant to survive even if full technological support is needed.[1] This is the concept of viability used by the United States Supreme Court in its landmark ruling, *Roe v. Wade*, in 1973.[2]

The typical definition of live birth in statutory law in the United States is expulsion of the fetus from the uterus and separation from the woman's body accompanied by signs of life. Consider:

> "Live birth" means the complete expulsion or extraction from its mother of a product of human conception, irrespective of the duration of pregnancy, which, after such expulsion or extraction, breathes or shows any other evidence of life such as beating of the heart, pulsation of the umbilical cord or definite movement of voluntary muscles, whether or not the umbilical cord has been cut or the placenta is attached.[3]

This is verbatim from the World Health Organization[4] and thus functions as an international definition.

In high-income countries, which can provide high-risk obstetric care as well as neonatal intensive care at the highest levels, viability occurs at about 24 (completed) weeks of gestation. Fetal physiology at a specified gestational age, like all human traits, displays variability. Tyson and colleagues identified five sources of such variability: gestational age, sex, birthweight, singleton pregnancy, and prenatal administration of steroids.[5] The Eunice Kennedy Shriver National Institute of Child Health and Human Development has incorporated the work of Tyson and colleagues into a calculator on its website.[6] The National Institute of Child Health and Human Development (NICHD) calculator sorts an individual into a population with similar characteristics and predicts mortality and morbidity for that population.

11.2 Periviable Birth

Periviable birth has been defined as "delivery occurring from 20 0/7 weeks to 25 6/7 weeks of gestation."[7,8] These numbers refer to completed weeks. Percent survival range from less than 5%–6% at 22 0/7–2 6/7 weeks to more than 70% at 25 0/7–25 6/7 weeks. A Japanese study reported a range of about 40% to more than 80% survival for the same gestational continuum.[7,9] These outcomes are affected to an unknown degree by variation in obstetric and neonatal practice and differences in population at 22 and 23 weeks but less so at higher gestational ages. Outcomes are improved when delivery occurs in a tertiary care center.

11.3 Professional Ethics in Perinatal Medicine

Deliberative clinical judgment about the obstetric and pediatric management of periviable birth should be based on evidence about outcomes with due caution about the limits of available evidence and the implications of professional ethics in perinatal medicine. The specialty of perinatal medicine combines maternal-fetal medicine, a subspecialty of obstetrics, and neonatology, a subspecialty of pediatrics. Professional ethics in perinatal medicine therefore needs to combine professional ethics in obstetrics with professional ethics in pediatrics. (See Chapter 2.) Professional ethics in perinatal medicine supports a preventive ethics approach to decision making about obstetric and pediatric clinical management of periviable birth.

In professional ethics in obstetrics the viable fetus is a patient when a pregnant woman is presented for clinical management to an obstetrician or other healthcare professional and there exist forms of clinical management that in deliberative clinical judgment are reliably predicted to result in net clinical benefit for the pregnant patient and the fetal patient. These are the medically reasonable alternatives for the clinical management of pregnancy after viability. In professional ethics in pediatrics a live-born infant is a patient when that infant is presented to a pediatrician or other healthcare professional and there exist forms of clinical management that in deliberative clinical judgment are reliably predicted to result in net clinical benefit for the pediatric patient. These are the medically reasonable alternatives for the clinical management of a neonatal patient.

The central task of deliberative clinical ethical judgment in perinatal medicine is to identity these medically reasonable alternatives and their limits. There is in professional ethics in perinatal medicine a prima facie autonomy-based ethical obligation to offer the medically reasonable alternatives for the management of the fetal patient's (obstetrics) or neonatal patient's (pediatrics) condition. When the limits of such treatment are reached and there is no longer net benefit but net disease-related and iatrogenic harm, there is a prima facie beneficence-based and nonmaleficence-based ethical obligation to recommend that life-sustaining treatment should not be initiated or, having been initiated, should be discontinued.

11.3.1 The Obstetric Component of Professional Ethics in Perinatal Medicine

Obstetricians and obstetric healthcare professionals have prima facie beneficence-based and prima facie autonomy-based obligations to the pregnant patient and prima facie beneficence-based obligations to the fetal patient. The ethical concept of the fetus as a patient requires that each of the three prima facie ethical obligations must be balanced against the others to reach a deliberative clinical ethical judgment about obstetric management. (See Chapter 2.) When the limits of beneficence-based deliberative clinical ethical judgment about fetal benefit are reached, non-aggressive obstetric management (no fetal monitoring, mode of delivery based on maternal indications only) should be recommended. The pregnant patient is the ultimate decision maker.

A preventive ethics approach to deliberative clinical ethical judgment in obstetrics comprises the following steps (See Table 11.1).

1. The obstetrician identifies the prima facie beneficence-based obligations to the pregnant patient, the strength of which varies by their evidence base.
2. The obstetrician identifies the prima facie autonomy-based obligations to the pregnant patient, the strength of which varies by her capacity to participate in decision making about the clinical management of her pregnancy.
3. The obstetrician identifies the prima facie beneficence-based obligations to the fetal patient, the strength of which varies by their evidence base.
4. The obstetrician considers these three prima facie obligations together in a deliberative clinical judgment about which of these obligations should have precedence when clinical reality or the decisions of the pregnant patient prevents these three obligations from being congruent (which they are almost all of the time). There is a crucial beneficence-based limitation: the pregnant woman is ethically obligated to take only reasonable clinical risks to herself for fetal and neonatal benefit.

11.3.2 The Pediatric Component of Professional Ethics in Perinatal Medicine

Pediatricians and pediatric healthcare professionals have prima facie beneficence-based and autonomy-based obligations to the pediatric patient based on the best interests of the child standard in professional ethics in pediatrics.[10,11] The best interests of the child standard is applied to an individual neonatal patient in beneficence-based clinical judgment, which creates the prima facie ethical obligation to provide clinical management that, in deliberative clinical judgment, is predicted to result in net clinical benefit for that patient.

The best interests of the child standard also applies to populations of neonatal patients. The ethical principle of healthcare justice in professional ethics in pediatrics creates the prima facie ethical obligation to prevent exploitation. Exploitation occurs in a population of patients when only a small percent receives net clinical benefit while a much larger percentage receives net clinical harm with no opportunity for offsetting benefit. Death is such a clinical harm. So, too, is survival with severe disease-related and iatrogenic physical and cognitive disabilities. For exploitation to be prevented, two conditions need to be satisfied. First, the majority should survive. Second, the majority of survivors should have less-than-severe disease-related and iatrogenic physical and cognitive disabilities so that the percent of such survivors is greater than that for survivors with severe disabilities. These two conditions are clearly met at 25 0/7–25 6/7 weeks gestational age.[6,8] They appear to be met at 24 0/7–24 6/7 weeks.[6,8] They appear not be met at 23 0/7–23 6/7 weeks.[6,8] We use the word "appear" to signal ongoing uncertainty about these prognostic judgments.

When exploitation does not apply clinically, deliberative clinical judgment should focus on the individual neonatal patient, taking into account the prognostic information provided by the NICHD calculator. When exploitation does apply, the permissibility of making an exception arises. One way to justify an exception is individualized deliberative clinical judgment about the implications of the best interests of the child standard. However, from the perspective of the general ethical principle of justice, like cases must be treated alike. This means that there are no exceptions but new subpopulations of patients who should be treated alike. Outcomes in populations created by exceptions may exhibit exploitation, in which case the burden of proof is on making exceptions. In this healthcare-justice–based context individualized beneficence-based deliberative clinical judgment is inadequate and should therefore not be used in isolation from the healthcare-justice–based ethical obligation to prevent exploitation.

When the limits of beneficence-based and healthcare-justice–based deliberative clinical ethical judgment are reached, not resuscitating an infant and not following up with neonatal intensive care should be recommended. The parents' role is to provide informed permission. (See Chapter 2.)

A preventive ethics approach to deliberative clinical ethical judgment in pediatrics comprises the following steps (See Table 11.2).
1. The pediatrician should identify prima facie beneficence-based obligations to the neonatal patient, the strength of which varies by their evidence base.
2. The pediatrician should determine whether there is a risk of exploitation of neonatal patients in a population that is resuscitated followed by neonatal intensive care.

11.4 The Continuum of Deliberative Clinical Judgment about the Clinical Management of Periviability

11.4.1 Intrapartum Management

As explained in Chapter 12, vaginal delivery is the default form of medically reasonable intrapartum management. This is because vaginal delivery fulfills the obstetrician's beneficence-based prima facie ethical obligations to the pregnant and fetal patients, especially the beneficence-based ethical prima facie ethical obligation to the pregnant patient to take only reasonable risk to the pregnant patient for fetal and neonatal benefit.

It follows that in deliberative clinical judgment cesarean delivery bears the burden of proof. This burden is met when there is a high level of evidence for the prediction that cesarean delivery will prevent serious, far-reaching, and irreversible harm to the fetal or neonatal patient. The risks to the pregnant woman in the current and future pregnancies should be considered reasonable in this clinical context. The burden of proof is not met when there is no or only low-level, weak evidence of fetal and neonatal benefit from cesarean delivery, because in this clinical context the risks to the pregnant woman in the current and future pregnancies should be considered unreasonable.

11.4.1.1 Consensus Statement from the American College of Obstetricians and Gynecologists and the Society for Maternal–Fetal Medicine

A recent Consensus Statement on periviable birth from the American College of Obstetricians and Gynecologists and the Society for Maternal–Fetal Medicine has presented evidence-based recommendations about mode of delivery that can be readily interpreted in the context of burden of proof for cesarean delivery.[7,9] As explained in Section 11.3.2, the conditions for absence of exploitation are clearly met at 25 0/7–25 6/7 weeks. The Consensus Statement's recommendation of cesarean delivery for fetal indications is ethically justified. Given the potential application of the healthcare-justice–based concept of exploitation, the Consensus Statement's position that cesarean delivery for fetal benefit should be "considered" at both 24 0/7–24 6/7 weeks and 23 0/7–232 6/7 weeks is ethically justified, because of the healthcare-justice–based prima facie ethical obligation to prevent exploitation. The Consensus Statement's position that cesarean delivery is "not recommended" for 20 0/7–21 6/7 and 22 0/7–22 6/7 is ethically justified because there is no evidence that cesarean delivery improves outcomes.

11.4.1.2 Limits of Deliberative Clinical Obstetric Judgment

It might at first appear that the NICHD calculator could be used to make a more refined deliberative obstetric clinical judgment about cesarean delivery for 24 0/7–24 6/7 weeks and 23 0/7–232 6/7 weeks. However, an evidence-based critical appraisal of the clinical components entered into the calculator has shown that the wide variability of these components makes a reliable prediction in deliberative obstetric clinical judgment unreliable.[12]

11.4.2 Evaluation of the Neonatal Patient for Clinical Application of Specified Concepts of Futility

Delivery of a live-born neonatal patient should be followed by evaluation of the newborn's condition in deliberative clinical judgment. If one or more of the specified concepts of futility described in Chapter 15 (terminal or irreversible condition, anatomic, physiologic, imminent-demise, or interactive-capacity) are considered applicable, there is a prima facie nonmaleficence-based ethical obligation not to initiate resuscitation, to prevent net disease-related and iatrogenic harm to the neonatal patient. In some cases, deliberative neonatal clinical judgment of the condition of the fetal patient supports a reliable prediction that one or more of the specified concepts of futility will apply at birth. In such circumstances, there is a prima facie nonmaleficence-based ethical obligation not to initiate resuscitation, to prevent net disease-related and iatrogenic harm to the neonatal patient.

11.4.3 Resuscitation as a Trial of Intervention

Resuscitation of an imperiled neonatal patient is undertaken with the physiologic goal of restoration of spontaneous circulation (ROSC). Resuscitation should be understood as a trial of intervention. When in deliberative clinical judgment the probability of achieving ROSC is very small, less than 3%, there is a prima facie beneficence-based ethical obligation to discontinue resuscitation for lack of efficacy and a prima facie nonmaleficence-based ethical obligation not to initiate resuscitation, to prevent net disease-related and iatrogenic harm to the neonatal patient. (See Chapter 15.)

11.4.4 Neonatal Critical Care as a Trial of Intervention

When resuscitation produces ROSC, it is physiologically effective. A trial of neonatal critical care begins with the short-term goal of preventing imminent death and the long-term goal of survival with at least some interactive capacity. (See Chapter 15.) When in deliberative clinical judgment the probability of achieving either goal is very small, less than 3%, because one or more of the specified concepts of futility, there is a prima facie beneficence-based ethical obligation to discontinue critical care management for lack of efficacy and a prima facie nonmaleficence-based ethical obligation to discontinue critical care management, to prevent net disease-related and iatrogenic harm to the neonatal patient.

11.5 A Multidisciplinary Team Approach to Counseling before Delivery

11.5.1 Clarifying Who Is the Decision Maker with the Perinatal Team

Prepartum counseling of the pregnant patient and her partner, as well as others whom she permits to participate, should be clear that (1) she is the ultimate decision maker about obstetric management and (2) both she and the other parent of the child have the authority to provide informed permission for the clinical management of their child who has become a neonatal patient. The role of other parties, especially family members, is to support the pregnant woman in her obstetric decision

Table 11.1 Preventive ethics approach to deliberative clinical ethical judgment in obstetrics.

1. Identify the prima facie beneficence-based obligations to the pregnant patient, the strength of which varies by their evidence base.
2. Identify the prima facie autonomy-based obligations to the pregnant patient, the strength of which varies by her capacity to participate in decision making about the clinical management of her pregnancy.
3. Identify the prima facie beneficence-based obligations to the fetal patient, the strength of which varies by their evidence base.
4. Consider these three prima facie obligations together in a deliberative clinical judgment about which of these obligations should have precedence when clinical reality or the decisions of the pregnant patient prevents these three obligations from being congruent, with a limitation: the pregnant woman is ethically obligated to take only reasonable clinical risks to herself for fetal and neonatal benefit.

Table 11.2 Preventive ethics approach to deliberative clinical ethical judgment in pediatrics.

1. Identify prima facie beneficence-based obligations to neonatal patient, the strength of which varies by their evidence base.
2. Determine whether there is a risk of exploitation of neonatal patients in a population that is resuscitated followed by neonatal intensive care.

making and the parents in their pediatric decision making.

11.5.2 A Multidisciplinary Approach

A multidisciplinary team should be assembled, including obstetrics, neonatology, nursing, social work, and pastoral/spiritual care.[7] When counseling the pregnant woman about obstetric clinical management, team members should think and speak like obstetric clinicians. The team should emphasize that the pregnant woman has no ethical obligation to her fetus or future child to accept more than reasonable risk to herself. When counseling prospective parents about neonatal clinical management, team members should think and speak like pediatric clinicians. Counseling should be based on the best interests of the child standard, including the need to prevent exploitation. The sequences of decision making described in Sections 11.3.1 and 11.3.2 – for obstetric decision making and pediatric decision making, respectively – should be followed. (See Tables 11.1 and 11.2.) Ethically justified recommendations should be made about mode of delivery, resuscitation, and neonatal critical care, including recommendations about setting clinically and ethically justified limits. The team should emphasize that accepting such limits will be consistent with being loving and good parents and that palliative care for the infant and support for the family will be provided.

11.6 Responding to Requests to "Do Everything"

11.6.1 A Preventive Ethics Approach

Chapter 15 provides a detailed account of how to respond to requests for inappropriate clinical management. The goal in responding to requests to "Do everything" is to support the pregnant patient in making an informed decision about cesarean delivery and parents in making informed decisions about resuscitation and neonatal critical care. Implementing requests that are not informed decisions creates a preventable threat to the professional virtue of integrity in professional ethics in obstetrics and gynecology.[13,14]

Counseling of the pregnant patient and prospective parents should already have introduced the concept that intrapartum management initiates neonatal management as a trial of intervention that sometimes reaches its limits to help the fetal or neonatal patient. Counseling should begin with this crucial concept and not permit it to become lost in subsequent conversation and, for religious individuals, in prayer and reflection for spiritual guidance.

11.6.2 Addressing Incomplete or Inaccurate Information

These requests are sometimes based on incomplete or inaccurate information. Team members should be alert to such mistaken beliefs and respectfully and consistently correct them. The professional virtue of integrity in professional ethics in obstetrics and in pediatrics creates a very strong ethical obligation not to allow mistaken beliefs to become the basis of deliberative clinical judgment and recommendations based on it.

11.6.3 Moral Theological Considerations

Most faith communities in their moral theologies accept as ethically permissible limitations of intrapartum and neonatal clinical management. Some do not. Responding to requests to "Do everything" based on such moral theologies requires the involvement of a religious adviser who has expertise about the moral theology of the faith community and who comes to the hospital to see the pregnant or neonatal patient and is willing to become well informed about the patient's condition and the deliberative clinical ethical judgment of the perinatal teams that setting limits on intrapartum or neonatal clinical management is justified. Hospital chaplains have an important role to play in this process, building on their relationships with local faith communities. Hospital policy should provide clear guidance for how to proceed in such cases. Hospital leadership have a professional integrity–based ethical obligation to fully support the implementation of such a policy and not make exceptions to it for reasons unrelated to patient care and respect for the faith community.

11.6.4 Hope and Coping with Loss

Almost all pregnant women who intend to complete their pregnancies, prospective parents, and parents have hopes for the future of their child. Hope has two components.[15] The first is the desire for a future state of affairs, in this case, the best for their child. The second is that this future state of affairs has a probability along the continuum of <1 and >0.

When the probability of a future state of affairs = 1, we expect it to occur, such as sunrise tomorrow. When the probability of a future state of affairs = 0, one cannot reasonably hope for it, because when the probability is 0 there are no evidence-based grounds for desiring it. This can be a harsh reality, a judgment that is a source of the common belief among physicians that it is a mistake to take hope away. Unfortunately, clinical reality and the limits of intrapartum management, resuscitation, and neonatal critical care can reduce the probability of survival to 0, e.g., when the specified concepts of anatomic, physiologic, or imminent demise futility apply. (See Chapter 15.)

When a pregnant woman, her partner, parents, and family members can no longer hope that a neonatal patient will survive, they begin to experience false hope, an agonizing experience that strongly interacts with impending loss of a child. They must be able to hope for something else. The perinatal team should emphasize that they will respect the dignity of their neonatal patient, provide excellent palliative care, and support parents and family members to begin coping with what they may experience as a catastrophic loss that is life-altering. Parents must be confident that the team saw to it that everything that should have been done for their child was done. The perinatal team should reassure them that this has been the case and will continue to be the case until death occurs. Offering the parents the opportunity to speak with a representative of the local Organ Procurement Organization about donating tissues and organs, when the neonatal patient has been determined to be an eligible source of tissues and organs, may offer the parents hope for the survival and health of another child. Parents who are members of a faith community should receive support from their spiritual advisor, especially concerning religious rites that should be performed before and after death has occurred.

References

1. Chervenak FA, McCullough LB, Levene MI. An ethically justified, clinically comprehensive approach to peri-viability: gynaecological, obstetric, perinatal, and neonatal dimensions. J Obstet Gynaecol 2007; 21: 3–7.

2. *Roe v. Wade*, 410 U.S. 113 (1973).

3. Oklahoma State Department of Health. Definition of Live Birth. Available at www.ok.gov/health/Birth_and_Death_Cert ificates/Birth_and_Death_Registration_(ROVER)/Stillbirth_R egistration_Training/Definition_of_Live_Birth.html (accessed March 1, 2019).

4. World Health Organization. 1950 definition of live birth. Available at www.gfmer.ch/Medical_education_En/Live_birt h_definition.htm (accessed March 1, 2019).

5. Tyson JE, Parikh NA, Langer J, et al. Intensive care for extreme prematurity – moving beyond gestational age. N Engl J Med 2008; 358: 1672–1681.

6. Eunice Kennedy Shriver National Institute of Child Health and Human Development. NICHD Neonatal Research Network (NRN). Extremely preterm birth outcome data. Available at www1.nichd.nih.gov/epbo-calculator/Pages/epbo_case.aspx (accessed March 1, 2019).

7. American College of Obstetricians and Gynecologists and the Society for Maternal-Fetal Medicine. Ecker JL, Kaimal A, Mercer BM, Blackwell SC, et al. Obstetric Care Consensus. #6 Periviable Birth. Obstet Gynecol 2017; 130: e187–e198.

8. Raju TNK, Mercer BM, Burchfield DJ, Joseph GF. Periviable birth. Executive summary of a joint workshop by the Eunice Kennedy Shriver National Institute of Child Health and Human Development, Society for Maternal–Fetal Medicine, American Academy of Pediatrics, and American College of Obstetricians and Gynecologists. Obstet Gynecol 2014; 123: 1083–1096.

9. American College of Obstetricians and Gynecologists and the Society for Maternal-Fetal Medicine. Obstetric Care Consensus, Number 6: Periviable Birth. Obstet Gynecol 2017; 130: 926–928.

10. American Academy of Pediatrics. Committee on Bioethics. Informed consent, parental permission, and assent in pediatric practice. Pediatrics 1995; 95: 314–317.

11. American Academy of Pediatrics. Katz AL, Webb SA, AAP Committee on Bioethics. Informed consent in decision-making in pediatric practice. Pediatrics 2016; 138: e20161485.

12. Skupski DW, McCullough LB, Levene M, Chervenak FA. Improving obstetric estimation of outcomes of extremely premature neonates: an evolving challenge. J Perinat Med 2010; 38: 19–22.

13. Brett AS, McCullough LB. When patients request specific interventions: defining the limits of the physician's obligation. N Engl J Med 1986; 315: 1347–1351.

14. Brett AS, McCullough LB. Addressing requests by patients for nonbeneficial interventions. JAMA 2012; 307: 149–150.

15. Whitney SN, McCullough LB, Frugé E, McGuire AL, Volk RJ. Beyond breaking bad news: the roles of hope and hopefulness. Cancer 2008; 114: 442–445.

Chapter 12: Intrapartum Management

GOAL
This chapter provides an ethical framework to guide decision making about intrapartum management.

OBJECTIVES
On completing study of this chapter, the reader will:

Identify a preventive ethics approach to cesarean delivery

Describe ethically justified intrapartum use of cephalocentesis

Describe an ethically justified response to refusal of cesarean delivery

Describe an ethically justified approach to decision making with, by, and for pregnant patients with mental disorders and illnesses

Explain how continuation of pregnancy in a patient in a permanent vegetative state and in a cadaver is an experiment

Describe ethically justified responses to requests for cesarean delivery

Describe an ethically justified response to the interest of pregnant patients in planned home birth

Apply the ethical framework to guide decision making about intrapartum management in clinical practice

TOPICS

12.1 The Continuum of Vaginal Delivery and Cesarean Delivery	149
12.2 Preventive Ethics for Cesarean Delivery	149
12.2.1 Preventive Ethics	149
12.2.2 The Goal of Preventive Ethics	149
12.2.3 The Informed Consent Process as Preventive Ethics	150
12.2.4 The Role of Recommendations	150
12.2.5 When Both Vaginal and Cesarean Delivery Are Medically Reasonable	150
12.3 Cephalocentesis	151
12.3.1 Isolated Fetal Hydrocephalus	151
12.3.2 Hydrocephalus with Severe Associated Abnormalities	151
12.3.3 Hydrocephalus with Other Associated Anomalies	152
12.4 Refusal of Cesarean Delivery	152
12.4.1 Refusal of Cesarean Delivery and Termination of Relationship with the Obstetrician	152
12.4.2 Refusal of Cesarean Delivery and Election of the Medically Reasonable Alternative of Vaginal Delivery	152
12.4.3 Refusal of Cesarean Delivery When It Is the Only Medically Reasonable Alternative: A Negative Right Coupled to a Positive Right	152

Section 3: Professionally Responsible Clinical Practice

        12.4.3.1 The Role of the Professional Virtue of Integrity in Professional Ethics in Obstetrics and Gynecology   152
   12.4.4 Antepartum Refusal   153
   12.4.5 Intrapartum Refusal   153
        12.4.5.1 Refusal of Cesarean Delivery for Well-Documented, Intrapartum, Complete Placenta Previa and for Severe Placental Abruption   153
        12.4.5.2 Refusal of Cesarean Delivery for Severe Fetal Distress and Prolapsed Umbilical Cord   154
   12.4.6 Court Orders for Forced Cesarean Delivery   154
12.5 Decision Making With, By, and For Pregnant Patients with Mental Disorders and Illnesses   154
   12.5.1 Managing Powerful Responses   154
   12.5.2 Informed Consent, Assisted Consent, and Surrogate Decision Making   155
        12.5.2.1 Assessment of Decision-Making Capacity   155
        12.5.2.2 The Informed Consent Process   155
        12.5.2.3 Assisted Decision Making   155
        12.5.2.4 Surrogate Decision Making   155
   12.5.3 Treatment Is Accepted by the Patient   155
   12.5.4 Treatment Is Not Accepted by the Patient   157
        12.5.4.1 Attempt Assent   157
        12.5.4.2 When Beneficence-Based Ethical Obligations Should Guide Clinical Management   157
12.6 Continuing a Pregnancy in a Patient in a Permanent Vegetative State and in a Cadaver   157
   12.6.1 Continuing Pregnancy Is an Experiment   157
12.7 Responding to Requests for Cesarean Delivery   158
   12.7.1 Preventing Involuntary Requests   158
12.8 Planned Home Birth   158
   12.8.1 Planned Home Birth Is Inconsistent with Patient Safety   158
   12.8.2 Implications for Counseling Women Who Express an Interest in a Planned Home Birth   159
        12.8.2.1 The Role of Recommendations   159
        12.8.2.2 Making Recommendations Supports, Not Impairs, Patient Autonomy   160

Key Concepts

Assent
Assisted decision making
Deliberative clinical judgment
Ethical concept of the fetus as a patient
Ethical concept of medicine as a profession
Ethical principle of beneficence in professional ethics in obstetrics
Ethical principle of nonmaleficence in professional ethics in obstetrics and gynecology
Ethical principle of respect for autonomy in professional ethics in obstetrics
Experiment
Informed consent process
Innovation
Medically reasonable
Pregnant patient
Professional ethics in obstetrics and gynecology
Research
Safety
Surrogate decision making
Ulysses contract

12.1 The Continuum of Vaginal Delivery and Cesarean Delivery

Most women deliver their babies vaginally. Vaginal delivery is clearly safer for the pregnant patient because no invasive clinical management is involved, even when fetal monitoring takes place. This clinical reality makes assisting vaginal delivery the default in clinical judgment, placing the burden of proof on justifying cesarean delivery. As a consequence, in traditional obstetric thinking, cesarean delivery is either indicated – the burden of proof is met – or nonindicated – the burden of proof is not met. When cesarean delivery is indicated, it should be recommended. When cesarean delivery is not indicated, it should not be offered, much less recommended.

As convenient and powerful as this traditional obstetric thinking has become, it is not clinically adequate. There are conditions in which both vaginal delivery and cesarean delivery are medically reasonable, i.e., technically possible and supported in beneficence-based clinical judgment. (See Chapters 1 and 2.) For example, after a previous low transverse incision both planned cesarean delivery and trial of labor after cesarean (TOLAC) in appropriately equipped and staffed hospitals are medically reasonable.[1] In the informed consent process the pregnant woman should be empowered with an account of both their clinical benefits and risks. The pregnant woman is free to authorize either, based on her values and beliefs.

There is therefore a continuum from vaginal delivery as the only medically reasonable alternative, which is most of the time, to both vaginal delivery and planned cesarean delivery as medically reasonable, to planned cesarean delivery as the only medically reasonable alternative.[1,2] For the two extremes of this continuum the obstetrician's clinical judgment is evidence based and beneficence based but not autonomy based. Counseling of the patient should be directive, in the form of a recommendation for vaginal delivery or planned cesarean delivery, respectively. For the mid-range of this continuum, the patient's values and beliefs are decisive. Shared decision making is a phrase without a fixed meaning.[3,4] Sometimes it is understood as a process that should start with the patient's values and beliefs and be guided throughout by respect for patient autonomy.[4,5] Inasmuch as directive counseling is justified when there is only one medically reasonable alternative for mode of delivery, shared decision making should not be understood to be a universal model for decision making about mode of delivery.[3,6] We therefore take a more clinically and ethically nuanced approach to the professional ethics of intrapartum management.

12.2 Preventive Ethics for Cesarean Delivery

12.2.1 Preventive Ethics

Cesarean delivery is invasive surgery and therefore entails clinical risks. Informed consent is therefore required,[6] as explained in Chapter 3. Leading an adequate informed consent process in the intrapartum period can be challenging, given the distractions of labor and the momentum for surgical intervention that can build as maternal or fetal indications justifiably come to dominate clinical judgment. There also can be insufficient time to meet the requirements of informed refusal (see Chapter 3), when a pregnant woman refuses to authorize cesarean delivery.

The best way to address this ethical challenge is with preventive ethics.[7] Preventive ethics uses the informed consent process to anticipate, prevent, and responsibly manage the potential for ethical conflict between the pregnant woman and her obstetrician. (See Chapter 3.) During prenatal visits, not taking a preventive ethics approach to decision making with pregnant patients about cesarean delivery should be understood as an unacceptable, missed opportunity. The obstetrician should aim to prepare the pregnant woman for a rush of decision making about cesarean delivery, so that it does not overwhelm her autonomy or birth experience.

12.2.2 The Goal of Preventive Ethics

The goal of a preventive ethics approach to informed consent for cesarean delivery is to empower the pregnant woman with information about cesarean delivery that she may need later. Given time and adequate support, pregnant women demonstrate the capacity to make informed, scientifically sophisticated decisions about their medical care, e.g., the use of invasive prenatal diagnosis on the basis of the results of non-invasive risk assessment to make decisions about invasive diagnosis in advance of the potential need for it.[8]

12.2.3 The Informed Consent Process as Preventive Ethics

An adequate informed consent process for cesarean delivery takes time. This process by its very nature requires the pregnant woman to give her attention to her obstetrician, listen carefully, think through and carefully assess the benefits and risks of cesarean delivery, and appreciate that, for maternal or fetal indications, cesarean delivery can become the only medically reasonable alternative for delivery. All of this takes time and a minimum of distraction, which are difficult to achieve under well-documented time constraints.[9] Obstetricians can and should take advantage of the fact that most pregnant women are seen prenatally, some even preconception, creating multiple opportunities for a preventive ethics approach to informed consent for cesarean delivery.

As part of routine prenatal care, every pregnant woman should be informed that cesarean delivery occurs in about one third of pregnancies.[10] Every pregnant woman should also appreciate that a low-risk pregnancy can change rapidly into a high-risk pregnancy during the intrapartum period and that cesarean delivery may become necessary for either maternal or fetal indications. The obstetrician should elicit the patient's attitudes about cesarean delivery and tailor subsequent information accordingly.

For some women, depending on their medical condition and informational needs, decisions about cesarean delivery require more than this general information that every pregnant women should receive. For these women, the obstetrician should explain that cesarean delivery is not always dichotomous,[1,2] as explained in Section 12.1. The obstetrician should explain that vaginal delivery is the default delivery mode in beneficence-based deliberative clinical judgment. The medical reasonableness of vaginal delivery, however, decreases as the evidence base in support of cesarean delivery increases. At some point the evidence for each might be in equipoise – a deliberative clinical judgment that the obstetrician should become uncertain about which is clinically superior.

12.2.4 The Role of Recommendations

The obstetrician should explain to pregnant women how the alternatives will be assessed in clinical judgment. When the evidence base for cesarean delivery is very strong, e.g., well-documented intrapartum complete placenta previa, there is no uncertainty about the relative clinical benefit of cesarean delivery. In such clinical circumstances, vaginal delivery becomes no longer medically reasonable. It follows that the obstetrician has a prima facie beneficence-based ethical obligation to recommend cesarean delivery. The strength of such recommendations should be directly proportional to the strength of the evidence base for relative clinical benefit of cesarean delivery.

The obstetrician should explain that sometimes planned cesarean delivery is justifiably recommended in advance of the intrapartum period, e.g., when there is a history of a previous classical cesarean delivery. The obstetrician should also explain that cesarean delivery is sometimes justifiably recommended during the intrapartum period, e.g., for newly diagnosed fetal distress, with the strength of the recommendation a direct function of the strength of evidence for the prediction of a poor neonatal outcome. Such discussion prepares the woman for the immediacy and urgency of both expected and unexpected intrapartum complications and lays the foundation for the rapid decision making that might become necessary during the intrapartum period.

12.2.5 When Both Vaginal and Cesarean Delivery Are Medically Reasonable

When the evidence base for cesarean delivery is not clear cut, e.g., previous low transverse cesarean delivery in a woman in her second pregnancy, both cesarean delivery and TOLAC are medically reasonable.[1,11,12] In such clinical circumstances, the obstetrician has the prima facie autonomy-based ethical obligation to offer both but refrain temporarily from making a recommendation until the pregnant woman has had the opportunity to think though both alternatives. This approach allows the pregnant woman to exercise her capacity for autonomous decision making without being unduly influenced by her obstetrician's views. If deliberative clinical judgment supports one alternative relative to the other, the obstetrician may then recommend it for the pregnant woman's consideration.

A preventive ethics approach to the informed consent process for cesarean delivery should at long last become an accepted component of routine obstetric care.[13] Taking a preventive ethics approach to the informed consent process for cesarean delivery should be expected to enhance the autonomy of pregnant women, by preparing them to cope more effectively with the complexity and urgency of decision making about cesarean delivery. A preventive ethics approach creates the opportunity to identify and resolve potential conflicts about cesarean delivery before the rush and intensity of the intrapartum period.[7]

12.3 Cephalocentesis

Cephalocentesis involves the drainage of an enlarged fetal head, secondary to hydrocephalus.[14,15] Fetal hydrocephalus is caused by obstruction of cerebrospinal flow and is diagnosed by such sonographic signs as dilatation of the atrium or body of the lateral ventricles.[16] In the third trimester, macrocephaly often accompanies the ventriculomegaly. In addition, sonography can diagnose hydrocephalus in association with gross abnormalities suggestive of poor prognosis, for example, hydranencephaly, microcephaly, encephalocele, alobar holoprosencephaly, or thanatophoric dysplasia with cloverleaf skull.[16] In the absence of defined anatomical abnormalities, however, diagnostic imaging is, at the present time, unable to predict the outcome. Although cortical mantle thickness can be measured with ultrasound, its value as a prognostic index is not established.[17]

Cephalocentesis should be performed under simultaneous ultrasound guidance so that needle placement into the cerebrospinal fluid is facilitated. An 18-gauge needle is used with subsequent collapse of the cranial bones, the endpoint for this procedure. Enough fluid is drained to permit reduction of the skull diameters so that passage through the birth canal is possible.[15,16] Cephalocentesis is a potentially destructive procedure. Perinatal death following cephalocentesis has been reported in more than 90% of cases.[14] The sonographic visualization of intracranial bleeding during cephalocentesis, and the demonstration of this hemorrhage at autopsy, further emphasize the morbid nature of the procedure. However, if decompression is performed in a controlled manner, the risk of mortality may be reduced.

12.3.1 Isolated Fetal Hydrocephalus

There is considerable potential for normal, sometimes superior, intellectual function for fetuses with even extreme, isolated hydrocephalus.[18–21] However, as a group, infants with isolated hydrocephalus experience a greater incidence of intellectual disability and early death than the general population. In addition, associated anomalies may go undetected, and a fetus may be incorrectly diagnosed as having isolated hydrocephalus.[17]

Given the outcomes of isolated hydrocephalus, there is no beneficence-based justification to undertake a potentially destructive procedure, the outcomes of which can be avoided by cesarean delivery. The probability of intellectual disability does not alter this judgment because it is impossible to predict which fetuses with isolated hydrocephalus will have cognitive disability and because the degree of cognitive disability cannot be reliably predicted in advance. The obstetrician therefore has a strong prima facie ethical obligation to recommend planned cesarean delivery as the medically reasonable alternative.

If the pregnant woman continues to refuse cesarean delivery and respectful persuasion (see Chapter 3) fails to gain her consent, the physician confronts tragic circumstances. If neither cesarean delivery nor cephalocentesis is performed, the woman is at risk for uterine rupture and death, and the fetal patient is at risk for death. There is a nonmaleficence-based prima facie ethical obligation to prevent these outcomes, because they result in serious, far-reaching, and irreversible harm to both the pregnant and the fetal patient. In the face of unyielding refusal to authorize cesarean delivery, the only way to fulfill this ethical obligation is to perform cephalocentesis in the least destructive way possible or to make an appropriate referral.

12.3.2 Hydrocephalus with Severe Associated Abnormalities

Some abnormalities that occur in association with fetal hydrocephalus are severe in nature for the child afflicted with them. "Severe" abnormalities are those that either are incompatible with continued existence, e.g., bilateral renal agenesis or thanatophoric dysplasia with cloverleaf skull, or compatible with survival in some cases but result in virtual absence of cognitive function, e.g., trisomy 13 or alobar holoprosencephaly.[17,22] In such clinical circumstances, the fetus' condition creates an unavoidable risk of serious, far-reaching, and irreversible harm. In nonmaleficence-based clinical judgment, performing cephalocentesis does not add a significant increment of such harm. Offering and performing cephalocentesis when the fetus has hydrocephalus with severe associated anomalies is ethically permissible. The obstetrician may justifiably recommend a choice between cesarean delivery and cephalocentesis to enable vaginal delivery.

12.3.3 Hydrocephalus with Other Associated Anomalies

On the continuum between the extreme cases of isolated hydrocephalus and hydrocephalus with severe associated abnormalities, there are cases of hydrocephalus associated with macrocephaly with other abnormalities with varying degrees of impairment of cognitive physical function. They range from hypoplastic distal phalanges to spina bifida to encephalocele.[17] Because these conditions have varying prognoses, it would be clinically inappropriate and therefore ethically misleading to treat this third category as homogeneous. Therefore we propose a working distinction between different kinds of prognoses. Some are "probably promising," by which we mean that there is a significant possibility the child will experience cognitive development with learning disabilities and physical handicaps that perhaps can be ameliorated to some extent. Some are "probably poor," by which we mean that there is only a limited possibility for cognitive development because of learning disabilities and physical disabilities that cannot be ameliorated to a significant extent.

When the clinical prognosis is probably promising, the obstetrician should be guided by the ethical reasoning about isolated fetal hydrocephalus described in Section 12.3.1. When the prognosis is probably poor, the obstetrician should be guided by the ethical reasoning about hydrocephalus with severe associated anomalies described in Section 12.3.2.

12.4 Refusal of Cesarean Delivery

Refusal of cesarean is a rare event. Some clinical circumstances are ethically significant even though rare and that is the case for refusal of cesarean delivery in professional ethics in obstetrics.

12.4.1 Refusal of Cesarean Delivery and Termination of Relationship with the Obstetrician

Sometimes a pregnant patient refuses clinical management that has been offered or recommended and terminates the physician–patient relationship. To fulfill the requirements of informed refusal, she should be informed about the risks that she is taking for herself and her pregnancy. The physician should implement the respectful persuasion process and ask her to reconsider. The physician should also assure her that she is free to return for care. (See Chapter 3.)

12.4.2 Refusal of Cesarean Delivery and Election of the Medically Reasonable Alternative of Vaginal Delivery

Sometimes a patient refuses one form of medically reasonable clinical management that has been offered and opts for another form of medically reasonable clinical management. This poses no ethical challenges, as her preferred course of care is a medically reasonable alternative because only medically reasonable alternatives should be offered in the informed consent process. (See Chapter 2).

12.4.3 Refusal of Cesarean Delivery When It Is the Only Medically Reasonable Alternative: A Negative Right Coupled to a Positive Right

Sometimes a patient refuses the only medically reasonable form of clinical management and remains a patient. This means that her refusal, the exercise of a negative right, is necessarily coupled with an implicit or explicit request for clinical management that is technically possible but in deliberative clinical judgment is reliably predicted to result in net clinical harm for the fetal and neonatal patient. To treat such refusal as simply the exercise of the patient's autonomy is both clinically and conceptually inaccurate. The nature of the positive right must be considered, as well as its limits, because positive rights always come with limits.[23]

12.4.3.1 The Role of the Professional Virtue of Integrity in Professional Ethics in Obstetrics and Gynecology

One limit in professional ethics in obstetrics and gynecology is the professional virtue of integrity.[24,25] This virtue requires a commitment to intellectual integrity, which is carried out by providing only clinical management that is medically reasonable. Failure to meet this requirement puts the patient at unnecessary, preventable clinical risk, which is incompatible with moral integrity and with the beneficence-based and nonmaleficence-based ethical obligation to prevent implementation of clinical management that in deliberative clinical judgment is reliably expected to result in net clinical harm.

The strength of these ethical obligations is a direct function of the evidence for the predictions of outcomes and gravity of harm. When the evidence is strong, the ethical obligation is strong and not fulfilling it bears a steep burden of proof. When the evidence is somewhat strong, the ethical obligation is strong and not fulfilling it bears a less-than-steep burden of proof. When the predicted harm is serious, far-reaching, and irreversible, the ethical obligation to prevent it is strong because failure to do so violates the ethical principles of beneficence and nonmaleficence in professional ethics in obstetrics. When the predicted harm is less than serious, not far-reaching, and manageable even when irreversible, not preventing it may be permissible.

12.4.4 Antepartum Refusal

Some pregnant women may express a preference against cesarean delivery, e.g., in their birth plans. The obstetrician should use the preventive ethics approach to cesarean delivery described in Section 12.2 to work with the pregnant woman to transform her request into an informed decision. Counseling should be directive and include explaining that, should cesarean delivery become the only medically reasonable alternative for intrapartum management, it will be recommended. Counseling should also include respectful persuasion, especially pointing out that cesarean delivery in such clinical circumstances will support the value that the woman places on a good outcome for her pregnancy for her child at acceptable risk to herself.

12.4.5 Intrapartum Refusal

Intrapartum refusal of cesarean delivery is a rare event because almost always the obstetrician and the pregnant woman agree that a cesarean delivery should be performed. Refusal is ethically significant in two clinical circumstances. The first is when cesarean delivery benefits the pregnant, fetal, and neonatal patient. The second is when cesarean delivery benefits the fetal and neonatal patients at reasonable risk to the pregnant patient.

12.4.5.1 Refusal of Cesarean Delivery for Well-Documented, Intrapartum, Complete Placenta Previa and for Severe Placental Abruption

For well-documented, intrapartum, complete placenta previa and severe placental abruption the probability of perinatal and maternal death can approach 100%. Death is a serious, far-reaching, and irreversible harm to the pregnant, the fetal, and the neonatal patient. The risk of this harm can be greatly reduced by cesarean delivery, because it essentially eliminates maternal mortality and greatly reduces perinatal mortality. The pregnant patient has a prima facie beneficence-based ethical obligation to take only reasonable risks to herself for fetal benefit; she surely has an ethical obligation to accept benefit to her for fetal benefit. For these two diagnoses, cesarean delivery results in no net risk of harm but unequivocal net clinical benefit for the pregnant patient. For these diagnoses, given this ethical analysis, refusal of cesarean delivery coupled with a request for vaginal delivery is not compatible with the professional virtue of integrity.

Her refusal should not be implemented. If she does not physically resist preparation for surgery the team should proceed. The obstetrician should explain what is being done and why but this should not be mistaken for the informed consent process or the informed refusal process, for neither of which is there adequate time. This approach does commit the team to ethically justified paternalism: interfering with the patient's autonomy for her clinical good. Ordinarily, paternalism faces a steep burden of proof. This burden can be met in cases like this, because her autonomy is already limited by her beneficence-based obligation to the fetal patient and because she has an undeniable, strong, and legitimate self-interest in preventing her own death. Those who would reject this line of ethical reasoning are implicitly committed to the view that the ethical principle of respect for autonomy in professional ethics in obstetrics is an absolute and not prima facie ethical principle that sweeps away the constraints of professional integrity.

This deprofessionalization of obstetrics bears a steep burden of proof,[26] which its proponents have not provided. George Annas, for example, assumes that such a reading of the ethical principle of respect for autonomy requires no ethical justification.[27] Howard Minkoff takes the same position, again without supporting argument.[28] Unfortunately for this view that the ethical principle of respect for autonomy is an absolute ethical principle, it has fatal flaws. This is ideology, not ethical reasoning.

12.4.5.2 Refusal of Cesarean Delivery for Severe Fetal Distress and Prolapsed Umbilical Cord

For severe fetal distress and prolapsed umbilical cord, the evidence base for a prediction of high probability of perinatal mortality and morbidity is strong. Cesarean delivery greatly reduces this probability. Cesarean delivery creates small but manageable risks of maternal morbidity. However, these risks should be considered reasonable in beneficence-based clinical judgment because in hospitals committed to patient safety and quality, these risks have been responsibly managed to a minimum. Cesarean delivery may also result in psychosocial benefit to the woman of reducing adverse neonatal outcomes.

Insisting that the patient accept cesarean delivery should be understood as ethically justified paternalism: imposing the judgment on the pregnant patient that she should want to accept the known, minimized risks of cesarean delivery for the benefit of reduced risk of perinatal mortality and morbidity to her soon-to-be born child. Objection to justified paternalism requires adopting respect for autonomy as an absolute ethical principle with its attendant ethical problems described in Section 12.4.5.1.

The obstetrician should respond to refusal of cesarean delivery with an abbreviated informed refusal process, informing the pregnant patient that the time window for potentially beneficial cesarean delivery is closing, and asking her to reconsider her refusal and authorize cesarean delivery while it is still supported in deliberative clinical judgment.

12.4.6 Court Orders for Forced Cesarean Delivery

In the scholarly literature of health law and bioethics, the justification for obtaining court orders in response to refusal of cesarean delivery is hotly disputed. The legal reality, however, is that, depending on the reason for cesarean delivery, some jurisdictions grant orders and some do not. There is a beneficence-based prohibition against increasing the risk of biopsychosocial harm that will fail to produce net clinical benefit. In jurisdictions in which court orders are highly unlikely to be forthcoming, they should not be mentioned and should not be sought. In jurisdictions in which a court order is likely to be forthcoming, there should be clear organizational policy setting out the procedure to be followed. Such a policy must be approved at the highest organizational levels, so that the obstetrics team can be confident that they will be fully supported when they implement such organizational policy.

12.5 Decision Making With, By, and For Pregnant Patients with Mental Disorders and Illnesses

Studies have reported that 2% of women have nonaffective psychotic disorders, and approximately half of these women give birth.[29,30] Given that this prevalence does not account for affective psychosis or agitation and that the age at onset for most of these illnesses is during late adolescence and early adulthood, it is not uncommon for obstetricians to encounter patients with major mental disorders at the time of delivery. Major mental disorders during pregnancy may be compounded by unrecognized medical problems, poor self-care, sexual exploitation, and victimization.[31,32] These women can also experience unstable living circumstances including homelessness, lack of supportive relationships including absentee fathers, lack of access to both mental health and obstetric care, and lack of integration of psychiatric and obstetric care.[33,34] Furthermore, the use of nicotine, alcohol, and cocaine is more common among women with major mental disorders, including schizophrenia, than in the general population.[33,34] Denial of pregnancy is a particular problem, not uncommon to this population, and related to a lack of antenatal care and precipitous deliveries.[35] Paranoia and agitation, in turn, can undermine a woman's ability to comply with obstetric recommendations, especially during the intrapartum period. Although women with major mental disorders often have normal pregnancies and deliveries, the risk of adverse obstetric events and outcomes is increased in this population.[36-39] In short, pregnant women with major mental disorders present obstetricians with a range of clinical challenges.[33]

12.5.1 Managing Powerful Responses

These clinical challenges, singly or in combination, can understandably evoke powerful responses, ranging from concern to frustration, foreboding, and even fear for the health and life of the pregnant, fetal, and neonatal patient.[33,40] These responses can be magnified when the patient presents in labor with a psychosis or agitation and there is limited time for decision making. These responses can bias clinical judgment and the obstetrician's capacity for professionally responsible decision making. To manage this bias, the obstetrician should deploy informed consent, followed by assisted consent and surrogate decision making, as needed. (See Chapter 3.)

12.5.2 Informed Consent, Assisted Consent, and Surrogate Decision Making

The concepts of informed consent, assisted consent, assent, and surrogate decision making described in Chapter 3 can be used to create an algorithm to guide decision making with pregnant patients with mental disorders and illnesses[41] (Figure 12.1).

12.5.2.1 Assessment of Decision-Making Capacity

The first step implements the presumption of decision-making capacity for this population of patients, who are at risk of impaired decision-making capacity from the chronically and variably impaired autonomy that is a distinguishing feature of major mental illness. Concern about the presumption of capacity may also be justifiably triggered by the woman's denial of pregnancy or refusal of recommended intrapartum management. Such clinically legitimate concerns do not defeat the presumption. The patient's decision-making capacity should be carefully assessed.

12.5.2.2 The Informed Consent Process

If the patient's decision-making capacity is intact, then decision making about intrapartum management should be guided by the informed consent process. The algorithm should be held in reserve to guide decision making in response to acute changes in decision-making capacity, such as sudden onset of paranoia or anxiety.

12.5.2.3 Assisted Decision Making

When patients are reliably judged to have significantly impaired decision-making capacity, assisted decision making should be attempted. One component is verbal interventions, such as reminding the woman about how her mental illness can impair her judgment. Verbal interventions can also include reminding her about long-standing values and preferences, including a good outcome to her pregnancy for herself, the fetal patient, and newborn, all of which may be reasonably presumed to be of value by virtue of having carried her pregnancy through to term. The obstetrician should appeal to these values, explain how proposed clinical management supports them, and ask the pregnant woman to accept the proposed clinical management. This is called respectful persuasion. (See Chapter 3.) Another component of assisted decision making is rapidly acting pharmacologic interventions that are relatively safe for the pregnant, fetal, and neonatal patients.[42] Medications, including benzodiazepines and antipsychotics, can be administered by mouth or by injection. It should be appreciated that these agents may, in the short term, not eliminate paranoia or anxiety or reverse denial of pregnancy. However, administering such medications may calm patients sufficiently to enable them to be successful at assisted decision making.

12.5.2.4 Surrogate Decision Making

When attempts at assisted decision making fail, surrogate decision making should be deployed. Decisions at this point will need to be made for the patient, guided in priority order by the substituted judgment standard, to actively incorporate the patient's preferences, and then by the best interests standard. Some patients may have consented to intrapartum management for maternal or fetal benefit in advance, which can be documented with what is known as a Ulysses contract. (See Chapter 3.) Endorsement by the surrogate decision making of such advance consent is ethically required, because it meets the substituted judgment standard of surrogate decision making. (See Chapter 3.) Often, the patient may not have available a legally designated surrogate. In such circumstances the obstetrician must become the patient's surrogate, with input from all team members aiming to make a deliberative surrogate decision, based on the substituted judgment or best interests standard as appropriate. Organizational policy governing decision making should explicitly identify and support this role.

12.5.3 Treatment Is Accepted by the Patient

If treatment is accepted, it should be implemented. We emphasize that the basis for this is not informed consent but rather the assent of the pregnant woman.

Section 3: Professionally Responsible Clinical Practice

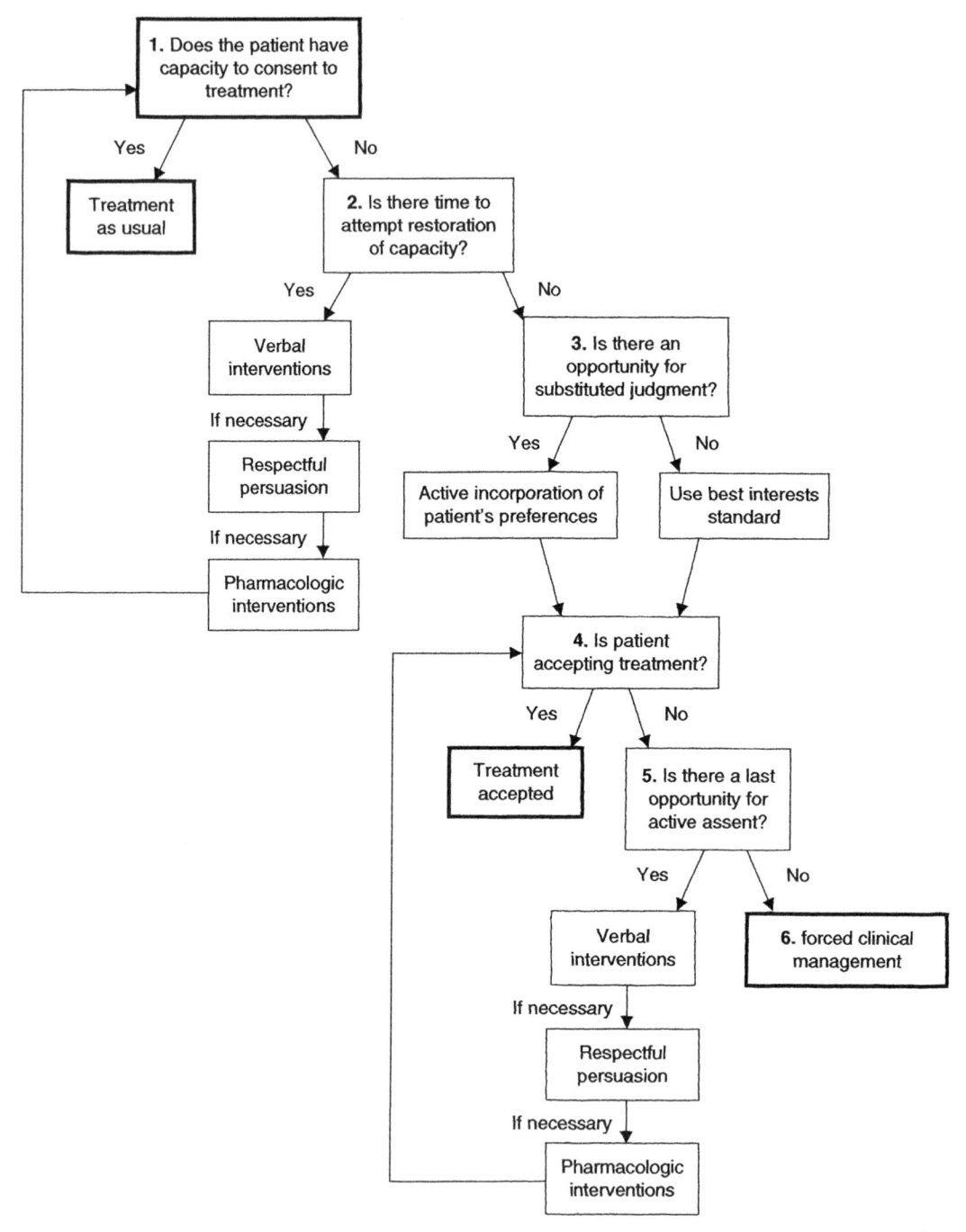

Figure 12.1 Algorithm for professionally responsible intrapartum management of patients with major mental disorders.[41]

12.5.4 Treatment Is Not Accepted by the Patient

12.5.4.1 Attempt Assent

Sometimes a patient who has significantly impaired decision-making capacity refuses treatment and attempts at respectful persuasion fail. The response should be one last attempt to obtain assent by recycling verbal and pharmacologic efforts to support assisted decision making and respectful persuasion. For example, the salutary effects on decision-making capacity of a short-acting medication may diminish or disappear during the course of prolonged labor. A change in caregiver may facilitate this last attempt to obtain assent. Documenting how the five questions in the algorithm were addressed should be incorporated into the obstetrician's post-delivery record entry.

12.5.4.2 When Beneficence-Based Ethical Obligations Should Guide Clinical Management

When all attempts at assisted decision making fail and the patient continues not to accept treatment, beneficence-based ethical obligations to the fetal patient become the guiding consideration. Postponing cesarean delivery may also increase the potential for maternal complications, especially from poorly controlled paranoia and anxiety. In such clinical circumstances, proceeding to cesarean delivery becomes ethically justified. This may be the ethically the least worst alternative – compared to nonintervention. The obstetrician should explain what is going to happen to minimize confusion, fear, and psychological trauma and proceed to coerced clinical management. The obstetrician and care team should be alert to signs and symptoms of postraumatic stress disorder in the months following delivery.[43]

12.6 Continuing a Pregnancy in a Patient in a Permanent Vegetative State and in a Cadaver

A permanent vegetative state is defined by the American Academy of Neurology (AAN) as an irreversible loss of awareness.[44] It is often the case that younger patients who have progressed to a permanent vegetative state after a brain injury or event do not require life-sustaining treatment. Such patients retain the physiological capacity to continue a pregnancy.

When a pregnant patient who has been on life-sustaining treatment has been determined to meet AAN brain-function criteria[45] and is therefore dead, it is possible to continue such treatment and retain a physiologic-technical capacity of the fresh cadaver to continue a pregnancy. This means that the first component of being a medically reasonable alternative, being technically possible, is satisfied.

The second condition, however, is not, because there is no evidence of net clinical benefit for the fetal and neonatal patient. There is no published evidence base to support in deliberative clinical judgment the prediction that continued pregnancy in a patient in a permanent vegetative state will result in net clinical benefit for the fetal and neonatal patient. A retrospective view of the outcomes of pregnancies sustained in cadavers indicates that the outcomes vary considerably and include fetal demise and neonatal mortality and morbidity.[46] There is therefore no evidence base to support in deliberative clinical judgment the prediction that continued pregnancy in a patient in a permanent vegetative state will result in net clinical benefit for the fetal and neonatal patient.

12.6.1 Continuing Pregnancy Is an Experiment

The two forms of obstetric management described in Section 12.6 must therefore be considered, not medically reasonable, but experimental. Either the experiment is undertaken to benefit an individual fetal and neonatal patient, in which case the experiment is planned innovation (see Chapter 17) or the experiment is undertaken to produce generalizable knowledge, in which case the experiment is research. (See Chapter 17.) There is an ethical obligation to obtain prior review and approval of planned innovation for its scientific, clinical, and ethical justification by a committee constituted for this purpose. (See Chapter 17.) There is an ethical and legal obligation to obtain prior review and approval of research by the Institutional Review Board for one's organization (See Chapter 17). It is not at all clear that such approval will be forthcoming.

The ethical judgment that continued pregnancy in these clinical circumstances should be classified as innovation or research means that it can never to be presented to a surrogate decision maker, organizational leaders, or the public as treatment, much less medically reasonable treatment. If approval is forthcoming, the informed consent process must make this very clear, along with its implication: there is never an ethical obligation for a surrogate decision maker to authorize an experiment. This means that refusing to authorize innovation or to enroll the patient or cadaver in a research protocol does not violate any beneficence-based ethical obligation to the fetal patient, when the fetus is a patient.

12.7 Responding to Requests for Cesarean Delivery

Cesarean delivery when it is not supported in beneficence-based deliberative clinical judgment cannot be justified by appeal to fetal and neonatal net clinical benefit. Claims that there is maternal benefit from protection of the pelvic floor should in deliberative clinical judgment be considered controversial. At the same time, the clinical risks of cesarean delivery performed in a hospital committed to patient safety and quality should be considered reasonable in deliberative clinical judgment. The perinatal and neonatal risks of cesarean delivery are not serious, far-reaching, and irreversible. It follows that the obstetrician should respond with a recommendation against nonindicated cesarean delivery and recommend vaginal delivery,[47] so that the pregnant patient becomes aware that nonindicated cesarean delivery is not medically reasonable.

These recommendations should be repeated. If they are still not accepted and the patient is well informed about the risks of cesarean delivery, implementing an informed decision for cesarean delivery that is not indicated is ethically permissible in professional ethics in obstetrics. We emphasize that a request that has not been transformed into an informed decision does not have this implication. The obstetrician should be clear in the patient's record and to her that the sole indication for cesarean delivery in such clinical circumstances is autonomy based.[48] If the patient's source of payment will not cover cesarean delivery that is solely autonomy based in its indication, the patient should be informed.

12.7.1 Preventing Involuntary Requests

This ethical reasoning also does not apply when the pregnant patient's decision-making process is involuntary. This occurs when she is subject to controlling influences or coercion (the use of force to control her decision making, accompanied by a threat of harm). The obstetrician should be alert to controlling influences and, especially, coercion and protect the pregnant patient from them so that she can make an informed *and* voluntary decision. If necessary to achieve this goal, the obstetrician should point out to those seeking such influence or control that their role is to support the pregnant patient's decision and not make decisions for her.

12.8 Planned Home Birth

12.8.1 Planned Home Birth Is Inconsistent with Patient Safety

Over the last decade there has been an increase in the United States of planned home births, although more recently the number of planned home births has leveled off. Planned home birth is one variant in the setting of childbirth; the hospital is another. The ethical permissibility of planned home birth is a function of whether planned home birth, as a variant of childbirth setting, is consistent with patient safety.

The commitment to the ethical concept of medicine as a profession requires all obstetricians to become and remain scientifically and clinically competent. To make and sustain this commitment, all obstetricians must commit to patient safety. Patient safety, therefore, becomes the required context for the assessment of absolute and relative risks of the processes and outcomes of patient care. Risk is defined as the potential of losing something of value, weighed against the potential to gain something of value. Valued states such as life and physical health can be gained or lost.[49] Risk assessment is more often than not expressed in relative risks (RR) rather than absolute risks.[50,51]

The concept of patient safety is directly linked to the commitment to quality of patient care, which is understood to be the responsible reduction of variation in the processes of patient care when that reduction improves outcomes. This is why the National Academy of Medicine (NAM) considers patient safety "indistinguishable from the delivery of quality health care."[52] The commitment to patient safety therefore requires the physician – and every other healthcare provider – to identify variations in the processes of patient care and to reduce variations when doing so results in improved outcomes, i.e., reduced relative risk of mortality and morbidity. Even when absolute risks are low, patient safety requires physicians and other healthcare providers not necessarily to reduce them to zero, but to responsibly and continuously minimize such risks. In the context of patient safety, the fact that absolute risks are very low does not by itself make these risks acceptable. Even when there are very low absolute risks, from the perspective of patient safety, a variant in the setting of childbirth should therefore be considered acceptable if and only if clinicians have responsibly minimized its very low absolute risks.

The concept of the paramount value of human life is at the heart of the commitment to patient safety. According to the Talmud: "... whoever saves a life, it is considered as if he saved an entire world ..."[53] Although this concept has ancient roots in Judaism, it has become a transreligious component of patient safety.

The focus on absolute risk is not a scientifically or clinically adequate basis for a determination that a clinical practice is consistent with the commitment to patient safety; relative risks must also be identified. Planned home births in the United States have been shown to be associated both with significantly increased absolute and relative risk of neonatal mortality and morbidity.[54-58] While absolute risks of total neonatal mortality in planned home births are low (1.26 per 1,000 live births), absolute risks of planned home births are significantly higher than midwife hospital births (1.26 versus 0.32/1,000 in midwife hospital births) with an elevated relative risk of 3.87.[54] Absolute risks for 5-minute Apgar score of zero in planned home births is also low (1.63/1,000) but significantly higher when compared to hospital midwives (1.63 vs. 0.09/1,000) with a relative risks of a 5-minute Apgar score of zero of 18.11.[55]

These data show that the increased relative risks of the birth-setting variant of planned home birth are preventable only by planned hospital birth, which includes birth in birthing centers directly attached to a hospital. This is because planned hospital birth eliminates an uncontrollable variable in planned home birth: the time for transfer, which far exceeds that which is accepted in deliberative clinical judgment in obstetrics.

The ethical concept of medicine as a profession requires a commitment to patient safety. The commitment to patient safety requires the reduction of variation when such reduction improves outcomes. Planned home birth, because of its preventable increased relative risks, is not consistent with the commitment to patient safety, because no improvement of planned home birth, including those proposed by the American Academy of Pediatrics,[59] can improve its safety given the unpreventable delay from transfer.

12.8.2 Implications for Counseling Women Who Express an Interest in a Planned Home Birth

Every obstetrician and other healthcare provider has a prima facie autonomy-based ethical obligation to communicate accurately and honestly with patients. To achieve accuracy, the provider should describe outcomes using both relative and absolute frequencies, to prevent confusion.[60] To achieve honesty, when the evidence is strong, the physician should engage in directive patient counseling in the form of making recommendations. Fulfilling this professional responsibility is essential for achieving patient safety in obstetrics and every other field of medicine. For example, healthcare professionals should: recommend immunization against influenza to all pregnant women; recommend screening for syphilis, HIV, and group B streptococcus during pregnancy; recommend cesarean delivery for placenta accreta,[61] advise against TOLAC after classic cesarean section[62]; recommend flu vaccination[63]; and advise against placentophagy.[64] Failure to undertake such directive counseling is an egregious clinical ethical error.

12.8.2.1 The Role of Recommendations

The evidence shows that planned home births have significantly increased absolute and relative risk of neonatal mortality and morbidity.[39-43] It is incompatible with the professional virtue of intellectual integrity to focus on low absolute risks and to ignore both increased relative and absolute risks and to not make recommendations against planned home births. The professional virtue of integrity creates the prima facie ethical obligation to respond with directive counseling of women who express an interest in planned home birth. Shared decision making is not appropriate. The obstetrician should make a strong recommendation against planned home birth, even though it has very low absolute risk, because these low absolute risks can be minimized with planned hospital births.

12.8.2.2 Making Recommendations Supports, Not Impairs, Patient Autonomy

Some take the view that making recommendations is incompatible with the ethical principle of respect for patient autonomy and they assert that recommendations discount patient values.[65,66] These objections should not be considered persuasive, because they assume that women are helpless pawns who will affirm whatever their obstetrician recommends. This assumption also profoundly disrespects the capacity of women to make their own healthcare decisions after having been empowered by their obstetricians with evidence-based clinical judgments and recommendations. Making a recommendation to improve outcomes does not diminish a woman's autonomy but empowers her to make an informed decision and still allows her to choose among options. Making recommendations is a mainstay of obstetric care and the obstetrician should not hesitate to engage in directive counseling when it is justified.[67]

References

1. Kalish RB, McCullough LB, Chervenak FA. Decision-making about caesarean delivery. Lancet 2006; 367: 883–845.
2. Nguyen MT, McCullough LB, Chervenak FA. The importance of clinically and ethically fine-tuning decision-making about cesarean delivery. J Perinat Med 2017; 45: 551–557.
3. McCullough LB. The professional medical ethics model of decisionmaking under conditions of uncertainty. Med Care Rev Res 2013; 70(1 Suppl): 141S–58S.
4. Kon AA. The shared decision-making continuum. JAMA 2010; 304: 903–904.
5. Chervenak FA, McCullough LB. The unlimited-rights model of obstetric ethics threatens professionalism. BJOG 2017; 124: 1144–1147.
6. Whitney SN, McGuire AL, McCullough LB. A typology of shared decision making, informed consent, and simple consent. Ann Intern Med 2003; 140: 54–59.
7. Chervenak FA, McCullough LB. Clinical guides to preventing ethical conflicts between pregnant women and their physicians. Am J Obstet Gynecol 1990; 162: 303–307.
8. Nicolaides KH, Chervenak FA, McCullough LB, et al. Evidence-based obstetric ethics and informed decision-making about invasive diagnosis after first-trimester assessment for risk of trisomy 21. Am J Obstet Gynecol 2005; 193: 322–326.
9. Salmeen K, Brincat C. Time from consent to cesarean delivery during labor. Am J Obstet Gynecol 2013; 209: 212.e1–6.
10. Martin JA, Hamilton BE, Ventura SJ, Osterman MJK, Wilson EC, Mathews TJ. Births: final data for 2010. U.S. Department of Health and Human Services. Centers for Disease Control and Prevention. National Vital Statistics Report. August 28, 2012; 61(1): 1–72. Available at www.cdc.gov/nchs/data/nvsr/nvsr61/nvsr61_01.pdf (accessed March 1, 2019).
11. National Institutes of Health consensus development conference statement: vaginal birth after cesarean: new insights, March 8–10, 2010. Obstet Gynecol 2010; 115: 1279–1295.
12. Chervenak FA, McCullough LB. An ethical framework for the informed consent process for trial of labor after cesarean delivery. Clin Perinatol 2011; 38: 227–231.
13. Chervenak FA, McCullough LB. Preventive ethics for cesarean delivery: the time has come. Am J Obstet Gynecol 2013; 209: 166–167.
14. Chervenak FA, Romero R. Is there a role for fetal cephalocentesis in modern obstetrics? Am J Perinatol 1984; 1: 170–173.
15. Chasen S, Chervenak FA, McCullough LB. The role of cephalocentesis in modern obstetrics. Am J Obstet Gynecol 2001; 185: 734–736.
16. Chervenak FA, Isaacson G, Campbell S. Anomalies of the cranium and its contents. In Textbook of Ultrasound in Obstetrics and Gynecology. Boston: Little, Brown, 1993: 825–852.
17. Chervenak FA, Berkowitz RL, Tortora M, et al. Management of fetal hydrocephalus. Am J Obstet Gynecol 1985; 151: 933–937.
18. Raimondi AJ, Soare P. Intellectual development in shunted hydrocephalic children. Am J Dis Child 1974; 127: 664.
19. McCullough DC, Balzer-Martin LA. Current prognosis in overt neonatal hydrocephalus. J Neurosurg 1982; 57: 378.
20. Sutton LN, Bruce DA, Schut L. Hydranencephaly versus maximal hydrocephalus: an important clinical distinction. Neurosurgery 1980; 6: 35.
21. Lorber J. The results of early treatment on extreme hydrocephalus. Med Child Neurol (Suppl) 1968; 16: 21.
22. Chervenak FA, McCullough LB. An ethically justified, clinically comprehensive management strategy for third-trimester pregnancies complicated by fetal anomalies. Obstet Gynecol 1990; 75: 311–316.
23. Chervenak FA, McCullough LB. Justified limits on refusing intervention. Hastings Cent Rep 1991; 21: 12–18.
24. Brett AS, McCullough LB. When patients request specific interventions: defining the limits of the physician's obligation. N Engl J Med 1986; 315: 1347–1351.
25. Brett AS, McCullough LB. Addressing requests by patients for non-beneficial interventions. JAMA 2012; 307: 149–150.
26. McCullough LB. Was bioethics founded on historical and conceptual mistakes about medical paternalism? Bioethics 2011; 25: 66–74.
27. Annas GJ. Protecting the liberty of pregnant patients. N Engl J Med 1987; 316: 1213–1214.
28. Minkoff H, Marshal MF, Liashenko J. The fetus and the "potential child," and the ethical obligations of obstetricians. Obstet Gynecol 2014; 123: 1100–1103.
29. DeSisto MJ, Harding CM, McCormick RV, et al. The Maine and Vermont three-decade studies of serious mental illness.

30. Howard LM, Kumar C, Leese M, et al. The general fertility rate in women with psychotic disorders. Am J Psychiatry 2002; 159: 991–997.

31. Miller LJ, Finnerty M. Sexuality, pregnancy, and childrearing among women with schizophrenia-spectrum disorders. Psychiatr Serv 1996; 47: 502–506.

32. Teplin LA, McClelland GM, Abram KM, et al. Crime victimization in adults with severe mental illness: comparison with the National Crime Victimization Survey. Arch Gen Psychiatry 2005; 62: 911–921.

33. McCullough LB, Coverdale JH, Chervenak FA. Ethical challenges of decision making with pregnant patients who have schizophrenia. Am J Obstet Gynecol 2002; 187: 696–702.

34. McCullough LB, Coverdale J, Bayer T, Chervenak FA. Ethically justified guidelines for family planning interventions to prevent pregnancy in female patients with chronic mental illness. Am J Obstet Gynecol 1992; 167: 19–25.

35. Miller LJ. Psychotic denial of pregnancy: phenomenology and clinical management. Hosp Community Psychiatry 1990; 41: 1233–1137.

36. Webb R, Abel K, Pickles A, Appleby L. Mortality in offspring of parents with psychotic disorders: a critical review and meta-analysis. Am J Psychiatry 2005; 162: 1045–1056.

37. Jablensky AV, Morgan V, Zubrick SR, Bower C, Yellachich L-A. Pregnancy, delivery, and neonatal complications in a population cohort of women with schizophrenia and major affective disorders. Am J Psychiatry 2005; 62: 79–91.

38. Schneid-Kofman N, Sheiner E, Levy A. Psychiatric illness and adverse pregnancy outcome. Int J Gynecol Obstet 2008; 101: 52–56.

39. Spielvogel A, Wile J. Treatment and outcomes of psychotic patients during pregnancy and childbirth. Birth 1992; 19: 131–137.

40. Coverdale JH, McCullough LB, Chervenak FA. Assisted and surrogate decision making for pregnant patients who have schizophrenia. Schizophr Bull 2004; 30: 659–664.

41. Babbitt KE, Bailey KJ, Coverdale JH, Chervenak FA, McCullough LB. Professionally responsible management of patients with major mental disorders. Am J Obstet Gynecol 2014; 210: 27–31.

42. American College of Obstetricians and Gynecologists. Use of psychiatric medications during pregnancy and lactation. ACOG Pract Bull 2008; 111: 1001–1020.

43. Ryding EL, Wijma B, Wijma K. Posttraumatic stress reactions after emergency cesarean section. Acta Obstet Gynecol Scand 1997; 76: 856–861.

44. Giacino JT, Katz DI, Schiff ND, Whyte J, et al. Practice guideline update recommendations summary: disorders of consciousness: Report of the Guideline Development, Dissemination, and Implementation Subcommittee of the American Academy of Neurology; the American Congress of Rehabilitation Medicine; and the National Institute on Disability, Independent Living, and Rehabilitation Research. Neurology 2018; 91: 450–460.

45. Russell JA, Epstein LG, MD, Greer DM, Kirschen M, et al., on behalf of the Brain Death Working Group. AAN Position Statement. Brain death, the determination of brain death, and member guidance for brain death accommodation requests. Neurology 2019; 92: 1–5.

46. Esmaeilzadeh M, Dictus C, Kayvanpour E, et al. One life ends, another begins: management of a brain-dead pregnant mother – a systematic review. BMC Medicine 2010; 8: 74.

47. American College of Obstetricians and Gynecologists. ACOG Committee Opinion Number 761. Cesarean delivery on maternal request. Obstet Gynecol 2019; 133: e.73–77.

48. Chervenak FA, McCullough LB. An ethically justified algorithm for offering, recommending, and performing cesarean delivery and its application in managed care practice. Obstet Gynecol 1996; 87: 302–305.

49. Kingwani P. Risk Management – An Analytical Study. IOSR Journal of Business and Management. February 2014, 83–89. Available at http://iosrjournals.org/iosr-jbm/papers/Vol16-issue3/Version-3/K016338389.pdf (accessed July 31, 2019).

50. Sheen JJ, Wright JD, Goffman D, et al. Maternal age and risk for adverse outcomes. Am J Obstet Gynecol 2018; 219: 390.e1–15.

51. Tita ATN, Jablonski KA, Bailit JL, et al. Neonatal outcomes of elective early-term births after demonstrated fetal lung maturity. Am J Obstet Gynecol 2018; 219: 296.e1–8.

52. Johnson JK, Miller SH, Horowitz SD. Systems-based practice: improving the safety and quality of patient care by recognizing and improving the systems in which we work. In Henriksen K, Battles JB, Keyes MA, et al., eds. Advances in Patient Safety: New Directions and Alternative Approaches (Vol. 2: Culture and Redesign). Rockville, MD: Agency for Healthcare Research and Quality (US); August 2008. Available at www.ncbi.nlm.nih.gov/books/NBK43731/ (accessed January 13, 2019).

53. Mishna Sanhedrin 4.9. Available at www.goodreads.com/author/quotes/14110064.Mishnah_Sanhedrin_4_9_Yerushalmi_Talmud_Tractate_Sanhedrin_37a_(accessed March 1, 2019).

54. Grünebaum A, McCullough LB, Sapra KJ, et al. Early and total neonatal mortality in relation to birth setting in the United States, 2006–2009. Am J Obstet Gynecol 2014; 211: 390.e1–7.

55. Grünebaum A, McCullough LB, Sapra KJ, et al. Apgar score of 0 at 5 minutes and neonatal seizures or serious neurologic dysfunction in relation to birth setting. Am J Obstet Gynecol 2013; 209: 323.e1–6.

56. Grünebaum A, McCullough LB, Brent RL, Arabin B, Levene MI, Chervenak FA. Perinatal risks of planned home births in the United States. Am J Obstet Gynecol 2015; 212: 350.e1–6.

57. Wax JR, Lucas FL, Lamont M, Cartin A, Blackstone J. Maternal and newborn outcomes in planned home birth vs planned hospital births: a metaanalysis. Am J Obstet Gynecol 2010; 203: 243.e1–8.

58. Snowden JM, Tilden EL, Snyder J, Quigley B, Caughey AB, Cheng YW. Planned out-of-hospital birth and birth outcomes. N Engl J Med 2015; 373: 2642–2653.

59. American Academy of Pediatrics: Policy Statement Planned Home Birth. Pediatrics 2013; 131: 1016–1020.

60. Gigerenzer G, Galesic M. Why do single event probabilities confuse patients? statements of frequency are better for communicating risk. BMJ; 2012; 344: e245.

61. Publications Committee, Society for Maternal-Fetal Medicine. Placenta accreta. Am J Obstet Gynecol 2010; 203: 430–439.

62. ACOG Practice bulletin no. 115: Vaginal birth after previous cesarean delivery. Obstet Gynecol 2010; 116: 450–463.

63. Rasmussen SA, Jamieson DJ, Uyeki TM. Effects of influenza on pregnant women and infants. Am J Obstet Gynecol 2012; 207: S3–8.

64. Farr A, Chervenak FA, McCullough LB, Baergen RN, Grünebaum A. Human placentophagy: a review. Am J Obstet Gynecol 2017; 218: 401.e1–11.

65. Ecker J. Minkoff home birth: what are physicians' ethical obligations when patient choices may carry increased risk? Obstet Gynecol 2011; 117: 1179–1182.

66. Minkoff H, Ecker J. A reconsideration of home birth in the United States. J Clin Ethics 2013; 24: 207–214.

67. Chervenak FA, McCullough LB. The unlimited-rights model of obstetric ethics threatens professionalism. BJOG 2017; 124: 1144–1147.

Chapter 13

The Perfect Baby

GOAL
This chapter provides an ethical framework for responding to an expectation of having a perfect baby.

OBJECTIVES
On completing study of this chapter, the reader will:
- Describe the perilous logic of the search for clinical perfection using "The Birth-Mark" by Nathaniel Hawthorne
- Identify preventive ethics as the antidote to the belief in control of human biology
- Describe an informed consent process designed to defuse the expectation of having a perfect baby
- Apply the ethical framework for responding to an expectation of having a perfect baby in clinical practice

TOPICS

13.1 The Perilous Logic of the Belief that Medicine Can Control Human Biology	164
13.1.1 The Quest for Control over Human Biology	164
13.1.2 A Perilous Logic	164
13.2 Creative Literature in Ethical Reasoning	164
13.3 The Perils of Belief in Control and Expectation of Perfection: A Cautionary Tale from American Literature	164
13.3.1 Nathaniel Hawthorne's "The Birth-Mark"	165
13.4 The Perils of the Logic of Belief in Control and Pursuit of Perfection	165
13.4.1 An Antidote: Preventive Ethics	165
13.4.2 The Interaction of Clinical and Social Conditions that Promote the Concept of the Perfect Baby	165
13.4.2.1 Fetal Imaging	165
13.4.2.2 Baby Pictures	165
13.4.2.3 Belief in Control over Human Biology	165
13.4.2.4 Consumer Rights Movement	166
13.5 Fashioning the Informed Consent Process to Defuse the Expectation That Medicine Can Control Human Reproductive Biology	166
13.5.1 No Guarantee of a Perfect Baby	167
13.5.2 What Obstetricians Should Know	167
13.5.3 What Patients Need to Know	167
13.5.4 Limits of Fetal Diagnosis	168
13.5.5 Experimental Maternal–Fetal Intervention	169
13.6 Perfection in Pregnancy Is Not Attainable	169

Section 3: Professionally Responsible Clinical Practice

Key Concepts	Informed consent process	Right
The clinical gaze	Patients' rights Preventive ethics	Therapeutic misconception

13.1 The Perilous Logic of the Belief that Medicine Can Control Human Biology

Patients sometimes present to their physicians requests for diagnostic tests and treatments, sometimes invasive tests and treatments. This is especially the case in obstetric practice. The prevalence with which pregnant women make requests of their obstetricians varies in different populations of pregnant women. However, obstetricians are familiar with – and are often challenged by – requests for diagnostic tests and for specific interventions, such as the detailed birth plans that some pregnant women present. These requests for clinical management reflect the values and priorities of pregnant patients and therefore should be taken seriously.

13.1.1 The Quest for Control over Human Biology

Sometimes, however, such requests reflect something more: the quest for control over human biology and the pursuit of perfection that such control should attain. Advances in modern medicine tend to encourage the belief that medicine can control human biology. There is an ethically significant logic of this belief: the expectation that medicine possesses an increasing capacity to control human biology implies that obstetrics can deliver the perfect baby.[1]

13.1.2 A Perilous Logic

This logic of the quest for control over human biology and expectation of perfection can become perilous. Sometimes this logic is expressed in requests that cause obstetricians to become uncomfortable, e.g., when a birth plan is internally inconsistent or sets conditions such as no analgesia or no cesarean delivery that, later, may not be consistent with treatment plans based on deliberative clinical judgment and its origins in beneficence-based and integrity-based ethical reasoning. The logic of expectations of control and perfection can also lead to parental rejection of resuscitation in the delivery room or of subsequent neonatal critical care for a premature newborn who was diagnosed as a fetus with an anomaly such as isolated Apert syndrome. Resuscitation and critical care management in such clinical circumstances prevent imminent death and result in preservation of interactive capacity. In such circumstances a parental refusal of resuscitation should not be implemented. (See Chapters 12 and 15.)

In short, the logic of the belief in biological control and the expectation of perfection that it generates for pregnant women with the belief are fraught with the potential for ethical conflict. In this chapter we identify some of the sources for this ethical conflict and propose a preventive ethics approach to replacing the logic of the expectations of control and perfection with more realistic and therefore more appropriate expectations.

13.2 Creative Literature in Ethical Reasoning

A distinctive feature of ethical reasoning in this chapter is its taking a work of creative literature as its point of departure. A short story, in the hands of a master writer, compactly and dramatically presents ethical challenges about the limits of the control that medical science is believed to have over human biology. In the global history of philosophy, few philosophers have left us such compelling writing. Plato's Dialogues come immediately to mind.

13.3 The Perils of Belief in Control and Expectation of Perfection: A Cautionary Tale from American Literature

We therefore start, not with Plato, but with the American writer Nathaniel Hawthorne (1804–1864). Hawthorne wrote one of the most compelling accounts of the perils of the logic of control and perfection in medicine, "The Birthmark."[2] It traces the tragic arc from belief in control of human biology and an expectation of perfection to pursuit of perfection.

13.3.1 Nathaniel Hawthorne's "The Birth-Mark"

Hawthorne relates the story of a woman renowned for her beauty, named Georgiana. Her beauty, however, appears incomplete: she has a birthmark in the shape of a hand on her cheek. Aylmer, her husband, comes to dislike his wife's birthmark. Georgiana, perhaps as a result of Aylmer's influence, comes to dislike her birthmark as well. Aylmer plans to use his scientific skills to eradicate the birthmark and make his wife's beauty complete, perfect. His thinking epitomizes the logic that leads inexorably from an exaggerated belief in scientific control over human biology to an expectation of its perfection.

Driven by this logic, Aylmer prepares a special liquid, a "chemical experiment," to rid her of the birthmark. His expectation of perfection has become a pursuit of it. He assures her: "The concoction of the draft has been perfect. … Unless all my science have failed me, it cannot fail." Despite concern for danger, Georgiana duly consumes the "powerful cosmetic." She falls into a sleep and her birthmark begins to disappear. Her first words on awakening are "My poor Aylmer." "'Poor? Nay, richest, happiest, most favored!' exclaimed he. 'My peerless bride, it is successful! You are perfect!'" But she is also dying and expires as her birthmark fades altogether from her cheek. The belief in scientific control over human biology and the expectation of perfection have transmuted into the pursuit of perfection that has exacted a terrible price.

13.4 The Perils of the Logic of Belief in Control and Pursuit of Perfection

13.4.1 An Antidote: Preventive Ethics

A directly parallel logic from belief in control of biology, to an expectation of perfection, and finally to the pursuit of perfection in pregnancy today can also exact a price, though, of course, not so terrible. The obstetrician should take a preventive ethics approach to the imperfect concept of a perfect baby. Preventive ethics has two components: identifying the conditions in clinical practice that can lead to ethical conflict; and using the informed consent process to address and defuse conditions that create the potential for conflict.[3] (See Chapter 3.)

13.4.2 The Interaction of Clinical and Social Conditions that Promote the Concept of the Perfect Baby

13.4.2.1 Fetal Imaging

Conditions in clinical practice can promote the concept of the perfect baby. These clinical conditions can interact with social conditions to encourage exaggerated beliefs and expectations about the ability of reproductive medicine to control biology. Modern fetal diagnosis and therapy feed public expectations of medicine's ability to control human reproductive biology. In a single generation, technological and interpretive advances have transformed fetal imaging. In high-income countries fetal imaging long ago left the world of grainy, bistable, static images that few physicians were competent to interpret. We now have four-dimensional, real-time ultrasound images that can be easily appreciated by the lay public, who have never before seen an ultrasound image of a developing fetus. Physicians, long accustomed to imaging technology, look on the results with a diagnostic eye, what Foucault called the "clinical gaze."[4] The clinical gaze appropriately medicalizes what it sees, because physicians are expected to diagnose and manage fetal abnormalities. One result is that the fetus may become a patient who can be diagnosed and treated, analogous to a newborn infant.[5] (See Chapter 2.) In the clinical gaze, the obstetrician analyzes images.

13.4.2.2 Baby Pictures

The lay or social gaze is not the same, because, as a rule, it is scientifically and clinically untrained. In the lay gaze patients and their families see a picture. Pictures, including "baby pictures," are not images of anatomy and physiology. Pregnant women and those involved in their pregnancies with them see an immediate and visually arresting picture of the fetus, sometimes with a coppery shimmer. Magnetic resonance pictures can be even more visually arresting, especially of the fetal head and facial features. The experience of "seeing" the fetus in pictures and videos can be a moving and bonding experience for the pregnant women and her partner.

13.4.2.3 Belief in Control over Human Biology

Given the intensity and power of fetal pictures, it is not unreasonable for lay persons to assume that the well-trained physician can see everything and therefore control human biology and thereby ensure perfection. This linking of a belief in control, an expectation of perfection, to the pursuit of perfection can feed the further expectation that medicine can predict human reproductive biology with little or no risk. After all, fetal images can be made routinely, simultaneously, and without risk. It is a small next step to the expectation that medicine can predict the perfect baby.

Invasive fetal diagnosis from chorionic villus sampling or amniocentesis results in karyotyping that is virtually certain in its ability to diagnose obvious aneuploidy. Karyotyping can encourage binomial thinking among some physicians that either there is a chromosomal abnormality or not, with the absence of abnormality resulting in reassurance.[6] The lay translation can be quite different: either something is wrong or everything is fine. What the physician thinks is simply reassurance can nonetheless encourage the expectation of perfection for the patient.

It is common knowledge that cesarean delivery can be life-saving for the fetus, e.g., from complete placenta previa or prolonged bradycardia. It is also common knowledge that cesarean delivery can reduce morbidity, e.g., from breech presentation. The recent introduction of steroid therapy to enhance fetal lung maturity has been shown to improve outcomes for infants born prematurely. Quality prenatal care that is initiated early in the pregnancy does not guarantee the prevention of prematurity. The administration of folic acid at 400 micrograms per day throughout pregnancy can markedly reduce the incidence of neural defects; however, it does not prevent all neural tube defects.[7,8] The introduction of $Rh_o(D)$ immune globulin (RhoGAM®) has markedly reduced the incidence of erythroblastosis fetalis. Intrauterine blood transfusion, though rarely needed for this condition, is the most well established form of invasive fetal therapy and can be life-saving for the fetus. More invasive forms of experimental fetal therapy, while performed only in a few centers, have been introduced. (See Chapter 17.) The publicity that can surround such surgery can give it an impact on public expectations that can be considerable, e.g., in the common use of "miracle" to describe such innovative fetal therapy.[9] Hospitals are not above encouraging such publicity, to market themselves in local, regional, national, and international markets. The drama of the publicity about such fetal therapy in the public arena obscures the rarity of its occurrence and clinical utility. The impression that fetal therapy is an expanding option encourages the belief in the ever-expanding power of medicine to control human reproductive biology.

13.4.2.4 Consumer Rights Movement

The consumer rights movement has appropriately encouraged patients, especially pregnant patients, to speak up for themselves. The discourse of patients' rights can be misused, especially when it encourages patients to make excessive demands on physicians, e.g., presenting detailed birth plans and requesting cesarean delivery in the absence of either fetal or maternal indications.[10] Sometimes implicit in these expressions of patients' rights is the belief that lay persons can set the standard of care for clinical practice. The failure of some physicians to adhere consistently to the discipline of evidence-based reasoning in obstetric practice has, ironically, supported this belief. It is a small step from the belief that lay persons can set the standard of care to the belief that patients can control human reproductive biology by making the right demands on their obstetricians.

Scientifically disciplined clinical judgment does not support the generalization from occasional success in clinical practice to uniform success. Lay thinking that is not scientifically disciplined can support this mistaken generalization. If patients have the belief that physicians can control human reproductive biology, bad outcomes must be the result of defective clinical judgment and practice, i.e., malpractice.

The safe, effective termination of pregnancy before viability can encourage the belief that a pregnant woman can control all the outcomes of pregnancy. This belief may mean that the errors of human reproduction can be detected through fetal diagnosis and eliminated through termination of pregnancy. The biological reality is that not all less-than-perfect outcomes can be detected prenatally.

13.5 Fashioning the Informed Consent Process to Defuse the Expectation That Medicine Can Control Human Reproductive Biology

The informed consent process should be used by obstetricians early in prenatal care as a preventive ethics tool to defuse expectations about the scientific and clinical ability to control human biology.[3] The first step in this informed consent is to provide patients with a succinct education about the

Table 13.1 Background reproductive risks.

Reproductive risk	Frequency
Immunologically and clinically diagnosed spontaneous abortions per million conceptions	350,000
Clinically recognized spontaneous abortions per million clinically recognized pregnancies	150,000
Genetic diseases per million births	110,000
Multifactorial or polygenic gene–environmental interactions, i.e., neural tube defects, cleft lip, hypospadius, hyperlipidemia, diabetes	90,000
Dominantly inherited disease, i.e., achondroplasia, Huntington's disease, neurofibromatosis	10,000
Autosomal and sex-linked genetic disease, i.e., cystic fibrosis, hemophilia, sickle-cell disease, thalassemia	1,200
Cytogenetic (chromosomal abnormalities), i.e., Down's syndrome, Fragile X syndrome, Turner's syndrome	5,000
New mutations of ova or sperm	3,000
Severe congenital malformations (due to all causes of birth defects: genetic, unknown, environmental per million births)	30,000
Prematurity/million	40,000
Fetal growth retardation/million	30,000
Stillbirths (>20 weeks)/million	4,000–20,900
Infertility	7% of couples

Modified from Brent.[11,12]

imperfections of human reproduction and the limits of medicine to alter these imperfections.[11,12] (See Table 13.1.)

13.5.1 No Guarantee of a Perfect Baby

No pregnant woman should begin her pregnancy with the idea that anyone can guarantee the birth of a normal baby. While there are some preventive measures, such as vaccination against German measles (Rubella vaccine), taking adequate amounts of folic acid (400 micrograms per day as a minimum),[13] excellent prenatal care, and women's self-care during pregnancy, some birth defects cannot be prevented. (See Table 13.2.) The concept to communicate is that the ability of medicine or a patient's behaviors to improve outcomes is limited. Therefore, obstetricians cannot guarantee that every birth will be normal. This information should be communicated as part of routine prenatal care.[3]

13.5.2 What Obstetricians Should Know

All obstetricians should be aware of the pertinent scientific information on background reproductive risks[11,12] and the etiology of congenital malformations.[11,12] (See Tables 13.1 and 13.3.) In addition, while there are high-risk conditions such as multiple gestation, prematurity with its complications such as cerebral palsy and bronchopulmonary dysplasia can occur in any pregnancy as well as in full-term newborns. (See Table 13.1.) The obstetrician should strive for a term pregnancy, although doing so is no guarantee that the risks usually associated with prematurity cannot occur in full-term newborns.

13.5.3 What Patients Need to Know

Patients do not need to be provided this information in detail but do need to be informed about the risks of birth defects, spontaneous miscarriage, and prematurity. Every pregnant woman should be told the following information (adjusted for the patient's educational level): "If you are healthy and have no personal or family history of reproductive or developmental defects, you began your pregnancy with a 3% risk of birth defects and once you knew you were pregnant, having missed your first menstrual period, you have a 15% risk of miscarriage.

Table 13.2 Prevention of congenital malformations.

1. Rubella vaccination.
2. Folic acid (400 μg/day) and vitamin B_6 (6 μg/day) supplementation.
3. Supplementation of iodide to deficient patients and populations.
4. Meticulous diabetic control.
5. Competent diagnosis and management of maternal hypothyroidism.
6. Screening for chromosome abnormalities and genetic disease.
7. Hepatitis B vaccination for at risk women.
8. HIV screening and treatment.
9. Screening for *N. gonorrhoeae*, *C. trachomatis*, group B streptococcus.
10. Vaccination of patients with group B streptococcus.
11. Maternal phenylalanine management for maternal phenylketonurics.
12. Management or discontinuation of oral use of anticoagulants, anticonvulsants, retinoids, thalidomide, and all known teratogens.
13. Recognize that new teratogens can be represented in the next new drug or chemical exposure: angiotensin converting enzyme (ACE) inhibitors, angiotensin II receptor blockers, mycophenolate, tumor necrosis factor (TNF) blockers.
14. Amniocentesis, chorionic villous sampling, maternal serum monitoring, ultrasound monitoring to diagnosis identifiable genetic diseases and serious birth defects in order for the parents to be informed about their options.
15. Maternal smoking and alcohol cessation.
16. Obesity control in itself reduces the risk of birth defects and decreases the risk of developing diabetes.
17. Immunization against known teratogenic infections. Botulinum toxin vaccine for the pregnant mother to prevent infant botulism.

Modified from Brent.[11,12]

There is also a risk of prematurity with its complications. These are background risks for all pregnant women." Obstetricians should be clear with patients that many congenital malformations have an unknown etiology so that, if a birth defect occurs, blame will not be inappropriately attributed to patients' behaviors, exogenous exposures, or obstetric management.[14,15] (See (Table 13.3.)

Ultrasound technology and genetic diagnosis can identify many anomalies. However, pregnant women need to be informed that, although obstetrics has made great advances in the past 50 years, we are not close to being able to diagnose or predict *every* genetic disease, anatomic malformation, or biochemical defect in each pregnancy and thus guarantee a normal pregnancy and its perfect outcome.

13.5.4 Limits of Fetal Diagnosis

Obstetricians need to be aware of the reasons why we cannot diagnose all developmental problems. Some genetic diseases and hereditary anatomic malformations are due to mutations that occur during oogenesis or spermatogenesis (the development of the ovum or sperm). (See Table 13.1.) Therefore, there is no family history of these diseases. Genome sequencing has the potential to identify thousands of genetic diseases and disorders, outstripping the current diagnostic capacity of karyotyping by amniocentesis or chorionic villus sampling.[16] However, even when genetic abnormalities or hereditary anatomic defects are discovered by diagnostic tests, there may be no information about the clinical significance of such findings. Many anatomic malformations may not be recognizable in utero and will not be able to be diagnosed for months, or even years, after the child is delivered. Autism, polycystic kidney disease, mental retardation, learning disability, schizophrenia, and many other serious behavior disorders are in this category. While many congenital malformations can be diagnosed in utero, attempts to treat the fetus with surgical or medical treatment are often experimental,

Table 13.3 Etiology of human congenital malformations observed during the first year of life.[a]

Suspected Cause	Percent of total
Unknown	65–75
Polygenic	
Multifactorial (gene–environment interactions)	
Spontaneous errors of development	
Synergistic interactions of teratogens	
Genetic	15–25
Autosomal and sex-linked inherited genetic disease	
Cytogenetic (chromosomal abnormalities)	
New mutations	
Environmental	10
Maternal conditions: Alcoholism, diabetes, endocrinopathies, phenylketonuria, smoking and nicotine, starvation, nutritional deficits	4
Infectious agents: Rubella, toxoplasmosis, syphilis, herpes simplex, cytomegalovirus, varicella-zoster, Venezuelan equine encephalitis, parvovirus B19	3
Mechanical problems (deformations): Amniotic band constrictions, umbilical cord constraint, disparity in uterine size and uterine contents	1–2
Chemicals, prescription drugs, high dose ionizing radiation, hyperthermia	1–2

[a]Modified from Brent.[11,12]

are not curative, and continue to have significant risks of mortality and morbidity. (See Chapter 17.)

13.5.5 Experimental Maternal–Fetal Intervention

Even if experimental maternal-fetal intervention is available, it is uncertain if it should be utilized. (See Chapter 17.) Once a developmental diagnosis had been confirmed, it is not an easy task to determine what can be done (termination of pregnancy, in utero therapy, or expectant management). Obstetricians should be aware that many couples are willing to embark on experimental intervention in the mistaken assumption that, in their case, it will work. Obstetricians should be prepared to disabuse pregnant women who believe that an experimental intervention will work and therefore do not appreciate its experimental nature, a confusion that is known as "therapeutic misconception."[17] Finally, it is important to emphasize that many pregnant patients are optimistic about advances in medicine and are confident that their physicians will solve all problems that could occur with their pregnancy. However, this version of the expectation of a perfect baby assumes powers of medicine to control human reproduction that medicine does not possess. There will almost certainly continue to be a significant percentage of anatomic birth defects that result from unpreventable developmental errors.

13.6 Perfection in Pregnancy Is Not Attainable

The obstetrician whose patient expresses the hope for a perfect baby should give this matter the serious and sensitive attention it deserves: a preventive ethics approach designed to educate the pregnant woman about the inherent errors of human reproduction, the highly variable clinical outcomes of these errors, the limited capacity of medicine to detect these errors, and the even more limited capacity to correct them. The message to convey is that perfection in pregnancy is not attainable now or even in the foreseeable future. Appropriate counseling of pregnant women, who may be influenced by the expectation of perfection and who therefore may believe that anything less is a disaster, can help them to realize that the fetus' condition and prospects are better than they think.

Physicians should keep in mind and help patients appreciate the ancient wisdom of the Hippocratic text, *The Art*,[18] which emphasizes that the power of the art and science of medicine to alter the course of disease and injury is always limited. When physicians ignore these limits, they experience a kind of "madness" from which Aylmer suffered, i.e., expecting more from medicine than its limited diagnostic and therapeutic capacities justify. In "The Birth-Mark" we can now see that Aylmer failed to meet the standards of preventive ethics and evidence-based reasoning when he said, "The concoction of the draft has been perfect. ... Unless all my science have failed me, it cannot fail."[2] Aylmer is thus an exemplar of what obstetricians should *not* do in response to the quest for the perfect baby.

In more contemporary terms, clinical judgment and counseling of pregnant women throughout their pregnancies should be disciplined by scientific information of the kind we have presented. The preventive ethics response in the search for the "perfect baby" should use the informed consent process to discipline the expectations of pregnant women to the greatest extent possible. We believe that this preventive ethics approach should be taken with every pregnant woman, to prepare her for the inherent uncertainties of pregnancy and its clinical management. Physicians should assume that, with adequate counseling and support, pregnant women are indeed capable of making scientifically disciplined decisions, if informed consent is appropriately evidence based, as has been shown for decision making about invasive prenatal diagnosis after first-trimester risk assessment.[19]

References

1. Chervenak FA, McCullough LB, Brent RL. The perils of the imperfect expectation of the perfect baby. Am J Obstet Gynecol 2010; 203: 101.e1–101.e5.
2. Hawthorne N. The Birth-Mark. 1843. www.online-literature.com/hawthorne/125/ (accessed March 1, 2019).
3. Chervenak FA, McCullough LB. Clinical guides to preventing ethical conflicts between pregnant women and their physicians. Am J Obstet Gynecol 1990; 162: 303–307.
4. Foucault M. Naissance de la Clinique: une archéologie du régard médical 1963. Translated as The Birth of the Clinic: An Archeology of Medical Perception. Sheridan Smith AM, trans. New York: Pantheon, 1973.
5. Chervenak FA, McCullough LB, Brent RL. The professional responsibility model of obstetric ethics: avoiding the perils of clashing rights. Am J Obstet Gynecol 2011; 205: 315.e1–5.
6. Brent RL. Saving lives and changing family histories: appropriate counseling of pregnant women and men and women of reproductive age, concerning the risk of radiation exposures during and before pregnancy. Am J Obstet Gynecol 2009; 200: 4–24.
7. Brent RL, Oakley GP. Triumph or tragedy: the present FDA program of enriching grains with folic acid. Pediatrics 2006; 117: 930–932,
8. Bell KN, Oakley GP Jr. Update on prevention of folic acid-preventable spina bifida and anencephaly. Birth Defects Res (Pt A) 2009; 85: 102–107.
9. Jones M. A miracle, and yet. New York Times Magazine. July 15, 2001. www.nytimes.com/2001/07/15/magazine/a-miracle-and-yet.html?scp=1&sq=A%20Miracle,%20and%20Yet&st=cse (accessed March 1, 2019).
10. Kalish RB, McCullough LB, Chervenak FA. Decision-making about cesarean delivery. Lancet 2006; 367(9514): 883–885.
11. Brent RL. Utilization of developmental basic science principles in the evaluation of reproductive risks from pre- and postconception environmental radiation exposures. Paper presented at the Thirty-third Annual Meeting of the National Council on Radiation Protection and Measurements. The Effects of Pre- and Postconception Exposure to Radiation, April 2–3, 1997, Arlington, Virginia. Teratology 1999; 59: 182–204.
12. Brent RL. Environmental causes of human congenital malformations: the pediatrician's role in dealing with these complex clinical problems caused by a multiplicity of environmental and genetic factors. Pediatrics 2004; 113(4 Suppl.): 957–968.
13. Brent RL, Oakley GP Jr. Commentary: The FDA must require the addition of more folic acid in "enriched" flour and other grains. Pediatrics 2005; 116: 753–755.
14. Brent RL. How does the physician avoid prescribing drugs and medical procedures that have reproductive and developmental risks? Medical legal issues in perinatal medicine. Clin Perinatol 2007; 34: 233–262.
15. Brent RL. Litigation-produced pain, disease and suffering: an experience with congenital malformation lawsuits. Teratology 1977; 16: 1–14.
16. Papp Z and International Academy of Perinatal Medicine. Ethical challenges of genomics for perinatal medicine: the Budapest Declaration. Am J Obstet Gynecol 2009; 201: 336.
17. Lidz CW, Appelbaum PS, Grisso T, Renaud M. Therapeutic misconception and the appreciation of risks in clinical trials. Soc Sci Med 2004; 58: 1689–1697.
18. Hippocrates. The Art. In WHS Jones, trans. Hippocrates, Vol. I. Cambridge, MA: Harvard University Press.
19. Nicolaides KH, Chervenak FA, McCullough LB, Avgidou K, Papageorghiou A. Evidence-based obstetric ethics and informed decision-making by pregnant women about invasive diagnosis after first-trimester risk assessment of risk of trisomy 21. Am J Obstet Gynecol 2005; 193: 322–326.

Chapter 14: Cancer and Pregnancy

GOAL
This chapter provides an ethical framework to guide decision making with patients about the management of pregnancy and concurrent cancer.

OBJECTIVES
On completing study of this chapter, the reader will:
- Distinguish congruent from noncongruent beneficence-based ethical obligations of the obstetrician
- Describe components of the informed consent process for the clinical management of pregnancy and concurrent cancer
- Apply the ethical framework to guide decision making with patients about the management of pregnancy and concurrent cancer in clinical practice

TOPICS

14.1 Ethical Challenges of Cancer and Pregnancy	172
14.2 Congruent and Noncongruent Beneficence-Based Ethical Obligations of the Obstetrician	172
14.2.1 Congruent Beneficence-Based Ethical Obligations to the Pregnant and the Fetal Patient	172
14.2.2 Noncongruent Beneficence-Based Ethical Obligations to the Pregnant and the Fetal Patient	172
14.3 The Informed Consent Process	173
14.3.1 The Informed Consent Process When the Fetus Is Previable	173
14.3.2 The Informed Consent Process When the Fetus Is Viable	173
14.3.2.1 Congruent Beneficence-Based Obligations to the Pregnant and the Fetal Patient	174
14.3.2.2 Noncongruent Beneficence-Based Obligations to the Pregnant Patient	174
14.3.2.3 Noncongruent Beneficence-Based Obligations to the Pregnant Patient and the Fetal Patient	174
The Previable Fetus	174
The Viable Fetus	175
The Viable Fetus before Lung Maturity	175
The Viable Fetus after Fetal Lung Maturity	176
14.4 Advance Directives	176

Section 3: Professionally Responsible Clinical Practice

Key Concepts

Advance directive
Double effect
Ethical concept of the fetus as a patient
Ethical principle of beneficence in professional ethics in obstetrics
Ethical principle of nonmaleficence in professional ethics in obstetrics and gynecology
Ethical principle of respect for autonomy in professional ethics in obstetrics
Informed consent process
Preventive ethics

14.1 Ethical Challenges of Cancer and Pregnancy

Cancer diagnosed during pregnancy presents the physician, pregnant woman, and her family with complex and difficult ethical challenges.[1] The conflicting concerns between the growing fetus and the dangers of cancer raise many ethical and clinical problems unique to the management of cancer during pregnancy. This chapter draws on professional ethics in obstetrics and its ethical concept of the fetus as a patient, to provide guidance for the responsible management of these ethical challenges.

Thirteen percent of cancers in women develop during the reproductive years and death due to cancer is second to accidents during that period.[2] Both in the United States and the United Kingdom, about 1 in 1,000 pregnancies are complicated by malignancy. This figure includes women who are pregnant and those six months postpartum. The incidence is expected to rise with the concomitant increasing age of childbearing. The scientific and clinical challenges of cancer and pregnancy have been explored in the literature. There has been particular attention to the clinical indications for and against treatment of cancer during pregnancy in terms of efficacy of treatment and risks to the pregnant woman and fetus.[3-6] The ethical challenges of cancer during pregnancy have received less attention.[7] The source of these ethical challenges is that the realities and limits of clinical management of pregnancy can create congruent and noncongruent beneficence-based ethical obligations of the obstetrician.

14.2 Congruent and Noncongruent Beneficence-Based Ethical Obligations of the Obstetrician

The ethical concept of the fetus as a patient requires that, in all cases, the obstetrician, oncologist, and other consultants and team members identify the implications of three prima facie ethical obligations: beneficence-based ethical obligations to the pregnant patient; autonomy-based ethical obligations to the pregnant patient, and beneficence-based ethical obligations to the fetal patient, when the fetus is a patient. (See Chapter 2.) The obstetrician has beneficence-based obligations to both the pregnant patient and to the fetal patient to reduce their risk of mortality and morbidity from cancer, and to keep cancer treatment to the minimum required to fulfill these ethical obligations.

14.2.1 Congruent Beneficence-Based Ethical Obligations to the Pregnant and the Fetal Patient

When treatment for the cancer in question reduces the woman's morbidity and mortality but does not increase the iatrogenic risk of mortality or morbidity for the fetal patient, there is congruence of the physician's obligations to treat the pregnant woman and to protect the fetal patient. (See Table 14.1.) In these cases, directive counseling – in the form of a recommendation of cancer treatment – is ethically justified. Nondirective counseling, or shared decision making, should not be deployed, because it may give the misleading impression that there is reason to be concerned about fetal patient safety. (See Chapter 3.)

14.2.2 Noncongruent Beneficence-Based Ethical Obligations to the Pregnant and the Fetal Patient

There are two clinical circumstances in which noncongruent beneficence-based obligations to the pregnant and fetal patient occur. (See Table 14.1.) The first clinical circumstance occurs when the beneficence-based ethical obligations to the

Table 14.1 Offering and recommending cancer treatment based on beneficence and respect for autonomy.

Beneficence-based obligations

Congruent

Cancer treatment reduces the woman's risk of mortality or morbidity and does not increase risk of iatrogenic mortality or morbidity for the fetus.

Noncongruent to the woman

Cancer treatment reduces the woman's risk of mortality or morbidity from her cancer but increases the iatrogenic risk of future infertility.

Noncongruent to the pregnant woman and fetus

Cancer treatment reduces the woman's risk of mortality or morbidity and increases the risk of iatrogenic mortality or morbidity for the fetus.

---

pregnant patient are not congruent, i.e., when treatment of the pregnant patient's cancer creates an iatrogenic risk of future infertility for her. The second clinical circumstance occurs when beneficence-based obligations to the pregnant woman and beneficence-based ethical obligations to the fetal patient are not congruent, i.e., when cancer treatment is reliably predicted to benefit the woman but create iatrogenic risk for the fetus. Professional ethics in obstetrics calls for the potential for noncongruent beneficence-based ethical obligations to be identified and managed in the informed consent process. The ethical concept of the fetus as a patient plays a major role in shaping the informed consent process.

14.3 The Informed Consent Process

The ethical concept of the fetus as a patient has implications for when the previable and viable fetus should be considered a patient, as explained in Chapter 3.

14.3.1 The Informed Consent Process When the Fetus Is Previable

For the previable fetus, the woman is free to confer, withhold, or having once conferred, withdraw the moral status of being a patient on or from the fetus. (See Chapter 2.) This is not a medical judgment for the obstetrician to make for the pregnant woman. As explained in Chapter 9, a maternal complication of pregnancy such as cancer creates an autonomy-based ethical obligation to offer induced abortion in a previable pregnancy. Counseling about termination of pregnancy by the obstetrician should therefore be nondirective. The obstetrician should not sugar-coat the patient's cancer, especially when it is late stage or metastatic, and its potential impact on the fetus. Such conversations are understandably uncomfortable, a response that should be managed by fidelity to the informed consent process.

The woman is free to give the fetus' health and life greater priority than her own health-related and other interests and vice versa. The obstetrician should make it clear to the pregnant woman that she is the ultimate decision maker. To protect the voluntariness of her decision-making process, if necessary, the obstetrician should explain to others involved in her decision making that everyone has the ethical obligation to respect and support her in her decision-making process. (See Chapter 3.)

14.3.2 The Informed Consent Process When the Fetus Is Viable

In professional ethics in obstetrics, the viable fetus is a patient when the pregnant woman presents for care. (See Chapter 2.) As a general rule, directive counseling for fetal benefit is ethically justified. It is also the case that recommending against clinical management of the pregnant woman's condition that could, on balance, be harmful to the fetal patient is also ethically justified. However, like all beneficence-based ethical obligations to the fetal patient, this ethical obligation is prima facie because the ethical concept of the fetus as a patient requires that the prima facie beneficence-based and nonmaleficence-based ethical obligation to prevent harm to a fetal patient must always be balanced against beneficence-based and autonomy-based obligations to the pregnant woman. Any such balancing must recognize that a pregnant woman is obligated only to take reasonable risks of medical interventions to her life, health, and future fertility that are reliably expected to protect the viable fetus or child later. (See Chapter 2.) Throughout the informed consent process in a viable pregnancy, the obstetrician has an important role to play in assisting the pregnant woman to evaluate alternatives on the basis of her values, especially concerning the risk she thinks she should be willing to take for life, health, and future fertility, and for the fetal and neonatal patient.

14.3.2.1 Congruent Beneficence-Based Obligations to the Pregnant and the Fetal Patient

When cancer treatment protects the pregnant patient's health and does not involve significant risk to her future fertility or risk to a future fetal patient, cancer treatment should be offered and recommended. Treatment will benefit the pregnant patient and she should be informed that initiating treatment during the pregnancy involves no significant risk to the fetus or future child. Squamous cell, basal cell, and malignant melanoma in situ of the skin pose no threat to the woman or fetus if treated during pregnancy. Patients who are pregnant and have a diagnosis of lymphoma in the second or third trimester can be safely treated with combination chemotherapy without deleterious effects to the fetus.[8] Throughout pregnancy, when cancer treatment is consistent with beneficence-based obligations of the obstetrician both to the pregnant patient and the fetal patient, the obstetrician should recommend cancer treatment in the setting of normal obstetric management. The physician should elicit any concerns that the woman may have about the safety of treatment and seek to reassure her that she can accept treatment consistent with her obligation to protect the fetal patient's and future child's health-related interests.

When the outcome of cancer treatment is not affected by a delay of several weeks, the obstetrician's beneficence-based obligation to the pregnant patient, to protect her life and health, and to the fetal patient, to protect its health by delaying treatment until fetal lung maturity, are congruent. The obstetrician should therefore recommend delay of treatment until the fetal patient achieves fetal lung maturity. A delay in treatment of cervical cancer has been the subject of many studies.[9–11] Most patients with pregnancy-associated cervical cancer present with early stage disease. Patients diagnosed after 24 weeks can be followed to fetal maturity. Pregnancy per se does not adversely affect the survival of women with invasive cervical cancer.[9]

14.3.2.2 Noncongruent Beneficence-Based Obligations to the Pregnant Patient

Noncongruent beneficence-based obligations to the pregnant patient occur when cancer treatment creates the risk of future infertility. Before pregnancy, the physician should provide the best evidence available about the medically reasonable alternatives to manage the cancer and the concomitant risk of iatrogenic infertility. When the woman's life is at stake, directive counseling for treatment is justified because in beneficence-based clinical judgment, premature death is a far greater harm than loss of fertility (even though loss of fertility is surely a significant harm). Although loss of fertility will result in the treatment of cervical cancer, early stage disease can be treated surgically with preservation of the ovaries. Advanced cervical cancer usually requires radiation, leaving the patient sterile and menopausal.

Delay of pregnancy until after completion of treatment for the woman's cancer should be recommended when it is supported by evidence. For example, the medical community is divided about allowing pregnancy after patients have been treated for Hodgkin's disease, melanoma, or breast cancer. However, over the last 50 years, there has been a change in the attitude about pregnancy in this group of patients. If these patients have gone three years without a recurrence, pregnancy is permitted after careful counseling on evidence-based oncology and what has been learned from systematic reviews. Abortion rates and anomaly rates do not seem higher than in the nonpregnant population used as controls. The fetuses produced do not seem to have a shortened longevity or acquire more diseases. The results for the next generation remain to be collected and studied.

14.3.2.3 Noncongruent Beneficence-Based Obligations to the Pregnant Patient and the Fetal Patient
The Previable Fetus

When the obstetrician's beneficence-based obligations to the pregnant patient and previable fetus are noncongruent, counseling should be nondirective and shared decision making deployed, for two reasons. First, the woman's autonomy is the sole basis for determining whether the previable fetus is a patient. She is therefore free to confer this status on her previable fetus or withhold or withdraw it. Second, given the uncertain nature of the risks of cancer treatment to the fetus and future fetal patient, she is free to make her own assessment about whether the risks should be taken in order for her to gain the benefit of cancer treatment. The obstetrician should offer the woman a choice among three medically reasonable alternatives. Because none is clinically superior in deliberative clinical judgment, no recommendation about which should be chosen should be made.

The first medically reasonable alternative is treatment with continuation of the pregnancy, with monitoring of the previable fetus for side effects of treatment and reconsideration of induced abortion before viability if such effects should occur. The estimated risks of malformations when a single agent is administered during the first trimester ranges from 7.5% to 17%, the teratogenic risk being estimated to increase when combination chemotherapy is being used. Spontaneous abortion usually occurs during the first month of gestation when cytotoxic agents are used but the risks of birth defects are most significant during the fifth to twelfth weeks of gestation during the time of organogenesis. Although brain and gonad development continues throughout pregnancy, there does not appear to be a major impact on childhood development. The second medically reasonable alternative is treatment preceded by induced abortion. The third medically reasonable alternative is treatment delay until fetal lung maturity, at which time it will be reasonably safe to deliver the fetal patient and reduce the risk of delaying treatment until full-term delivery should the fetal patient be affected by treatment of the pregnant woman's cancer.

If cancer is diagnosed in the late second trimester, clinical judgment concerns whether the pregnancy can be carried to viability or whether immediate intervention is indicated. If the data so indicate, it may be justified to wait for viability of the fetus if this is the woman's preference. Respecting that preference is consistent with the physician's beneficence-based obligations to the pregnant woman and fetal patient, a status she confers by her preference to continue her pregnancy to viability.

The concept of "double effect" will be relevant to the first option for women who accept independent moral status of the previable fetus (which they are free to do, as the basis for conferring the status of being a patient and for other purposes, as well). This concept was created in Roman Catholic moral theology to deal with situations in which an intrinsically good act, in this case cancer treatment, had both a good effect (treatment of the cancer with subsequent health-related benefits for the woman) and a bad or evil effect (the death of the fetus). Invasive cervical cancer treated with radiation therapy will result in fetal demise and usually a spontaneous abortion. The bad effect is permitted so long as it is not the cause of the good effect and the proportionate good outweighs the harm.[12] For example, under this concept, radiation therapy for cervical cancer and surgical management of uterine cancer during pregnancy are both permitted as part of treatment for uterine cancer because the surgery has both a good and bad effect, the good is proportionately greater, and the death of the fetus is not the means for producing the good of saving the woman's life. Death is therefore understood to be a foreseen, but not intended effect. The causal independence of the two effects is crucial for the application of this concept. It would certainly be appropriate to involve religious counselors or ethics consultants familiar with this concept and its clinical applications to assist the woman to think through the permissibility of termination of her pregnancy, so that she can be assured that such a decision can be made in good conscience.

The Viable Fetus

Because the viable fetus is a patient the obstetrician's counseling role is shaped by beneficence-based obligations to the fetal patient as well as beneficence-based obligations to the pregnant patient. A major ethical consideration for both the obstetrician and the pregnant patient concerns delay of treatment until fetal lung maturity, after which time early delivery of the fetal patient is consistent with beneficence-based obligations to the fetal and the neonatal patient. Counseling about cancer treatment when the fetus is viable therefore needs to take gestational age into account. Breast cancer is the most common tumor occurring during the reproductive years and although not common in pregnancy, presents special management problems. Survival stage for stage 1 is identical to the nonpregnant patient. However, diagnosis is usually delayed in the pregnant patient. The treatment modality should be based on current guidelines.[4-6]

The Viable Fetus before Lung Maturity

When cancer treatment can be safely delayed for the pregnant patient and when her treatment has potential risk for the fetal patient, counseling should be directive for fetal benefit by recommending delay of treatment. When treatment cannot be safely delayed, the obstetrician should offer the two medically reasonable alternatives: cancer treatment preceded by delivery and treatment delay with delivery until fetal lung maturity has been achieved No recommendation should be made because neither is clinically superior in deliberative clinical judgment. The pregnant patient should be offered assistance in weighing risks of each option to herself and to the fetal patient. This nondirective counseling, shared decision making is required because, in beneficence-based clinical judgment, the physician has no expertise to decide which life is more important.

The Viable Fetus after Fetal Lung Maturity

When cancer treatment can be safely postponed for the pregnant patient and treatment has the potential of risk to the fetal patient, the physician should recommend delay with a duration determined by maternal risk. This is because fetal risks of cancer treatment are substantially reduced by the end of the pregnancy. When delay is not justified, early delivery is consistent with protection of the fetal patient.

14.4 Advance Directives

Chapters 3 and 15 provide additional guidance on advance directives. Supported both by health law and professional ethics in obstetrics and gynecology, and in medicine generally, an advance directive permits a patient, in advance of a time at which she will no longer have decision-making capacity, to make her own decisions about the clinical management of a terminal or irreversible condition or to assign a surrogate decision maker to act for her.

Four aspects of the ethical principle of respect for autonomy in professional ethics in obstetrics and gynecology provide the ethical justification for advance directives.

1. A patient may exercise her autonomy now in the form of a refusal of or request for life-prolonging interventions.
2. Autonomy-based refusal, expressed in the past and left unchanged, remains in effect for any future time during which the patient loses decision-making capacity.
3. That past autonomy-based refusal or request should therefore translate into physician obligations at the time the patient becomes unable to participate in the informed consent process.
4. In particular, refusal of life-prolonging medical intervention should translate into the withholding or withdrawal of such interventions.

It is obvious, but bears repeating, that terminally or irreversibly ill patients who are able to participate in the informed consent process retain their autonomy to make their own decisions. The obstetrician should regard advance directives as powerful, practical tools for implementing a preventive ethics approach to decisions about limiting life-sustaining treatment when the pregnant patient can no longer participate in decision making. Some states do not permit implementation of an advance directive for pregnant patients. Hospital policy should be based on applicable law and provide for how to proceed. This policy should be as clear as possible about the legal permissibility of induced abortion or feticide before life-sustaining treatment is discontinued. Questions about these legal matters should be addressed to hospital legal counsel.

References

1. Chervenak FA, McCullough LB, Knapp RC, Caputo TA, Barber HRK. A clinically comprehensive ethical framework for offering and recommending cancer treatment before and during pregnancy. Cancer 2004; 100: 215–222.
2. Jemal A, Thomas A, Murray T, et al: Cancer statistics, 2002. CA, A Cancer Journal for Clinicians 2002; 52: 34–35.
3. Barber HRK. Malignant disease in pregnancy. J Perinat Med 29; 2001: 97–106.
4. Botha MH, Rajaram R, Karunaratne K. Cancer in pregnancy. In J Gynecol Obstet 2018; 143 (Suppl. 2): 137–142.
5. Salani R, Billingsley CC, Crafton SM. Cancer and pregnancy: an overview for obstetricians and gynecologists. Am J Obstet Gynecol 2014; 211: 7–14.
6. Albright CM, Wenstrom KD. Malignancies in pregnancy. Best Pract Res Clin Obstet Gynecol 2016; 33: 2–18.
7. Thorny S, McCullough LB, Chervenak FA. Ethical and spiritual considerations for treatment decision associated with cancer in pregnancy. Cancer Bull 1994; 5: 391–394.
8. Sood AK, Sorosky JI. Invasive cervical cancer complicating pregnancy. How to manage the dilemma. Obstet Gynecol Clin North Am 1998; 2: 343–352.
9. Zemlickis D, Lishner M, Degendorfer P, et al. Maternal and fetal outcome after invasive cervical cancer in pregnancy. J Clin Oncol 1991;9:1956–61.
10. Berek J, Hacker NF, eds. Practical Gynecologic Oncology. Philadelphia: Lippincott Williams & Wilkins, 2000.
11. Weisz B, Schiff E, Lishner M. Cancer in pregnancy: maternal and fetal implications. *Hum Reproduct* Update 2001; 7: 390–393.
12. Aulisio MP. Double effect, principle or doctrine of. In Jennings B, ed. Encyclopedia of Bioethics, 4th ed. Farmington Hills, MI: Gale, Cengage Learning 2014, 889–894.

Chapter 15
Setting Ethically Justified Limits on Life-Sustaining Treatment

GOAL
This chapter provides an ethical framework for setting justified limits on life-sustaining treatment.

OBJECTIVES
On completing study of this chapter, the reader will:
   Identify an historical perspective on ethical challenges of setting limits on life-sustaining treatment
   Describe an algorithm for setting ethically justified limits on life-sustaining treatment
   Explain why the Groningen Protocol for infant euthanasia should be rejected
   Describe ethically justified responses to inappropriate requests for life-sustaining treatment
   Apply the ethical framework for setting justified limits on life-sustaining treatment in clinical practice
   Apply the algorithm for setting ethically justified limits on life-sustaining treatment in clinical practice

TOPICS

15.1 Two Goals of Life-Sustaining Treatment	178
15.2 Beneficence-Based and Autonomy-Based Limits of Life-Sustaining Treatment	178
15.3 Historical Perspective	179
15.3.1 The Hippocratic Tradition of Declaring Gravely Ill Patients Incurable and Abandoning Them	179
15.3.2 John Gregory's Reversal of the Hippocratic Tradition of Abandoning Dying Patients	179
15.3.3 The Influence of Enthusiasm in American Critical Care	180
15.3.4 The Influence of American Common Law	180
15.3.5 An Emerging Consensus	180
15.3.6 The Influence of a Landmark Article	180
15.4 An Algorithm for the Role of the Obstetrician-Gynecologist in Decision Making about Setting Ethically Justified Limits on Life-Sustaining Treatment	181
15.4.1 Steps of the Algorithm	182
Step 1: Invoking Applicable Advance Directive Law	182
Step 2: Invoking Anatomic Futility	182
Step 3: Invoking Physiologic Futility	182
Step 4: Invoking Imminent-Demise Futility	182
Step 5: Invoking Interactive-Capacity Futility	182
Step 6: Invoking Quality-of-Life Futility	183
Step 7: Managing Trends toward Ethically Justified Limits on Life-Sustaining Treatment	183
15.4.2 Preventing Unacceptable Opportunity Costs to Other Patients	183
15.5 Why the Groningen Protocol Should Be Rejected in Professional Ethics in Perinatal Medicine	184

Section 3: Professionally Responsible Clinical Practice

15.6 A Preventive Ethics Approach to Setting Ethically Justified Limits on Life-Sustaining Treatment — 184
15.7 Responding to Inappropriate Requests for Life-Sustaining Treatment — 185
    15.7.1 The Role of the Professional Virtue of Integrity in Professional Ethics in Obstetrics and Gynecology and in Perinatal Medicine — 185
    15.7.2 Why Requests to "Do Everything" Are Made: A Hypothesis from Qualitative Research on End-of-Life Surrogate Decision Making — 185
    15.7.3 Responding to Requests to "Do Everything" — 185
    15.7.4 The Essential Role of Hospital Policy and Commitment to It by Hospital Leadership — 186

Key Concepts

Advance directive
Anatomic futility
Decision-making capacity
Enthusiasm
Ethical principle of beneficence in professional ethics in gynecology
Ethical principle of beneficence in professional ethics in obstetrics
Ethical principle of healthcare justice in professional ethics in obstetrics and gynecology
Ethical principle of respect for autonomy in professional ethics in gynecology
Ethical principle of respect for autonomy in professional ethics in obstetrics
Futility
Groningen Protocol
Imminent demise futility
Informed consent process
Interactive capacity futility
Opportunity cost
Physiologic futility
Professional virtue of compassion
Professional virtue of integrity
Quality of life
Quality-of-life futility
Surrogate decision making
Unacceptable opportunity cost
Vitalism

15.1 Two Goals of Life-Sustaining Treatment

Sometimes a patient's condition has deteriorated to such a degree that in deliberative clinical judgment the prediction of imminent death becomes reliable. When death is imminent patients are transferred to a critical care unit in which they receive life-sustaining treatment. Life-sustaining treatment deploys a range of interventions, including physical intervention such as cardiopulmonary resuscitation; intravenous administration of drugs, fluids, and nutrition; and mechanical devices such as circulation devices, extracorporeal membrane oxygenation, dialysis, and ventilators. These interventions are designed to support or replace organ functions in the absence of which the risk of mortality will rapidly approach 100%.

Prevention of imminent death is not the only goal of critical care medicine. In the history of global medical ethics one cannot find the view that medicine is committed to the preservation of human life without qualification (known as vitalism) but to the preservation of human life when there is interactive capacity, however small, that supports human development and the meaning individuals give to their lives.[1] Indirect evidence for the view that medicine is not vitalist exists in the index of the most comprehensive scholarly work on the global history of medical ethics: that index does not include "vitalism."[2]

There is a prima facie beneficence-based ethical obligation in the professional ethics of medicine and therefore in the professional ethics of obstetrics and gynecology to pursue *both* goals of critical care management: prevention of imminent death and survival with at least some interactive capacity. There are both beneficence-based and autonomy-based limits on the pursuit of the two goals of critical care management in obstetrics and gynecology.

15.2 Beneficence-Based and Autonomy-Based Limits of Life-Sustaining Treatment

Like all prima facie ethical obligations, the beneficence-based ethical obligation to prevent imminent death can reach ethically justified limits. Either imminent death cannot be prevented or, when imminent death can be prevented in deliberative clinical judgment the patient is reliably expected to survive but to have lost interactive capacity. There is also an autonomy-based limit: when in the informed consent process the patient refuses life-sustaining treatment, directly or through an advance directive, or the patient's surrogate decision maker refuses life-sustaining treatment. (See Chapter 3.) When beneficence-based limits have been reached, there is strong consensus in health law and the professional ethics of medicine that it is ethically and legally permissible either not to initiate or to discontinue life-sustaining treatment. If the patient is experiencing pain, distress, or suffering that cannot be mitigated by even aggressive palliative care, then it becomes ethically obligatory in beneficence-based deliberative clinical judgment not to initiate or to discontinue life-sustaining treatment because such clinical management is resulting in net clinical harm for the patient.

There is also strong consensus in health law and the professional ethics of medicine that every adult patient with intact decision-making capacity has the autonomy-based right to refuse offered or recommended clinical management, including especially life-sustaining treatment, and that this negative right can be exercised for patients without decision-making capacity by their legally designated surrogate decision maker. (See Chapter 3.) When the outcome of the informed consent process with the patient or the patient's surrogate is refusal of life-sustaining treatment, there is a prima facie autonomy-based ethical obligation to discontinue life-sustaining treatment.

The obstetrician-gynecologist has the professional autonomy-based ethical obligation to empower the patient or surrogate with clinically relevant information and recommendations. (See Chapter 3.) This chapter provides an algorithm to guide this process regarding setting ethically justified limits on life-sustaining treatment. In addition, this chapter provides guidance for how to respond to inappropriate requests for life-sustaining treatment.

15.3 Historical Perspective

15.3.1 The Hippocratic Tradition of Declaring Gravely Ill Patients Incurable and Abandoning Them

The Hippocratic texts address the physician's role in the care of those with grave illness or injury. Such patients should be considered to be "overmastered" by their disease or injury and a physician who does not recognize the limits of medicine (Hippocratic physicians were therapeutic minimalists) to alter the course of a serious disease or injury has gone willfully mad.[3] Put in more modern terms, such a physician abandons his or her intellectual integrity. To prevent these unacceptable outcomes, the Hippocratic texts call for physicians to learn to distinguish conditions for which their ministrations hold the promise of relief (curable conditions) from conditions before which they stand as helpless as the sick person (incurable conditions). Physicians should declare the sick in the latter group as incurable and leave off their care.

Abandoning incurable, dying patients to their fate put the physician in a position to blame nature's overwhelming power for the patient's death. Doing so prevented gaining a reputation for doing things that result in the patient's death. Such a reputation would have surely undermined a physician's chances of economic survival in what was then a highly competitive, unregulated (there was no licensure, for example, much less peer review for safety and quality or government oversight) market that rewarded failure to gain and hold market share with poverty.

15.3.2 John Gregory's Reversal of the Hippocratic Tradition of Abandoning Dying Patients

The Hippocratic practice of abandoning the incurable became a self-interested, not patient-centered, practice during the next two millennia. It functioned as the equivalent of a standard of care until John Gregory's (1724–1773) professional ethics in medicine. Gregory, one of the inventors of professional ethics in medicine (See Chapter 1), called for the end of abandoning the gravely ill and dying to their own devices: "Let me here exhort you against the custom of some physicians, who leave their patients when their life is despaired of, and when it is no longer decent to put them to farther expence. It is as much the business of a physician to alleviate pain, and to smooth the avenues of death, when unavoidable, as to cure diseases."[4, p. 35] Gregory and his contemporaries were committed to the view that diseases were caused by pathologies but they were well aware that they did not yet have a science of pathology. They were, however, keen observers and symptoms, which they could relieve or "cure" in the discourse of eighteenth-century British medicine. Curing diseases did not mean fighting death at all costs but recognizing the limits of medicine and conducting responsible research to expand those limits. Notice that pain relief is among the physician's ethical obligations when attending to dying patients, as well as the obligation to "smooth the avenues of death, when unavoidable."[4, p. 35] This created an ethical justification for the liberal use of laudanum, which was readily available as there was no state agency to limit access of the sick to this liquid form of opium. Smoothing the avenues of death is now known as comprehensive palliative care.

15.3.3 The Influence of Enthusiasm in American Critical Care

With the creation of mechanical ventilation in the middle of the twentieth century, it became possible to prevent the deaths of patients who otherwise would have died. A dramatic reduction of mortality resulted, in adult, pediatric, and neonatal critical care in the United States and other resource-rich countries. During the middle third of the twentieth century in the United States, enthusiasm – clinical beliefs that lack an evidence base – drove the subsequent development and deployment of critical care interventions. Enthusiasm in this case took the form of the belief, not that death could be defeated at all costs, but that death could be defeated at little or no cost to the patient. The origin of this belief was a simple clinical reality: intensivists did not provide longitudinal care for the "graduates" of their units. One exception were groups of neonatologists and pediatric intensivists who ran continuity clinics for their patients, largely because other pediatricians and adult medicine specialists did not consider themselves qualified to manage such complex cases. These intensivists directly observed the costs to some of their graduates: chronic severe disability in the forms of technological dependency and severe and profound physical and cognitive disability. By the 1990s physicians, nurses, and family members began to take seriously the beneficence-based view that not all incremental reductions in mortality were worth such chronic, severe, and profound disability.[5,6]

15.3.4 The Influence of American Common Law

The common law of the United States contributed to this change in clinical judgment. The New Jersey Supreme Court ruled in 1976 that the father of a patient named Karen Ann Quinlan could make the decision to discontinue her respirator after she had been diagnosed to be in a "persistent chronic vegetative state," which is now called a permanent vegetative state or an irreversible loss of awareness. The Court determined that the state did not have a compelling interest – the prerogative to use its police powers to protect Ms. Quinlan's interests by ordering medical treatment – because she was not expected to return to a "cognitive, sapient state."[7] In other words, that she would survive with continued critical care intervention was not enough; she had to survive with some capacity to experience the world and continue to develop as a human being.[1]

15.3.5 An Emerging Consensus

A consensus began to emerge in the 1980s and 1990s: evidence-based, ethically justified limits needed to be set that took account of risks of *both* mortality and morbidity, not mortality alone.[8] Unwittingly, the ethics of end-of-life decision making recovered the core of Gregory's view: the dying patient should neither be abandoned nor subject to treatment without limit. The clinical ethical concept of futility played a major role in translating this consensus into clinical practice. In general terms, a form of clinical management becomes futile when in deliberative clinical judgment it is predicted to have a high rate of failure in achieving the goal for which it was created. To be clinically useful, this general concept must be specified, in two steps. The ethical justification for setting limits must include a justification of what should count as an acceptable failure rate. The goal of each form of critical care must be clearly stated.

15.3.6 The Influence of a Landmark Article

In a landmark article, "Must we always use CPR?" Leslie Blackhall completed the first step.[9] The failure rate should be set high, she maintained, because invoking limits on critical care interventions will almost always result in the patient's death. Beneficence-based clinical judgment requires that the failure rate should be conservative. Blackhall proposed a 97%–100% failure rate.

The second step specifies clearly the overall and specific goals of critical care interventions. Because both mortality and morbidity must be taken into account, the overall goal of critical care is to prevent imminent death with an acceptable functional status among survivors. Acceptable functional status is understood in beneficence-based deliberative clinical judgment to mean at least some, minimal interactive capacity.[1] When interactive capacity ceases to exist, the patient cannot use her survival to engage in any of the life tasks that human beings value. Such patients do not have a poor quality of life (engaging in valued life tasks and deriving satisfaction from doing so); they do not have the capacity for any quality of life. Acceptable functional status in autonomy-based deliberative clinical judgment means that the patient has some interactive capacity that is also enough to support engaging in valued life tasks (as defined by the patient) and gaining satisfaction from doing so (as judged by the patient). From the patient's perspective – and *only* from the patient's perspective – the patient's functional status supports an acceptable quality of life. When this is not the case, the patient has – from the patient's perspective and only from the patient's perspective – an unacceptable quality of life.

In beneficence-based deliberative clinical judgment the goals of specific forms of critical care intervention can be reliably specified. The goal of cardiopulmonary resuscitation is the restoration of spontaneous circulation. The goal of mechanical circulation is to maintain blood circulation. The goal of mechanical ventilation is to maintain adequate oxygenation levels, which is also the objective of extracorporeal membrane oxygenation. The goal of using pressors and other medication is to maintain adequate heart function. The goal of dialysis is to remove toxins from the blood. The goal of total parenteral nutrition is to provide nutrients that cannot be obtained by masticating, swallowing, and digesting foodstuffs.

15.4 An Algorithm for the Role of the Obstetrician-Gynecologist in Decision Making about Setting Ethically Justified Limits on Life-Sustaining Treatment

We propose an end-of-life decision-making algorithm based on the two goals of critical care. Neonatal, pediatric, and adult critical care have both a short-term and a long-term goal. The short-term goal is to prevent imminent death. Intensivists and the vast array of interventions at their command are very effective in achieving this goal. As a result, the likelihood of dying in a critical care unit is very remote. The long-term goal is survival with an acceptable functional status. Acceptable functional status can be understood from a clinical, beneficence-based perspective: at least some interactive capacity. This is a deliberately conservative concept, again, because the patient's life is at stake. Acceptable functional status can also be understood from the patient's perspective: an unacceptable quality of life given predicted functional status.

We do not share the skepticism of others about invoking the discourse of futility as the basis for setting ethically justified limits on a trial of critical care management.[10] This is because, as demonstrated in Section 15.3.5, the general concept of futility can be clearly stated and its specifications can be clearly stated. These specifications can be organized into an ethically justified, clinically applicable stepwise algorithm.[11] This algorithm is designed to guide the obstetrician-gynecologist in making recommendations to discontinue life-sustaining treatment when either of its goals is reliably predicted not to be met and its limits therefore met. (See Table 15.1.)

Table 15.1 End-of-life decision-making algorithm.

Step 1: Invoking applicable advance directive law based on deliberative clinical judgment about the patient's condition
Step 2: Invoking the specified concept of anatomic futility
Step 3: Invoking the specified concept of physiologic futility
Step 4: Invoking the specified concept of imminent-demise futility
Step 5: Invoking the specified concept of interactive-capacity futility
Step 6: Invoking the specified concepts of quality-of-life futility
Step 7: Managing trends toward ethically justified limits on life-sustaining treatment

15.4.1 Steps of the Algorithm

Step 1: Invoking Applicable Advance Directive Law

The first step of the end-of-life decision-making algorithm invokes the patient's condition: Does the patient have a terminal, irreversible, or other condition, as defined in the applicable advance directives legislation, in the deliberative clinical judgment of the patient's attending physician? The answer to this step should be based on the definitions in applicable law and hospital policy, which should be based on applicable law. If the answer in deliberative clinical judgment is yes, then discontinuing life-sustaining treatment becomes medically reasonable and should be recommended, especially to respect the adult patient's autonomy as expressed in her advance directive or as expressed by a surrogate decision maker. Advance directive law typically allows parents to make decisions for their infant or minor child.

The subsequent steps of the end-of-life decision-making algorithm invoke sequential specifications of the general concept of futility.

Step 2: Invoking Anatomic Futility

Does deliberative clinical judgment support the prediction of a 97–100% rate of failure to achieve the anatomic goal of maintaining or restoring adequate anatomy? If the answer in deliberative clinical judgment is yes, the beneficence-based ethical obligation to continue intervention ends, because of anatomic futility. Anatomic futility plays a major role in gynecologic surgery, e.g., when the patient's tumor is so large and invasive that not all of it can be removed. Anatomic futility means that imminent death cannot be prevented. As a result, the long-term goal of continued critical care intervention cannot be achieved. The beneficence-based limits of the critical care intervention have been reached. Both not initiating and discontinuing life-sustaining treatment become medically reasonable and should be recommended to protect the patient from iatrogenic morbidity that confers no offsetting clinical benefit.

Step 3: Invoking Physiologic Futility

Does deliberative clinical judgment support the prediction of a 97–100% failure rate to achieve the physiologic goal of a critical care intervention? The outcome appropriate to each critical care intervention should be stated precisely, as noted in Section 15.3.6.

It is crucial not to confuse a physiologic effect, e.g., transient heart beat during resuscitation, with the physiologic goal. If the answer to the aforementioned question in deliberative clinical judgment is yes, the beneficence-based ethical obligation to continue intervention ends, because of physiologic futility. Physiologic futility means that imminent death cannot be prevented. As a result, the short-term goal of continued critical care intervention cannot be achieved. The beneficence-based limits of the critical care intervention have been reached. Both not initiating and discontinuing life-sustaining treatment become medically reasonable and should be recommended to protect the patient from iatrogenic morbidity that confers no offsetting clinical benefit.

Step 4: Invoking Imminent-Demise Futility

Does deliberative clinical judgment support a prediction that intervention will be physiologically effective for a short period of time (days to weeks) but then result in death (in the critical care unit) with a 97%–100% rate and without any interactive capacity before death occurs? If the answer in deliberative clinical judgment is yes, the beneficence-based ethical obligation to continue intervention ends, because of imminent-demise futility. Imminent-demise futility means that imminent death can at best be postponed. Moreover, the long-term goal of continued critical care intervention cannot be achieved and the short-term goal will soon become unachievable. The beneficence-based limits of the critical care intervention have been reached. Both not initiating and discontinuing life-sustaining treatment become medically reasonable and should be recommended to protect the patient from iatrogenic morbidity that confers no offsetting clinical benefit.

Step 5: Invoking Interactive-Capacity Futility

Does deliberative clinical judgment predict that the intervention will be physiologically effective, prevent imminent demise, but with a 97%–100% rate result in irreversible loss of interactive capacity? If the answer in deliberative clinical judgment is yes, the beneficence-based ethical obligation to continue intervention ends, because of interactive-capacity futility. Interactive-capacity futility means that imminent death can be postponed for a short time but not prevented altogether. As a result, the long-term goal of continued critical care intervention cannot be achieved because the outcome is unacceptable from a clinical perspective. The beneficence-based limits of the critical care intervention have been reached. Both not initiating and discontinuing life-sustaining treatment become medically reasonable and should be recommended to protect the patient from iatrogenic morbidity that confers no offsetting clinical benefit.

Step 6: Invoking Quality-of-Life Futility

Does deliberative clinical judgment predict that the intervention will be physiologically effective, prevent imminent demise, and preserve at least interactive capacity but the patient considers the resulting quality of life unacceptable from the patient's – and *only* from the patient's – perspective? If the answer in deliberative clinical judgment is yes, the autonomy-based ethical obligation to continue intervention ends, because of quality-of-life futility. The short-term goal of critical care management can be achieved. However, the long-term goal of continued critical care intervention cannot be achieved because the outcome is unacceptable from the patient's perspective. The autonomy-based limits of the critical care intervention have been reached. Both not initiating and discontinuing life-sustaining treatment become medically reasonable and should be recommended to protect the patient from iatrogenic morbidity that confers no offsetting clinical benefit.

We emphasize that quality-of-life futility cannot be invoked with neonatal patients. Infants do not have the capacity to identify valued life goals or to have the concept of sufficient satisfaction with achieving valued life goals. This means that current quality of life of an infant cannot be invoked. No one can reliably predict what life tasks a future child and adult will value or how he or she will make judgment about sufficient satisfaction. Moreover, some studies show no difference between disabled children and non-disabled children in self-reported quality of life.[12] This means that future quality of life of an infant cannot be invoked. We make this point fully aware that current or predicted poor quality of life, especially for infants with physical or cognitive disabilities, is sometimes invoked. Current or future disabilities cannot be invoked in setting ethically justified limits on life-sustaining treatment of neonatal patients.

There is evidence that physicians are at risk for underestimating the quality of life of adult patients when compared to self-reports.[13] The professional virtue of integrity in professional ethics in obstetrics and gynecology creates an ethical obligation of physicians not to make quality-of-life judgments about their adult patients. By contrast, surrogate decision makers who fulfill the substituted judgment standard, by making a decision based on the patient's values, beliefs, and preferences, can make reliable estimates of the patient's current and projected quality of life.

Step 7: Managing Trends toward Ethically Justified Limits on Life-Sustaining Treatment

The patient, for whom none of these concepts of futility apply but appears to be on a course to a condition in which one or more may apply, should be carefully monitored. The surrogate decision maker should be informed that the trial of critical care management is being continued but with new attention to whether clinically and ethically justified limits might have to be set and that, if this should turn out to be the case, there will be future discussion focused on recommending ethically justified limits.

15.4.2 Preventing Unacceptable Opportunity Costs to Other Patients

The ethical justification for recommending discontinuation of life-sustaining treatment becomes stronger when one or more steps of the end-of-life decision-making algorithm apply and continuing life-sustaining treatment creates an unacceptable opportunity cost to another patient. An opportunity cost exists when the use of a limited resource blocks access to that resource by others. The concept of an opportunity cost is not the same as the financial costs of a patient's care; it is about resource use and its effects on other patients, not on financial cost. If the current use of the limited resource is ethically justified, the opportunity cost is acceptable. However, when one or more steps of the end-of-life decision-making algorithm apply, the use of a critical care bed, personnel, and equipment is not supported in beneficence-based deliberative clinical judgment or, in the first and last steps of the end-of-life decision-making algorithm, autonomy-based clinical judgment. When the use of limited clinical resources for a patient is reliably predicted not to benefit that patient clinically and that use also blocks access to those limited clinical resources by a patient reliably predicted to benefit from the use of those resources, an unacceptable opportunity cost exists.

In the circumstances of an unacceptable opportunity cost, the obstetrician-gynecologist's beneficence-based ethical obligations to his or her patient have reached their limits. The patient receiving critical care is not equal in need with the patient who could benefit from critical care. This creates a healthcare-justice–based ethical obligation to give the second patient priority for critical care admission. If the recommendation to discontinue life-sustaining treatment is not accepted, then hospital policy should permit – and support – unilateral discharge to hospice and palliative care to free up the critical care resources for the patient reliably predicted to benefit from their use. The Society of Critical Care Medicine has supported the position that "Patients who are not expected to benefit from intensive care ... should not be placed in the intensive care unit."[14] This implies that such patients should not continue to be placed in an intensive care unit. Unilateral discharge should be contemplated if and only if there is a clear hospital policy that provides for it and this policy is supported by the hospital's senior leadership.

15.5 Why the Groningen Protocol Should Be Rejected in Professional Ethics in Perinatal Medicine

Eduard Verhagen and Pieter J. J. Sauer reported on the Dutch experience with euthanasia in newborns under current Dutch law and medical practice and proposed a protocol, called the Groningen Protocol, to guide the decision making.[15] The protocol has two parts. The first addresses "requirements that must be fulfilled," including diagnosis and prognosis that are "certain," presence of "hopeless and unbearable suffering," and confirmation of the diagnosis and prognosis by an independent physician. The second addresses "information needed to support and clarify the decision about euthanasia" that covers five domains: diagnosis and prognosis; "euthanasia decision"; consultation; implementation; and "steps taken after death." The Protocol also presents a medical and legal justification for the protocol and clinical practice based on it.

The Protocol develops this justification by referring to twenty-two cases of disabled newborns, all but one of them diagnosed with spina bifida.[16] Neither "hopeless suffering" nor the other clinical criteria cited in the Protocol apply to spina bifida in infants. This failure to adhere to the professional virtue of integrity in professional ethics in pediatrics is not explained.

In addition, the justification the Protocol offers is woefully inadequate. It relies on appeals to the concepts of "hopeless and unbearable suffering," the "best interests of the patient," and "medical-ethical values,"[15] but it never explains these concepts, and it gives no ethical argument for their clinical application. In addition, the Protocol invokes the concepts of current quality of life and predicted quality of life, which, as shown earlier, cannot be applied to neonatal patients.

The Groningen Protocol fails to meet the basic requirement of ethical analysis, as explained in Chapter 1: getting as clear as possible about concepts considered relevant to a topic. The Groningen Protocol should therefore be rejected as the basis for perinatal and neonatal practice in the Netherlands and throughout the world.[17–19]

15.6 A Preventive Ethics Approach to Setting Ethically Justified Limits on Life-Sustaining Treatment

As explained in Chapter 3, preventive ethics deploys the informed consent process to anticipate ethical challenges and prevent them from evolving into ethical conflict that has the potential to paralyze deliberative clinical judgment. Preventive ethics has particular application to adult patients who have survived an admission to a critical care unit and are being prepared for transfer to another service or discharge. There should be a discussion with the patient or surrogate of the prognosis of anatomic, physiologic, imminent-demise, interactive-capacity, or quality-of-life futility and the implication of each for clinical management during the next admission. The obstetrician-gynecologist should emphasize that patients who do not make clear decisions about life-sustaining treatment and do not communicate those decisions to others, either orally or in the form of a completed advance directive, put themselves at risk of receiving life-sustaining treatment by default.[20] The physician should recommend that the patient give this risk serious consideration and support the patient to make and communicate clear decisions. Documenting such decisions can play a major role in ensuring that the patient's wishes guide the healthcare team on the next admission. The physician should offer assistance to the patient in the completion of advance directives to patients who express an interest in learning more about them.

In the perinatal setting when counseling prospective parents about the implications of fetal anomalies for neonatal critical care, the obstetrician and neonatologist should work with them to increase their understanding of the concepts of anatomic, physiologic, imminent-demise, and interactive-capacity and how they would be applied to set ethically justified limits on neonatal critical care. The physician should explain the concept of quality-of-life futility and why it does not create a justification for limiting neonatal critical care. This approach differs considerably from a recently proposed autonomy-based approach, in which parents of a newborn are simply given options and their requests implemented.[21] This proposed approach is inconsistent with professional ethics in pediatrics and its core beneficence-based concept of the best interests of the child.[22,23]

15.7 Responding to Inappropriate Requests for Life-Sustaining Treatment

The obstetrician-gynecologist should take a preventive ethics approach to responding to requests for inappropriate life-sustaining treatment by pursuing two goals: transforming the request into an informed decision and protecting the patient from inappropriate life-sustaining treatment. The following ethical considerations set the stage for pursuing these two goals.

15.7.1 The Role of the Professional Virtue of Integrity in Professional Ethics in Obstetrics and Gynecology and in Perinatal Medicine

A request for life-sustaining treatment is the exercise of a positive right, the justified claim to the resources of others as the means to protect and promote one's interests. All positive rights come with limits; ethical justification therefore focuses on which limits should be set.[24] The professional virtue of integrity in professional ethics in obstetrics and gynecology sets a justified beneficence-based limit. When life-sustaining treatment is technically possible but is not in deliberative clinical judgment reliably predicted *not* to result in net clinical benefit, it is not a medically reasonable alternative. Providing clinical management that is not medically reasonable is incompatible with the professional virtue of integrity, because this virtue creates a prima facie ethical obligation not to provide clinical management that is not going to help the patient clinically.[25,26] Put another way, the professional virtue of integrity protects the obstetrician-gynecologist from functioning as a mere technician. When clinical management that is not medically reasonable is in deliberative clinical judgment predicted to result only in net clinical harm for the patient – mortality, morbidity, pain, distress, or suffering, the ethical principles of beneficence and nonmaleficence as well as the professional virtue of compassion in professional ethics in obstetrics and gynecology combine to create a prima facie ethical obligation to recommend discontinuation of life-sustaining treatment.

15.7.2 Why Requests to "Do Everything" Are Made: A Hypothesis from Qualitative Research on End-of-Life Surrogate Decision Making

There is qualitative research that helps to understand why such requests might be made.[27] This research suggests the hypothesis that a request for inappropriate life-sustaining treatment is made by a surrogate decision maker when he or she confronts two synergistic uncertainties: conflicting prognoses from members of the care team, which understandably creates uncertainty about discontinuation of life-sustaining treatment; and uncertainty about what the patient would want, making it very difficult to fulfill the substituted judgment standard of surrogate decision making. This standard requires the surrogate decision maker to make a decision based on reliable beliefs about the patient's values and beliefs and preferences based on them. (See Chapter 3.) In this qualitative study surrogate decision makers reported that they managed the resulting overwhelming stress by requesting that "everything be done."

15.7.3 Responding to Requests to "Do Everything"

This research suggests that it is mistake to label a surrogate decision maker who requests that everything be done as irrational and therefore impossible to persuade to reconsider.[28] Instead, the obstetrician-gynecologist should canvas the care team and consultants for the prognoses they have offered. There will be one of two outcomes.

If it is discovered that this prognostic information has been inconsistent, the obstetrician-gynecologist should meet with the team and consultants with the goal of reaching consensus on the patient's prognosis. If in deliberative clinical judgment there are evidence-based reasons for disagreement about prognosis, continuation of life-sustaining treatment as a trial of management remains a medically reasonable alternative. The surrogate decision maker should be informed that continuation of the trial of management is medically reasonable and be informed that the trial will be periodically reviewed to make a judgment about whether a continuing trial of management is still helping the patient.

If it is discovered that there is a consistent prognosis of a high probability of failure to achieve the goals of critical care management, the end-of-life decision-making algorithm should be deployed with the care team and consultants to reach agreement on which one or more of the specified concepts of futility apply. The obstetrician-gynecologist should meet with the surrogate decision maker and ask him or her what he or she understands the patient's prognosis to be. The obstetrician-gynecologist should then explain that the team and consultants have met and agreed on the patient's prognosis. The nature of the prognosis should be presented along with the consensus clinical reasoning that supports it. The obstetrician-gynecologist should support the surrogate decision maker to process and accept this information.

The obstetrician-gynecologist should then explain the steps of the end-of-life decision-making algorithm that the team and consultants believe apply. The obstetrician-gynecologist should support the surrogate decision maker to process and accept this information. The obstetrician-gynecologist should then recommend that the surrogate agree that it is time to accept limits on life-sustaining treatment because it is no longer predicted to help the patient. The obstetrician-gynecologist should support the surrogate decision maker to process this information and ask him or her to accept the recommendation to discontinue life-sustaining treatment. To support the surrogate decision maker through this momentous process, the obstetrician-gynecologist should be sure to include colleagues such as social workers who have the skillset to help family members cope with stressful and momentous decisions. In addition, for religious patients, a chaplain or religious advisor who is experienced in these discussions should also be present. It will be very important for the chaplain or religious advisor to be able and willing to inform the surrogate decision maker that accepting the recommendation to discontinue life-sustaining treatment is supported by the family's faith community.

The response to inappropriate requests for life-sustaining treatment should be addressed in a process that starts with deliberative clinical judgment about the patient's prognosis and continues with the deliberative clinical application of the end-of-life decision-making algorithm, recommendations based on its results, and sustained psychosocial and spiritual support for the surrogate decision maker and other family members. The Society of Critical Care Medicine supports a process-based response to these requests.[10] The goal should be to transform an inappropriate request into an informed decision.

15.7.4 The Essential Role of Hospital Policy and Commitment to It by Hospital Leadership

Hospital policy should provide clear and unequivocal support for this or a similar stepwise approach[10] to responding to requests for inappropriate life-sustaining treatment. In addition, hospital policy should describe how to respond when the recommendation to discontinue life-sustaining treatment is not accepted. Some states address this matter in their advance directives legislation or common law. Other states do not. Nonetheless, it is essential that hospital policy provide needed direction and that senior leadership are fully committed to using the hospital's resources to support the obstetrician-gynecologist and other team members when a surrogate decision maker rejects the recommendation and reiterates the request for inappropriate life-sustaining treatment. Failure to create and fully support such hospital policy undermines the professional virtue of integrity in professional ethics in obstetrics and gynecology and in all other medical specialties, which no hospital leader is ethically free to do. (See Chapter 16.)

References

1. McCormick RA. To save or let die: the dilemma of modern medicine. JAMA 1974; 229: 172–176.
2. Baker RB, McCullough LB. The Cambridge World History of Medical Ethics. New York: Cambridge University Press, 2009.

3. Hippocrates. The Art. In Reiser SJ, Dyck AJ, Curran WJ, eds. Ethics in Medicine: Historical Perspectives and Contemporary Concerns. Cambridge, MA: MIT Press, 1977: 6.
4. Gregory J. Lectures on the Duties and Qualifications of a Physician. London: W. Strahan and T. Cadell, 1772. Reprinted in McCullough LB, ed. John Gregory's Writings on Medical Ethics and the Philosophy of Medicine. Dordrecht, the Netherlands: Kluwer Academic Publishers, 1998: 161–248.
5. Placencia FX, McCullough LB. The history of ethical decision making in neonatal intensive care. J Intensive Care Med 2011; 26: 368–384.
6. Placencia FX, McCullough LB. Biopsychosocial risks of parental care for high-risk neonates: implications for evidence-based parental counseling. J Perinatol 2012; 32: 381–386.
7. In re Quinlan. 70 N.J. 10; 355 A.2d 647 (1976).
8. Rabeneck L, McCullough LB, Wray NP. Ethically justified, clinically comprehensive guidelines for percutaneous endoscopic gastrostomy tube placement. Lancet 1997; 349: 496–498.
9. Blackhall, L. Must we always use CPR? N Engl J Med 1987; 317: 1281–1285.
10. Kon AA, Shepard EK, Sederstrom NO, Swoboda SM, et al. Defining futile and potentially inappropriate interventions: a policy statement from the Society of Critical Care Medicine Ethics Committee. Crit Care Med 2016; 44: 1679–1774.
11. McCullough LB, Jones JW. Postoperative futility: a clinical algorithm for setting limits. Brit J Surg 2001; 88: 1153–1154.
12. Saigal S, Tyson J. Measurement of quality of life of survivors of neonatal intensive care: critique and implications. Semin Perinatol 2008; 32: 59–66.
13. Leplège A, Hunt S. The problem of quality of life in medicine. JAMA 1997; 278: 47–50.
14. Consensus statement of the Society of Critical Care Medicine's Ethics Committee regarding futile and other possibly inadvisable treatments. Crit Care Med 1997; 25: 887–891.
15. Verhagen E, Sauer PJJ. The Groningen Protocol: euthanasia in severely ill newborns. N Engl J Med 2005; 352: 959–962.
16. Verhagen AAE, Sol JJ, Brouwer OF, Sauer PJ. Actieve levensbeendiging bij pasgeborenen in Nederland, Een analyse can alle meldingen van 1997–2004. Ned Tijdschr Geneeskd 2005; 149: 183–188.
17. Chervenak FA, McCullough LB, Arabin B. Why the Groningen Protocol should be rejected. Hastings Cent Rep 2006; 36: 30–33.
18. Kon AA. Neonatal euthanasia is unsupportable: the Groningen Protocol should be abandoned. Theor Med Bioeth 2007; 28: 453–463.
19. Kodish E. Paediatric ethics: a repudiation of the Groningen Protocol. Lancet 2008; 371: 892–893.
20. Braun UK, McCullough LB. Preventing pathways to life-sustaining treatment by default. Ann Fam Med 2011; 9: 250–256.
21. Lantos JD. Ethical problems in decision making in the neonatal ICU. N Engl J Med 2018; 379: 1851–1860.
22. American Academy of Pediatrics. Committee on Bioethics. Informed consent, parental permission, and assent in pediatric practice. Pediatrics 1995; 95: 314–317.
23. Katz AL, Webb SA. Committee on Bioethics. American Academy of Pediatrics. Informed consent in decision-making in pediatric practice. Pediatrics 2016; 138: pii: e20161485.
24. Chervenak FA, McCullough LB. Justified limits on refusing intervention. Hastings Cent Rep 1991; 21: 12–18.
25. Brett A, McCullough LB. When patients request specific interventions: defining the limits of the physician's obligations. N Engl J Med 1986; 315: 1347–1351.
26. Brett AS, McCullough LB. Addressing requests by patients for non-beneficial interventions. JAMA 2012; 307: 149–150.
27. Braun UK, Beyth RJ, Ford ME, McCullough LB. Voices of African American, Caucasian, and Hispanic surrogates on the burdens of end-of-life decision-making. J Gen Intern Med 2008; 23: 267–274.
28. Braun UK, Naik AD, McCullough LB. Reconceptualizing the experience of surrogate decision making: reports vs genuine decisions. Ann Fam Med 2009; 7: 249–253.

Section 4 — Professionally Responsible Leadership

Chapter 16

Leadership

GOAL
This chapter provides an ethical framework to guide leadership of obstetrics and gynecology in healthcare organizations.

OBJECTIVES
On completing study of this chapter, the reader will:
- Identify the implications of professional virtues in professional ethics in obstetrics and gynecology for leadership
- Describe the concept of organizational culture
- Describe progressive stages of dysfunction of organizational culture
- Describe the role of leadership in managing guild interests of obstetrician-gynecologists
- Apply the ethical framework to guide leadership of obstetrics and gynecology in healthcare organizations in leadership roles

TOPICS

16.1 Ethical Challenges in Organizational Leadership	190
16.2 Leadership as a Philosophy	190
16.2.1 Plato on Leadership	191
16.2.2 Peter Drucker on Leadership	191
16.2.3 John Gregory and Thomas Percival on Professional Virtues in Leadership	191
16.2.3.1 The Professional Virtue of Self-Effacement	191
16.2.3.2 The Professional Virtue of Self-Sacrifice	192
16.2.3.3 The Professional Virtue of Compassion	192
16.2.3.4 The Professional Virtue of Integrity	192
16.2.3.5 The Professional Virtue of Humility	192
16.3 Gregory and Percival on Organizational Culture	192
16.3.1 Professional Treatment of Colleagues	192
16.3.2 Professional Resource Management	193
16.3.2.1 The Perils of a Utilitarian Organizational Culture	193
16.3.2.2 The Perils of a Libertarian Organizational Culture	193
16.3.3 Professional Use of Power	193
16.3.3.1 Thomas Hobbes on Power	193
16.3.3.2 Monopoly Power and Monopsony Power	193
16.3.4 Organizational Dysfunction: A Progressive Disorder	194

16.3.4.1	Machiavellian Organizational Culture	194
16.3.4.2	A Cynical Organizational Culture	194
16.3.4.3	A Wonderland Organizational Culture	194
16.3.4.4	A Kafkaesque Organizational Culture	194
16.3.4.5	A Postmodern Organizational Culture	194
16.3.4.6	Common Signs of Progressive Organizational Dysfunction	195

16.4 Managing Guild Interests — 195
   16.4.1 Guild Interests: An Insidious Threat to a Professional Organizational Culture — 195
   16.4.2 Two Potentially Insidious Incentives — 196
      16.4.2.1 Productivity Incentives — 196
      16.4.2.2 Regulatory and Compliance Demands — 196
   16.4.3 A Powerful Antidote: An Organizational Culture that Subordinates Guild Interests to Professionalism — 196
      16.4.3.1 Setting Reasonable Limits on Self-Sacrifice — 197
      16.4.3.2 Preventing Incremental Subordination of Professionalism to Guild Self-Interest — 197

16.5 Navigating the Perilous Waters of Scylla and Charybdis — 197

Key Concepts

Cynical organizational culture
Guild
Guild self-interest
Kafkaesque organizational culture
Libertarian justice
Machiavellian organizational culture
Monopoly power
Monopsony power
Organizational Culture
Postmodern organizational culture
Power
Profession of medicine as a public trust
Professional virtue of compassion
Professional virtue of humility
Professional virtue of integrity
Professional virtue of self-effacement
Professional virtue of self-sacrifice
Utilitarian justice
Wonderland organizational culture

16.1 Ethical Challenges in Organizational Leadership

Obstetrician-gynecologists in leadership positions confront ethical challenges on a daily basis. These range from making decisions about improving patient safety,[1-3] managing disruptive physician behavior,[4] the allocation of organizational resources,[5] securing cooperation from reluctant colleagues for the use of evidence-based guidelines,[3] and obtaining vital resources from organizational leaders who promise prompt action and then obfuscate and delay.[6] These challenges require effective management, which includes attention to the ethical issues at the core of many of these leadership challenges. Professional ethics in obstetrics and gynecology provides obstetrician-gynecologist leaders with guidance for identifying and managing common leadership challenges.[7,8]

16.2 Leadership as a Philosophy

Leadership in healthcare depends on a philosophy grounded in professional ethics in obstetrics and gynecology. Leadership as a philosophy includes the ability to articulate a vision and implement strategies requisite for accomplishing the mission, managerial competence, and, especially, appropriate ethical values. Competence, comprising management knowledge and skills, is an essential component of leadership. It cannot be overstated that healthcare organizations are no exception to the general managerial dictum that revenues must exceed expenses. In the absence of excess revenues, no physician leader can capitalize an organization's future and the organization's viability will decline. In addition, obstetrician-gynecologist leaders must develop, implement, and enforce policies and practices that ensure both the quality and service in a cost-efficient manner. Obstetrician-gynecologist leaders must not lose sight of the fact that medicine is not primarily a business but they also must be committed to the competent management of the business aspects of medicine.[9]

16.2.1 Plato on Leadership

The core component of leadership as a philosophy is appropriate ethical values. Ethical values should shape mission and requisite strategy and guide management decisions. Plato (424 BCE–348 BCE) articulated perhaps the most influential philosophy of leadership in the Western tradition in his classic work, *Republic*.[10] For Plato, the best leader is the philosopher king, someone who has been rigorously trained for years in the life of service to those subordinate to his power. This is a demanding way of life, in which the philosopher king understands his own interests entirely in terms of the interests of the citizens of the republic, who are subordinate to his power. In the technical language of ethics, the philosopher king has and is shaped by the responsibility to protect and promote the interests of subordinates and keep self-interest systematically secondary.[11] This commitment provides direction and purpose to the leadership role. Without this commitment to the life of service and the direction it provides, Plato rightly feared that leaders will become predatory and subordinates unacceptably harmed.[10,11] The commitment to the protection and promotion of those subordinate to one's power makes one a moral fiduciary, i.e., someone who can be trusted.[9]

16.2.2 Peter Drucker on Leadership

A recent expression of Platonic leadership philosophy can be found in the work of one of the most highly regarded scholars of management science, Peter Drucker (1909–2005). Drucker succinctly summarized leadership as a philosophy in a way that Plato would instantly recognize: "Leadership without direction is useless ... As the pace of change in our world continues to accelerate, strong basic values become increasingly necessary to guide leadership behavior."[12] The values that should guide healthcare leadership derive from the ethical concept of medicine as a profession.

16.2.3 John Gregory and Thomas Percival on Professional Virtues in Leadership

John Gregory (1724–1773) and Thomas Percival (1740–1804) invented professional ethics in medicine,[13–16] based on the ethical concept of medicine as a profesion. (See Chapter 1.) Percival was perhaps the first in modern Western medical ethics to address organizational ethics. Percival was concerned about the fierce competition among the physicians, surgeons, and apothecaries at the Royal Infirmary of Manchester, England, which at times resulted in profound organizational dysfunction. He called for the creation of an organizational culture of professionalism, based on the mutual, evidence-based accountability of physicians and surgeons, who were still separate and highly competitive guilds (known as the Royal Colleges), to improve the quality of the processes and outcomes of patient care based on sustained cooperation. He also called for organizational resources to be based primarily on the ethical principle of beneficence and not primarily on economics. A distinctive feature of the professional ethics in medicine created by Percival and Gregory is the central role of the professional virtues. (See Chapter 1.) The professional virtues of self-effacement, self-sacrifice, compassion, humility, and integrity apply directly to the leadership role of the obstetrician-gynecologist.[8,9]

16.2.3.1 The Professional Virtue of Self-Effacement

Self-effacement creates the prima facie beneficence-based ethical obligation of leaders to be unbiased. Leaders should not show favoritism to their own specialties or friends in a healthcare organization or on the basis of gender or shared academic pedigree. Nor should leaders show favoritism in decisions about resources in a merged institution, in which they were formerly in a leadership position in one of the components.[8,9] It may be obvious, but must still be emphasized, that self-effacement rules out as ethically impermissible prejudice of all kinds (including racial, religious, gender, sexual orientation, first language spoken) and sexual harassment.

16.2.3.2 The Professional Virtue of Self-Sacrifice

Self-sacrifice creates the prima facie beneficence-based ethical obligation to be willing to risk individual and organizational self-interest, especially in the economic domain. Leaders must pay attention to the bottom-line – no margin, no mission – but they should not focus exclusively on the bottom line. They should, instead, value economics as a tool rather than an overriding value. The organization's mission to create and sustain an organizational culture of professionalism should be the guiding value. Self-sacrifice creates the prima facie ethical obligation to take risks for the organization's legitimate fiscal self-interest when necessary to accomplish a mission, e.g., in securing funding for essential clinical services that do not make a profit.[8,9]

16.2.3.3 The Professional Virtue of Compassion

Compassion creates the prima facie beneficence-based ethical obligation of leaders to become aware of and respond with appropriate support to the distress of colleagues and staff. To fulfill this obligation, leaders should routinely ask, "What can I do to help?"[8,9]

16.2.3.4 The Professional Virtue of Integrity

The fourth, and bedrock, virtue is integrity, which creates the prima facie beneficence-based ethical obligation of leaders to make management decisions on the basis of intellectual and moral excellence. Intellectual excellence requires clinical care, research, and education to have a strong evidence base incorporated into deliberative clinical judgment. Moral excellence requires putting the interests of patients first and keeping individual and organizational self-interest systematically secondary. Adherence to self-effacement, self-sacrifice, and compassion is the key to achieving moral excellence. Indicators of integrity in physician leaders, by which they should be judged, include open and honest communication, accessibility, and accountability.[8,9]

16.2.3.5 The Professional Virtue of Humility

Leaders should cultivate the professional virtue of humility as an antidote to the arrogance of power. The power of physician leaders over subordinates is considerable, e.g., setting salaries, determining promotion and advancement, and assigning colleagues to subordinate leadership positions, e.g., appointment of division chiefs. Humility helps to keep the focus on the well-being of the organization rather than the self-interests of the leader. A good leader should promote the accomplishments of colleagues and give them credit when credit is due. Self-aggrandizing in the form of taking credit that belongs to others is incompatible with the professional virtue of humility, especially publicly taking credit that rightly belongs to others.

16.3 Gregory and Percival on Organizational Culture

Organizational culture is complex. It includes the organization's stated mission and core values, policies and practices, judgments about attitudes and behaviors that are to be promoted and rewarded, judgments about attitudes and behaviors that are to be discouraged and punished, and what is tolerated. There is also an informal organizational culture of what is perceived by employees, patients, and the community to be its "real" mission and core values, what it promotes and discourages, what it tolerates, and what it tolerates that should not be tolerated.

Gregory and, to a much greater extent, Percival recognized that physicians should not be expected to sustain their commitment to the ethical concept of medicine as a profession in the absence of an organizational culture committed to this concept as the basis for all that it does. Obstetrician-gynecologist leaders therefore bear the responsibility for creating sustainable cultures of organizational professionalism, permeated by the effects of routinely fulfilling the obligations of the professional virtues of physician leaders.[8,9] There are specific steps that obstetrician-gynecologist leaders should take to create a professional organizational culture.

16.3.1 Professional Treatment of Colleagues

Professional treatment of colleagues requires that they be treated with respect. The moral philosophy of Immanuel Kant (1724–1804) is essential for understanding what "respect" means. Kant's enduring contribution to the global history of moral philosophy is his categorical imperative.[17] This perhaps forbidding phrase means that we should treat each other as ends and not simply as means to achieving one's own or an organization's interests. When leaders treat colleagues as ends and not mere means, leaders show respect for each colleague as a person. In healthcare organizations, the end that all should seek for themselves is professionalism, which has received great emphasis in the medical literature.[18] Physician leaders can implement the categorical imperative by supporting and rewarding professional colleagues and staff in routinely fulfilling their commitments to patient care, research, and education and keep the leader's and organization's self-interest systematically secondary.[19] Respect for colleagues and staff as persons includes fulfilling leadership commitments and accepting enforcement of such commitments. The familiar management tool of securing "buy in" becomes ethically significant only when the organization's leaders make respect for persons a reality rather than a slogan.

16.3.2 Professional Resource Management

Obstetrician-gynecologist leaders should manage organizational resources on the basis of healthcare justice. (See Chapters 1 and 2.) Resource allocation should be directed to the prima facie healthcare-justice–based ethical obligation to see to it that each patient receives medically reasonable clinical management.

16.3.2.1 The Perils of a Utilitarian Organizational Culture

This approach will function as an antidote to a utilitarian organizational culture. Utilitarian justice in a healthcare organization endorses policies and practices that advance the organization's mission without reference to professionalism.[20] This narrow commitment can result in inequality of burdens, such as "taxes" that divert resources from teaching, patient care, and research.[8,9,11] This diversion can undermine the healthcare-justice–based ethical obligation to treat patients equally: seeing to it that each patient receives medically reasonable clinical management. Unfortunately, outcomes incompatible with healthcare justice can occur routinely in a utilitarian organizational culture, because such outcomes are acceptable in the logic of utilitarian justice. Obstetrician-gynecologist leaders should prevent adoption of a utilitarian organizational culture by implementing the healthcare-justice–based ethical obligation to maintain equality of access to medically reasonable clinical management of all patients.

16.3.2.2 The Perils of a Libertarian Organizational Culture

Libertarian justice defines unfairness or inequity in terms of the processes of decision making and therefore emphasizes fairness of process.[20] Fair processes of organizational decision making identify and address the obligations and interests of all stakeholders. Fair processes are consistent with wide differences in resource allocation for salaries and space. Libertarian justice also supports privileges and power based on the generation of revenue streams. The problem with libertarian justice is that it disadvantages individuals and clinical services that do not generate large revenues or margins but are essential to the organization's healthcare-justice–based mission to meet the clinical needs of all of its patients. Healthcare justice creates a prima facie ethical obligation to protect economically weak and vulnerable organizational units that are essential to the organization's mission.[20] Obstetrician-gynecologist leaders should prevent adoption of a libertarian organizational culture, by preventing the distorting effects of claims to special privilege and power by fiscal "rainmakers."

16.3.3 Professional Use of Power

Obstetrician-gynecologist leaders, by virtue of their position, exercise power, the ability to make and implement decisions, directly or through others.

16.3.3.1 Thomas Hobbes on Power

Thomas Hobbes (1588–1679) was the political philosopher par excellence of power.[21] Hobbes lived through the English civil war, in which power was exercised without constraint. Hobbes called for power to be constrained by a social contract, because the alternative was a life that would be "solitary, poor, nasty, brutish, and short."[21] The deployment of organizational power should be directed to sustaining a professional organizational culture.[22,23] Two kinds of power merit attention: monopoly power and monopsony power.[24]

16.3.3.2 Monopoly Power and Monopsony Power

Monopoly power is wielded by sellers with a dominant position in a market, such as a medical school with a closed staff. Monopsony power is the dominance of a market by a single buyer, such as an independent hospital that is a primary affiliate of a medical school. Monopoly and monopsony power both can affect the mission of creating a sustainable culture of professionalism by exploitation. Exploitation occurs when power is used to advance self-interest by unfairly shifting financial burdens onto others whose interests are harmed without the opportunity for offsetting benefit, e.g., leadership issuing unfunded mandates to physicians or clinical services for quality improvement or patient satisfaction. Exploitation is not permitted by the ethical principle of healthcare justice.

In a professional organizational culture obstetrician-gynecologist leaders should constrain monopoly or monopsony power so that they do not distort or undermine a professional organizational culture. Failure to do so will promote the exercise of raw power, power that cannot demonstrate a connection to a professional organizational culture, such as penalizing clinical services for failing to meet completely unrealistic revenue expectations. Hobbes helps us to understand the result: the "war of all against all"[21] that tears a healthcare organization apart. The war of all against all that follows inevitably from exercising raw power is not benign; it is toxic to professional organizational cultures. Obstetrician-gynecologist leaders should be on the alert to exercises of raw power and stop them.

16.3.4 Organizational Dysfunction: A Progressive Disorder

A key component of physician leaders' responsibility for creating sustainable organizational cultures of professionalism is the prevention and effective management of organizational dysfunction. Organizational dysfunction is a progressive disorder,[6] the stages of which we now identify. Obstetrician-gynecologist leaders should deploy preventive ethics in response, to identify, arrest, and reverse progression.

16.3.4.1 Machiavellian Organizational Culture

The political philosopher Niccolo Machiavelli (1469–1527) contributed an eponymous adjective to the English language, Machiavellian, which connotes actions based on cunning or, worse, bad faith.[25] Dysfunctional organizational cultures can exhibit Machiavellian tendencies when the appearance of professionalism masks the neglect or absence of professionalism. Physician leaders, by fulfilling their obligation to create sustained professional organizational cultures, can obviate the need to cultivate the cunning skills of the Machiavellian physician.

16.3.4.2 A Cynical Organizational Culture

A cynical organizational culture exhibits a deteriorating connection between organizational rhetoric and reality and a defensive posture of leadership in response to criticism.[6] For example, a dean may extol the virtues of teaching but leave unchanged a long-standing promotion system that ignores teaching in favor of research and publication. In such a culture, physicians committed to the ethical concept of medicine as a profession find each other and form moral enclaves that provide strength and support for efforts to confront and reform the deterioration of professionalism.

16.3.4.3 A Wonderland Organizational Culture

The next stage of deterioration is a Wonderland culture in which organizational rhetoric becomes self-deceptive when used by leaders, who expect subordinates to embrace self-deception.[6] For example, the mission statement emphasizes honest business practice, when it is common knowledge that the organization has systematic shortcomings in this area. Response to criticism takes the form of denial and accusations of disloyalty. In such a culture, physicians committed to the ethical concept of medicine as a profession strengthen their moral enclaves and vigorously seek to resist and expose self-deception as antithetical to this commitment.

16.3.4.4 A Kafkaesque Organizational Culture

Named for the Bohemian writer Franz Kafka (1883–1924), the next stage of deterioration is a Kafkaesque culture, in which organizational rhetoric and reality become dissociative.[6] For example, a department chairman strongly publicizes the appointment of a new associate chairman for patient safety and quality and then provides a budget that is entirely inadequate to improve patient safety. The response of leaders to criticism is threats, for example, in the form of, "You might be happier elsewhere." In such a culture, physicians committed to professionalism strengthen their moral enclaves against organizational assault on professional integrity, recognizing the futility and grave personal danger of attempts to change the culture.

16.3.4.5 A Postmodern Organizational Culture

Unfortunately, things can get much worse; an organization can devolve into a postmodern culture.[6] The connection between organizational rhetoric and reality, as well as the response of leaders to criticism, becomes incoherent and unpredictable in its variation. Truth is no longer valued. For example, a physician leader is able with aplomb to make incompatible promises to different constituencies and then expresses surprise and dismay about the inability of the different constituencies to work together for the good of the organization. In such a culture physicians committed to professionalism form moral fortresses until there is a change of leadership that recognizes and seeks to treat a very sick culture; otherwise such physicians quit.

16.3.4.6 Common Signs of Progressive Organizational Dysfunction

There are two common signs of progressive organizational dysfunction: strategic procrastination and strategic ambiguity.[26] Strategic procrastination of organizational leaders is evidenced by delays in making and implementing decisions about funding and other vital aspects of the organization's mission, as well as responding slowly to inquiries about such matters. Strategic ambiguity of organizational leaders can take several forms. Leaders can make financial or other promises without a detailed documentation of the promise and commitment to a plan of implementation. Leaders can order a subordinate to terminate someone's employment and then express perplexity about why the termination occurred. Leaders can also use the rhetoric of organizational excellence without offering policies and budgets that make the rhetoric actionable. Strategic procrastination and ambiguity are used by leaders to preserve their power for its own sake and to avoid resolution of organizational challenges and problems, transparency and accountability – behaviors toxic to an organizational culture based on professional responsibility. Obstetrician-gynecologists in leadership positions who are committed to an organizational culture of professionalism should never deploy strategic procrastination or ambiguity. They should also be alert to their incremental appearance and use their position of power to reverse these symptoms of organizational dysfunction.

16.4 Managing Guild Interests

16.4.1 Guild Interests: An Insidious Threat to a Professional Organizational Culture

Among leadership responsibilities is the development and implementation of organizational policies and practice to responsibly manage conflicts of interest. (See Chapter 5.) Proposals have been put forth for how to responsibly manage conflicts of interest with industry,[27-30] to teach professionalism in obstetrics and gynecology,[31] to assess professionalism in learners in obstetrics and gynecology,[32,33] and to promote trust as an essential component of professionalism.[34] A crucial topic has been overlooked: Other powerful, insidious incentives[35,36] now exist that could subordinate professionalism to guild self-interest, the group self-interests of physicians, depending on how physicians respond to those incentives. How obstetrician-gynecologist leaders and their colleagues respond to these incentives will therefore determine whether guild self-interests will define our specialty.

Guild self-interests have deep roots in the history of medicine. In his masterful biography of Hippocrates, Jacques Jouanna argues that the oath was created because not enough sons of the Hippocratic physicians wanted to become physicians, making it necessary to recruit strangers. The problem was that strangers could not be counted on to keep the secrets of Hippocratic physicians and so the new recruits had to sign a "written covenant" of loyalty.[37] The oath was a loyalty oath to the group and its interests. A group of physicians organized around their shared interests is the definition of a "guild." In short, the Hippocratic oath should be understood to be a guild oath. (See Chapter 1.)

During the next two millennia physicians in Europe formally organized themselves into merchant guilds, to protect their *collective* economic, social, and political interests in ways that they could not accomplish as individuals. Gregory and Percival, the coinventors of the ethical concept of medicine as a profession, explicitly rejected the concept of a guild and replaced it with the concept of medicine as a profession. (See Chapter 1.) Gregory attacked what he called the "Corporation spirit," referencing the royal corporations or Colleges that fiercely protected the group self-interests of their members from competition, an essential purpose of a guild.[14] Percival identified the antidote: creating and sustaining medicine as a "public trust."[16] Medicine should no longer be considered a guild that protects group interests but a profession that serves patients and society. Gregory and Percival aimed to subordinate guild interests to professionalism in medicine.

16.4.2 Two Potentially Insidious Incentives

Two incentives loom large in creating mounting pressure to subordinate professionalism to guild self-interest.[38] The first is to meet and exceed productivity incentives and the second is to respond to ever-increasing regulatory and compliance demands. These are valuable management tools that become insidious incentives.

16.4.2.1 Productivity Incentives

Productivity incentives can create an incentive for obstetrician-gynecologists to depart from evidence-based patient care, in order to increase the group's revenue. Consider the use of a group's laboratory. There is no question that groups that have a fiscal interest or ownership in any type of laboratory benefit financially if the laboratory is very successful, because most of the funds are comingled with patient care revenue and then distributed to the members.

Consider the following examples, reported to us, of productivity incentives for use of an in-house laboratory. Group A requires all members to order bone density scans on all women over age 60 regardless of their complaints and to have the group's bone density laboratory perform all of these tests. This policy was ordered by the physician administrator/owner of the group because the laboratory was losing money. This physician's proposed justification was that this new policy would be a preventive health measure to help identify osteoporosis early. Group B established the policy of routinely ordering metabolic profiles and other blood studies on all patients, with all such studies to be performed in the group's laboratory, whether they are indicated or not, as a method of increasing revenue under the cover of preventive medicine.

Consider an example, also reported to us, about the establishment of time limits on patient encounters based on maximizing revenue. A very good young physician was dropped from the large practice she had recently joined because "she took too much time with her patients." Unfortunately, young physicians today are being hired into practices where the emphasis is on how many patients one can see and how quickly, not on how you can deliver high-quality patient care.

16.4.2.2 Regulatory and Compliance Demands

Payers continue to deploy well-known and economically damaging tactics such as denial and delayed payment of claims, forcing obstetrician-gynecologists to divert resources of time and money in response. Obstetrician-gynecologists ignore these ever-mounting pressures at their extreme peril. One widely adopted response has been for obstetricians in small private practices to band together into larger groups, because large groups have more power than smaller groups or individuals to respond to these pressures. Efficient large groups can lower per capita administrative costs, resulting in net increased income for everyone in the group. Large-group practice brings survival-positive advantages that outweigh the attractions of solo or small-group practice. This organizational change creates the risk of increased emphasis on group self-interest.

16.4.3 A Powerful Antidote: An Organizational Culture that Subordinates Guild Interests to Professionalism

Obstetrician-gynecologist leaders should create and sustain an organizational culture that aims to subordinate guild self-interest to professionalism. The key to doing so is Percival's concept of the profession of medicine as a public trust.[16]

The fund of knowledge and skillset of every obstetrician-gynecologist is surely a product of the years of study and training that it took to produce them; that knowledge and those skills surely belong to the obstetrician-gynecologist. Percival's ethical point in using the phrase "public trust" is that the knowledge and skills of an obstetrician-gynecologist do not belong *solely* to that obstetrician-gynecologist. They also belong to society, which has invested considerable resources into medical education and biomedical research. They also belong to future physicians and their patients. To use a colloquial expression, obstetrician-gynecologists have the professional responsibility to "pay it forward." This means that each obstetrician-gynecologist should pass the profession of medicine as a public trust on to the next generation of physicians in an improved condition. Keeping guild self-interests secondary to professionalism is essential for fulfilling this professional responsibility, because doing so prevents bias that can undermine professionalism and professional integrity from within.

Obstetrician-gynecologist leaders should be alert to the expression of guild self-interests. Leaders should educate colleagues about the concept of guild self-interests, to avoid the deadly trap of self-deception. This education should emphasize that all guild self-interests, however strongly felt, pose a potential threat to professionalism. The professional virtues should play a major role in shaping an organizational culture whose immune system can encapsulate and thereby reduce the influence of guild self-interest.

16.4.3.1 Setting Reasonable Limits on Self-Sacrifice

A sound business model is essential for the success of private practice, because "No margin, no mission" applies to everyone. An unsound business model will undermine professionalism. So will failure to maintain ethically justified limits on self-sacrifice, because excessive self-sacrifice can promote the primacy of guild self-interest.

Consider two examples. The terms of a contract that has been offered by an insurance company may present the opportunity to expand the group's practice significantly, perhaps into new areas, but may also contain terms that are reliably predicted to result in persistent loss of revenue during the life of the contract. This could result in excessive economic self-sacrifice for the group. Excessive self-sacrifice creates fertile ground for guild self-interest becoming dominant. Excessive self-sacrifice undermines the primacy of excellence in patient care. The contract should be vigorously negotiated to provide fair compensation or rejected.

Second, in settings where reimbursement does not distinguish simple from complex cases, a group may adopt the practice of routinely referring out complex and therefore time-consuming cases that the group is fully qualified to manage, to preserve group productivity and subsequent reimbursement. The group should not make such referrals and modify its business model to support the time and effort to deal with the more complicated cases, even if that means manageable lost revenues for the group.

16.4.3.2 Preventing Incremental Subordination of Professionalism to Guild Self-Interest

Some guild self-interests threaten professionalism incrementally and therefore can be difficult to detect and responsibly manage. This is because threats accumulate in small increments over time until they cross a ruinous threshold. For example, one obstetrician-gynecologist in a group decides to start referring out a small number of complex cases, as a way to incrementally enhance productivity, and succeeds after several months, without this change being detected by inattentive leadership. He tells colleagues what he has done and the practice spreads without leadership becoming aware. The culture of the group has shifted subtly to one in which over time guild self-interests have come to dominate.

A transparent organizational culture is the antidote. To achieve transparency, the entire group should prospectively monitor practice patterns to detect and address incremental drift away from excellence in patient care to the predominance of guild self-interest. Failure to do so results in the subordination of professionalism to guild self-interest.

16.5 Navigating the Perilous Waters of Scylla and Charybdis

The challenges physician leaders confront today call to mind Odysseus' challenge to steer his fragile ship successfully on a very narrow path between the two disastrous options of Scylla and Charybdis, sea monsters that threatened to destroy him and his crew.[39] The modern Scylla takes the form of ever-increasing pressures to provide more resources for professional liability, compliance, patient satisfaction, central administration, and a host of other demands. The modern Charybdis takes the form of ever-increasing pressures to procure resources when fewer are available and competition for them is unrelenting, including managed care, hospital administration, payers, employers, patients who are uninsured or underinsured, research funding, and philanthropy. Professional ethics in obstetrics and gynecology guides obstetrician-gynecologist leaders by proving an explicitly ethical set of responses. The failure to implement the kind of responses that we have identified means that physician leaders will tolerate what professionalism prohibits: undermining professional responsibility by allowing the emergence of organizational cultures that are antithetical to the life of service to patients first articulated by Plato and translated into professional medical ethics by Gregory and Percival. Such organizational cultures would be devoid of moral worth occupied by "physician leaders" who, in the words of T.S. Eliot, would be "hollow men" and "stuffed men" working in the "dead land."[40]

Section 4: Professionally Responsible Leadership

References

1. Knox GE, Simpson KR. Perinatal high reliability. Am J Obstet Gynecol 2011; 204: 373–377.
2. Pettker CM, Thung SF, Raab CA, Donahue KP, Copel JA, Lockwood CJ, Funai EF. A comprehensive obstetrics patient safety program improves safety climate and culture. Am J Obstet Gynecol 2011; 204: 216.e1–6.
3. Grünebaum A, Chervenak F, Skupski D. Effect of a comprehensive patient safety program on compensation payments and sentinel events. Am J Obstet Gynecol 2011; 204: 97–105.
4. Rosenstein AH. Managing disruptive behavior in the health care setting: focus on obstetric services. Am J Obstet Gynecol 2011; 204: 187–192.
5. Schuchat A. Reflections on pandemics, past and present. Am J Obstet Gynecol 2011; 204 (6 Suppl 1): S4–6.
6. Chervenak FA, McCullough LB. The diagnosis and management of progressive dysfunction of health care organizations. Obstet Gynecol 2005; 105: 882–887.
7. Chervenak FA, McCullough LB, Brent RL. The professional responsibility model of obstetric ethics: avoiding the perils of clashing rights. Am J Obstet Gynecol 2011; 205: 315.e1–5.
8. Chervenak FA, McCullough LB, Brent RL. The professional responsibility model of physician leadership. Am J Obstet Gynecol 2013; 208: 97–101.
9. Chervenak FA, McCullough LB. The moral foundation of medical leadership: the professional virtues of the physician as fiduciary of the patient. Am J Obstet Gynecol 2001; 184: 875–880.
10. Plato. Republic. In Cooper JM, Hutchinson DS, eds. Plato Complete Works. Indianapolis, IN: Hackett, 1997.
11. Brent RL. The changing role and responsibilities of chairmen in clinical academic departments: the transition from autocracy. Pediatrics 1992; 90: 50–57.
12. Hesslebein F, Goldsmith M, Beckhard R, eds. The Drucker Foundation: The Leader of the Future. San Francisco: Jossey-Bass, 1997.
13. McCullough LB. John Gregory and the Invention of Professional Medical Ethics and the Profession of Medicine. Dordrecht, Netherlands: Kluwer Academic, 1998.
14. Gregory, J. Lectures on the Duties and Qualifications of a Physician. London: W. Strahan and T. Cadell, 1772. Reprinted in McCullough LB, ed. John Gregory's Writings on Medical Ethics and Philosophy of Medicine. Dordrecht, the Netherlands: Kluwer Academic, 1998: 161–245.
15. McCullough LB. The ethical concept of medicine as a profession: its origins in modern medical ethics and implications for physicians. In Kenny N, Shelton W, eds. Lost Virtue: Professional Character Development in Medical Education. New York: Elsevier, 2006: 17–27.
16. Percival T. Medical Ethics, or a Code of Institutes and Precepts, Adapted to the Professional Conduct of Physicians and Surgeons. London: Russell and Johnson, 1803. Reprinted in Pellegrino ED, ed. The Classics of Medicine Library. Birmingham, AL: Gryphon Editions, 1985.
17. Kant I. Groundwork of the Metaphysics of Morals. 1785. Paton HJ, trans. New York: Harper and Row, 1964.
18. ABIM Foundation. American Board of Internal Medicine. ACP-ASIM Foundation; American College of Physicians-American Society of Internal Medicine; European Federation of Internal Medicine. Medical professionalism in the new millennium: a physician charter. Ann Intern Med 2002; 136: 243–246.
19. Chervenak FA, McCullough LB. An ethical framework for identifying, preventing, and managing conflicts confronting leaders of academic health centers. Acad Med 2004; 79: 1056–1061.
20. Chervenak FA, McCullough LB. Professionalism and justice: ethical management guidelines for leaders of academic medical centers. Acad Med 2002; 77: 45–47.
21. Hobbes T. *Leviathan*. Oakeshot M, ed. New York: Oxford University Press, 1947.
22. Chervenak FA, McCullough LB, Baril TE Sr. Ethics, a neglected dimension of power relationships of physician leaders. Am J Obstet Gynecol 2006; 195: 651–656.
23. Chervenak FA, McCullough LB. The identification, management, and prevention of conflict with faculty and fellows: a practical ethical guide for department chairs and division chiefs. Am J Obstet Gynecol 2007; 197: 572e1–572.e5.
24. Chervenak FA, McCullough LB. Responsibly managing the medical school – teaching hospital relationship. Acad Med 2005; 80: 690–693.
25. Machiavelli N. The Prince: A Revised Translation. Adams RM, trans. New York: Norton, 1992.
26. Chervenak FA, McCullough LB. Physicians and hospital managers as co-fiduciaries: rhetoric or reality? J Healthc Manag 2003; 48: 172–180.
27. Rothman DJ, McDonald WJ, Berkowitz CD, et al. Professional medical associations and their relationships with industry: a proposal for controlling conflicts of interest. JAMA 2009; 301: 1367–1372.
28. Kahn NB, Lichter AS. The new CMSS code for interactions with companies managing relationships to minimize conflicts. J Vasc Surg 2011; 54: 34S–40S.
29. Shalowitz DI, Spillman MA, Morgan MA. Interactions with industry under the Sunshine Act: an example from gynecologic oncology. Am J Obstet Gynecol 2016; 214: 703–707.
30. Thompson JC, Vople KA, Bridgewater LK, et al. Sunshine Act: shedding light on inaccurate disclosures at a gynecologic annual meeting. Am J Obstet Gynecol 2016; 215: 661.e1–661.e7.
31. Mejia RB, Shinkunas LA, Ryan GL. Ethical issues identified by obstetrics and gynecology learners through a novel ethics curriculum. Am J Obstet Gynecol 2015; 213: 867.e1–867.e11.
32. Sullivan ME, Frishman GN, Vrees RA. Showing your public face: does screening social media assess residency applicants' professionalism? Am J Obstet Gynecol 2017; 216: 619–620.
33. Patterson BR, Kimball KJ, Walsh-Covarrubias JB, Kilgore LC. Effecting the sixth core competency: a project-based curriculum. Am J Obstet Gynecol 2008; 199: 561.e1–6.
34. Callegari LS, Aiken AR, Dehlendorf C, Cason P, Borrero S. Addressing potential pitfalls of reproductive life planning with patient-centered counseling. Am J Obstet Gynecol 2017; 216: 129–134.

35. von Gruenigen VE, Powell DM, Sorboro S, McCarroll ML, Kim U. The financial performance of labor and delivery units. Am J Obstet Gynecol 2013; 209: 17–19.
36. Lagrew DC Jr, Jenkins TR. The future of obstetrics/gynecology in 2020: a clearer vision: finding true north and the forces of change. Am J Obstet Gynecol 2014; 211: 617–622.
37. Jouanna J. *Hippocrates*. DeBevoise MB, trans. Baltimore, MD: Johns Hopkins University Press, 1999.
38. Chervenak FA, McCullough LB, Hale RW. Guild interests: an insidious threat to professionalism in Obstetrics and Gynecology. Am J Obstet Gynecol 2018; 2019: 581–584.
39. Homer. *The Odyssey*. Feagles R, trans. Knox B, intro. and notes. New York: Penguin Books, 1997.
40. Eliot T. The hollow men. In Untermeyer L, ed. Modern American Poetry. New York: Harcourt Brace & World, 1962: 395–396.

Section 5 Professionally Responsible Innovation and Research

Chapter 17

Clinical Innovation and Research in Obstetrics and Gynecology

GOAL

This chapter provides an ethical framework to guide clinical innovation and research in obstetrics and gynecology.

OBJECTIVES

On completing study of this chapter, the reader will:

Define maternal–fetal intervention

Describe ethically justified criteria for maternal–fetal innovation and research for fetal benefit and for the transition into clinical practice

Describe ethically justified criteria for maternal–fetal innovation and research for maternal benefit and for the transition into clinical practice

Identify an ethical framework to guide clinical innovation and research for maternal benefit with pregnant patients with mental illnesses and disorders

Apply the ethical framework to guide clinical innovation and research in obstetrics and gynecology to clinical innovation and research in obstetrics and gynecology

TOPICS

17.1 Clinical Innovation and Research	202
17.2 Maternal–Fetal Intervention	202
17.2.1 The Role of Animal Models	203
17.2.2 Prospective Oversight of Maternal–Fetal Innovation: The Perinatal Innovation Review Committee	203
17.2.3 Prospective Oversight of Maternal–Fetal Research by the Institutional Review Board	203
17.2.4 Professionally Responsible Transition to Clinical Practice	205
17.3 The MOMS Clinical Trial: A Model for Maternal–Fetal Research	205
17.4 Minimizing Risk to the Fetal Patient of Maternal–Fetal Research for Fetal Benefit	205
17.5 The Transition into Clinical Practice	206
17.6 Ethically Justified Criteria for Maternal–Fetal Innovation and Research and for the Transition to Clinical Practice	206
17.6.1 Ethically Justified Criteria for Maternal–Fetal Innovation and Early-Phase Maternal–Fetal Clinical Research for Efficacy and Safety for Fetal Benefit	206
17.6.2 Ethically Justified Criteria for Randomized Controlled Trials for Fetal Benefit	206
17.6.3 Ethically Justified Criteria for the Professionally Responsible Transition to Clinical Practice	207
17.6.4 The Informed Consent Process	207
17.7 Research with Pregnant Patients with Mental Illnesses and Disorders	207
17.7.1 Guidance from the Council for International Organizations of Medical Societies	208

17.7.1.1	Balance of Benefits and Risks to the Pregnant Patient	208
17.7.1.2	Balance of Benefits and Risks to the Fetal Patient	208
17.7.1.3	Balance of Benefits and Risks to the Neonatal and the Pediatric Patient	209
17.7.1.4	Overall Ethical Evaluation	209
17.7.2	Ethically Justified Study Design	210
17.7.2.1	Phase of Study	210
	Ethically Justified Criteria for Innovation and Early Phase Research for Maternal Benefit	210
	Ethically Justified Criteria for Randomized Controlled Trials for Maternal Benefit	210
17.7.2.2	The Informed Consent Process	210

Key Concepts

Beneficence-based ethical obligation
Decision-making capacity
Ethical concept of the fetus as a patient
Ethical principle of beneficence in professional ethics in obstetrics
Ethical principle of respect for autonomy in professional ethics in obstetrics
Evidence-based equipoise
Experiment
Institutional Animal Care and Use Committee
Informed consent process
Institutional Review Board
Innovation
Maternal–fetal intervention
Minimal risk
Minimized risk
Perinatal Innovation Review Committee
Research

17.1 Clinical Innovation and Research

Improving the quality of obstetric and gynecologic care depends on clinical innovation and research. Innovation and research are both experimentation.[1,2] An experiment occurs when in deliberative clinical judgment the outcomes of a clinical intervention cannot be reliably predicted.

Innovation in gynecology is an experiment performed on a female patient for her clinical benefit. Innovation in obstetrics is performed on both the pregnant patient and the fetal patient, either for maternal or fetal benefit. Clinical research is an experiment performed on a group of human subjects who are also patients with the goal of creating generalizable knowledge that is intended to benefit future patients. It is a mistake to equate human experimentation with human subjects research, because human experimentation also includes clinical innovation.

Clinical innovation cannot produce generalizable knowledge because clinical outcomes from a clinical innovation on a single female patient or pregnant patient–fetal patient pair constitute a single set of data points. A single set of data points is not sufficient in scientific methodology to test a hypothesis. Clinical innovation can establish the initial feasibility of hypotheses. A feasible hypothesis should then be tested in early phase research for efficacy and safety. To maintain clarity about the scientific and ethical relationship between clinical innovation and clinical research, clinical innovation should be organized as pre-research that aims to generate hypotheses to be investigated in subsequent phases of human subjects research.

17.2 Maternal–Fetal Intervention

Maternal–fetal intervention is performed on two patients, the pregnant patient and the fetal patient.[3] More complex interventions may occur in a "Fetal Center." In response to developments in the United States, the American College of Obstetricians and Gynecologists and the American Academy of Pediatrics published joint recommendations for fetal centers. These include ethically significant topics such as informed consent, the oversight of fetal centers, and the need to gather data on outcomes.[4]

In its early stages surgery for fetal benefit was often characterized by "fetal surgery." In time, this nomenclature came to be understood as problematic, because surgery for fetal benefit is necessarily also surgery on the pregnant woman for fetal benefit.[5] "Maternal–fetal intervention" is now the preferred nomenclature and encompasses pharmacologic management, minimally invasive surgery, and invasive surgery. "Maternal" in the hyphenated phrase is required because all forms of intervention must go through the pregnant woman's body. "Maternal" is also required by the ethical concept of the fetus as a patient, which includes not only beneficence-based ethical obligations to the fetal patient but also beneficence-based ethical obligations to the pregnant patient. Medical maternal–fetal intervention occurs when the pregnant woman is given medication that can cross the placenta and thus affect fetal physiology. For example, medications can be given to the pregnant woman to manage fetal arrhythmias.

17.2.1 The Role of Animal Models

When there are appropriate animal models, maternal–fetal innovation and research should be preceded by animal research, with the review and approval of the investigators' Institutional Animal Care and Use Committee. When such research is promising or when there is no appropriate animal model, clinical innovation with patients and clinical research with human subjects may be undertaken, to initiate the process to create an evidence base in human subjects research for the professionally responsible introduction of new techniques of maternal–fetal surgery into clinical practice for fetal benefit or for maternal benefit.

17.2.2 Prospective Oversight of Maternal–Fetal Innovation: The Perinatal Innovation Review Committee

The Society of University Surgeons has proposed that the era of planned surgical innovation without peer review should come to an end, because of its mixed record of success and failure. Instead, clinical innovation in surgery should become accountable for its scientific, clinical, and ethical integrity, rather than follow the sometimes haphazard approach of the past. Surgical departments should provide oversight of planned clinical innovation through prospective review and approval by a Surgical Innovation Committee.[6] For maternal–fetal intervention Fetal Centers should create and support the Perinatal Innovation Review Committee.[7]

Physicians considering a planned maternal–fetal innovation for maternal or for fetal benefit should prepare a proposal that describes the scientific and clinical justification for the innovation; its prior use in animal models (when feasible) and in cases reported in the peer-reviewed literature (when they exist); the clinical benefit intended for the patient (including reduction of the risks of mortality, morbidity, and disability); the short-term and long-term risks of mortality, morbidity, and disability for both the pregnant and fetal patients; the informed consent process; and what will be considered successful outcomes and their measurement. The informed consent process should make clear to the pregnant woman and those whom she wishes to be involved in the decision with her that the proposed clinical innovation is an experiment: its outcomes for both the fetal and pregnant patients cannot be reliably predicted and are therefore unknown. The physician leading the informed consent process should emphasize that the proposed clinical innovation is not accepted clinical practice and therefore it should not be expected by the pregnant woman to result in certain fetal and neonatal benefit. The informed consent process should emphasize that the short-term and long-term outcomes for the fetal, neonatal, and pregnant patients are unknown. The pregnant woman has a beneficence-based ethical obligation to the fetal patient to take only reasonable risks to herself for fetal benefit. Inasmuch as the maternal risks of innovation are unknown, the pregnant woman has no ethical obligation to accept them. She should therefore be informed that she should not consider herself ethically obligated to her fetus or future child to undergo the risks to her of the proposed innovative maternal–fetal intervention.

17.2.3 Prospective Oversight of Maternal–Fetal Research by the Institutional Review Board

Without exception, proposed maternal–fetal research must receive prospective review and approval by an Institutional Review Board (IRB) in the United States or, in other countries, a Research Ethics Committee (REC). The protocol must address the nature of the maternal–fetal intervention; why (on the basis of previous animal models and case reports of clinical innovation) it should be considered to have scientific and clinical merit; why it has an acceptable benefit/risk ratio for the pregnant patient in this and subsequent pregnancies, as well as for the fetal and neonatal patient; and the informed consent process. The informed consent process should make clear to the pregnant woman that the proposed clinical research is an experiment: its outcome for both the fetal and pregnant patients cannot be reliably predicted. The physician leading the informed consent process should emphasize that the proposed clinical research is not accepted clinical practice. The pregnant woman should be informed that she therefore has no ethical obligation to her fetus or future child to undergo the proposed maternal–fetal medical or surgical research. The pregnant woman, as explained in Chapter 2, is ethically obligated to take only reasonable risk to herself for fetal benefit. Because research is an experiment, fetal benefit is unknown. The pregnant woman has no ethical obligation therefore to take risk to herself, although she is free to do so. This should serve as an important consideration for those pregnant women who say that they would be willing to do anything that will help their baby.

The Common Rule (45 CFR 46) comprises federal regulations governing research with human subjects in the United States. (See Table 17.1.) These regulations should be followed for all clinical gynecologic research. 45 FCR 46.204 requires paternal consent when maternal–fetal research is undertaken with "the prospect of direct benefit solely to the fetus" (45 CFR 46.204(e)). Because the pregnant woman is the ultimate decision maker, as explained in Chapter 2, this requirement is not compatible with professional ethics in obstetrics. Nonetheless, clinical investigators must obtain paternal consent in these limited clinical circumstances and IRBs should enforce this legal requirement.

Table 17.1 46.204 Research involving pregnant women or fetuses.

Pregnant women or fetuses may be involved in research if all of the following conditions are met:

(a) Where scientifically appropriate, preclinical studies, including studies on pregnant animals, and clinical studies, including studies on nonpregnant women, have been conducted and provide data for assessing potential risks to pregnant women and fetuses;

(b) The risk to the fetus is caused solely by interventions or procedures that hold out the prospect of direct benefit for the woman or the fetus; or, if there is no such prospect of benefit, the risk to the fetus is not greater than minimal and the purpose of the research is the development of important biomedical knowledge which cannot be obtained by any other means;

(c) Any risk is the least possible for achieving the objectives of the research;

(d) If the research holds out the prospect of direct benefit to the pregnant woman, the prospect of a direct benefit both to the pregnant woman and the fetus, or no prospect of benefit for the woman nor the fetus when risk to the fetus is not greater than minimal and the purpose of the research is the development of important biomedical knowledge that cannot be obtained by any other means, her consent is obtained in accord with the informed consent provisions of subpart A of this part;

(e) If the research holds out the prospect of direct benefit solely to the fetus then the consent of the pregnant woman and the father is obtained in accord with the informed consent provisions of subpart A of this part, except that the father's consent need not be obtained if he is unable to consent because of unavailability, incompetence, or temporary incapacity or the pregnancy resulted from rape or incest;

(f) Each individual providing consent under paragraph (d) or (e) of this section is fully informed regarding the reasonably foreseeable impact of the research on the fetus or neonate;

(g) For children as defined in §46.402(a) who are pregnant, assent and permission are obtained in accord with the provisions of subpart D of this part;

(h) No inducements, monetary or otherwise, will be offered to terminate a pregnancy;

(i) Individuals engaged in the research will have no part in any decisions as to the timing, method, or procedures used to terminate a pregnancy; and

(j) Individuals engaged in the research will have no part in determining the viability of a neonate.

45 CFR 46.204, available at www.ecfr.gov/cgi-bin/retrieveECFR?gp=&SID=83cd09e1c0f5c6937cd9d7513160fc3f&pitd=20180719&n=pt45.1.46&r=PART&ty=HTML#se45.1.46_1204 (accessed March 1, 2019)

Because of the rarity of the conditions for which maternal–fetal surgery is being developed, multicenter cooperative trials will be essential for the advancement of the field. Such trials could also help to address variation from center to center or even from surgeon to surgeon within large centers in how maternal–fetal surgeries are performed. This variation can affect outcomes. The antidote is multicenter research in which there are comparative trials of potentially clinically significant variable surgical techniques. The North American Fetal Therapy Network (NAFTNet) has been established to support and provide scientific and ethical review of such multicenter collaborative maternal–fetal research.[2]

17.2.4 Professionally Responsible Transition to Clinical Practice

The results of maternal–fetal research should be introduced into clinical practice when the outcomes of research support the deliberative clinical ethical judgment that the intervention is reliably predicted to result in net short-term and long-term clinical benefit for the female patient or for fetal and neonatal patients and acceptable short-term and long-term risk to the pregnant, fetal, and neonatal patient. Long-term neonatal risks include effects on cognitive and motor development, as well as the need for corrective surgery, for example, spinal cord tethering after in utero repair of spina bifida. Long-term maternal risks will be especially important to assess, e.g., in subsequent pregnancies after maternal–fetal intervention that includes cesarean delivery. Maternal–fetal intervention, when it meets these conditions, should be considered medically reasonable. When such maternal–fetal intervention has become medically reasonable for a complication of pregnancy, it should be offered to the pregnant woman in the informed consent process described in Chapter 3.

17.3 The MOMS Clinical Trial: A Model for Maternal–Fetal Research

Maternal–fetal research on surgical management of fetal spina bifida provides a case study of how the transition from research to clinical practice should occur. This maternal–fetal surgery was shown in a multicenter, National Institutes of Health–funded, randomized controlled trial (RCT), known as the Management of Myelomeningocele Study (MOMS), to be clinically beneficial for children and acceptably risky for the fetal and pregnant patients in a population defined by rigorous inclusion and exclusion criteria.[8] Maternal–fetal surgery decreased rates of disability and the need for shunting for hydrocephalus in children when compared to expectant obstetric management followed by neonatal surgical repair, with acceptable rates of maternal morbidity and fetal mortality and morbidity. Maternal–fetal surgery for repair of spina bifida for pregnant patients who meet the MOMS criteria has become medically reasonable. All pregnant women whose fetus has been diagnosed to have spina bifida and who meet the MOMS criteria should therefore be offered both maternal–fetal surgery and expectant obstetric management followed by neonatal surgery. When spina bifida is diagnosed before fetal viability, there is an autonomy-based prima facie ethical obligation to offer induced abortion. (See Chapter 9.)

The obstetrician has the professional responsibility to ensure that reasonable efforts have been made to educate the pregnant woman so that she understands the in-utero repair to be maternal–fetal surgery, the nature of the procedure, its morbidity risks for the pregnant woman in her current and future pregnancies, and the mortality and morbidity risks for the fetal patient and future child. The physician should also make a reasonable effort to ensure that the pregnant woman's decision-making process is free of internal or external controlling influences.

17.4 Minimizing Risk to the Fetal Patient of Maternal–Fetal Research for Fetal Benefit

For maternal–fetal research for fetal benefit, 45 CFR 46.204(b) and (c) call for minimizing risk to the fetus. Baruch Brody (1943–2018) explains that this is not the same as "minimal" risk.[9] 45 CFR 46.102(j) defines "minimal risk": "*Minimal risk* means that the probability and magnitude of harm or discomfort anticipated in the research are not greater in and of themselves than those ordinarily encountered in daily life or during the performance of routine physical or psychological examinations or tests" (emphasis in original). (See also Table 17.1.) Investigators should be clear that they are using the concept of minimizing risk in the protocols that they submit to the IRB with jurisdiction.

205

17.5 The Transition into Clinical Practice

A comprehensive ethical framework that addresses clinical ethical judgment about the initiation of innovation, early phase research, randomized controlled clinical trials, and the responsible transition to clinical practice is available.[1] The distinctive feature of this approach is that the criteria are based on the ethical concept of the fetus as a patient. (See Chapter 2.) The clinical application of this ethical concept requires the identification and balancing of beneficence-based obligations to the fetal patient, beneficence-based obligations to the pregnant patient, and autonomy-based obligations to the pregnant patient. Taking all three obligations into account means that the pregnant woman has a beneficence-based ethical obligation to the fetal patient to take only reasonable risks to herself for fetal benefit. These criteria are designed to take account of the risks of mortality, morbidity, and disability to pregnant, fetal, and neonatal patients.

17.6 Ethically Justified Criteria for Maternal–Fetal Innovation and Research and for the Transition to Clinical Practice

Improving the health of pregnant and fetal patients is a direct function of planned clinical innovation and clinical research.[10]

17.6.1 Ethically Justified Criteria for Maternal–Fetal Innovation and Early–Phase Maternal–Fetal Clinical Research for Efficacy and Safety for Fetal Benefit

The ethical concept of the fetus as a patient supports criteria for clinical innovation and early phase clinical investigation that focus on minimizing the risks of mortality and the risks of morbidity, injury, and disability to both the pregnant and the fetal patient. We emphasize that the ethical concept of the fetus as a patient requires that criteria for innovation and research for fetal and neonatal benefit must be based on *both* beneficence-based ethical obligations to the fetus and beneficence-based ethical obligations to the pregnant patient because they are both patients who have become research subjects. Like all beneficence-based clinical ethical criteria, the proposed criteria are clinically conservative in that they put the burden of proof on the innovator or investigator.

1. The proposed fetal intervention is reliably expected on the basis of previous animal studies either to be lifesaving or to prevent serious and irreversible disease, injury, or disability for the fetal patient.
2. Among possible alternative designs, the intervention is designed in such a way as to involve the least risk of mortality and morbidity to the fetal patient.
3. On the basis of animal studies and analysis of theoretical risks both for the current and future pregnancies, the mortality risk to the pregnant woman is reliably expected to be low and the risk of disease, injury, or disability to the pregnant woman is reliably expected to be low or manageable for current and future pregnancies.[1, p. 46]

17.6.2 Ethically Justified Criteria for Randomized Controlled Trials for Fetal Benefit

It is permissible to refer a patient to an RCT when in deliberative clinical judgment the evidence about outcomes of two or more forms of clinical management requires the physician to become uncertain about which is clinically superior. The initiation of an RCT therefore requires what is known as evidence-based equipoise: a comprehensive, evidence-based evaluation of the outcomes of animal-model research and early phase investigation in deliberative clinical judgment requires the physician to become uncertain about the relative clinical benefit of the maternal–fetal intervention versus expectant obstetric management and neonatal intervention.[11] The beneficence-based criteria generated by the ethical concept of the fetus as a patient center on continued minimization of the risks of mortality and the risks of morbidity, injury, and disability to both the pregnant and the fetal patient. We emphasize that the ethical concept of the fetus as a patient requires that criteria for innovation and research for fetal and neonatal benefit must be based on *both* beneficence-based ethical obligations to the fetus and beneficence-based ethical obligations to the pregnant patient because they are both patients who have become research subjects. Like all beneficence-based clinical ethical criteria, the proposed criteria are clinically conservative in that they put the burden of proof on the innovator or investigator.

1. Early phase (I or II) research indicates that the proposed fetal intervention is reliably expected either to be lifesaving or to prevent serious and irreversible disease, injury, or disability for the fetal patient.
2. Among possible alternative designs, the intervention continues to involve the least risk of morbidity and mortality to the fetal patient.
3. Early phase research indicates that the mortality risk to the pregnant woman is reliably expected to be low and the risk of disease, injury, or disability to the pregnant woman, including for future pregnancies, is reliably expected to be low or manageable.[1, p. 46]

17.6.3 Ethically Justified Criteria for the Professionally Responsible Transition to Clinical Practice

The beneficence-based criteria generated by the ethical concept of the fetus as a patient center on the clinical ethical judgment that the outcomes of either early phase research (when an RCT is infeasible) or of an RCT support an expectation of significant fetal benefit and acceptable risks of mortality, morbidity, injury, and disability for both the pregnant and the fetal patient. We emphasize that the ethical concept of the fetus as a patient requires that criteria for innovation and research for fetal and neonatal benefit must be based on *both* beneficence-based ethical obligations to the fetus and beneficence-based ethical obligations to the pregnant patient because they are both patients who have become research subjects. Like all beneficence-based clinical ethical criteria, the proposed criteria are clinically conservative in that they put the burden of proof on making the transition to clinical practice.

1. The maternal or fetal intervention has positive results, that is, it has a significant probability of being life-saving or of preventing serious or irreversible disease, injury, or disability for the pregnant woman or fetal patient.
2. The maternal or fetal intervention involves low mortality and low or manageable risk of serious and irreversible disease, injury, or disability to the fetal patient.
3. The mortality risk to the pregnant woman is low and the risk of disease, injury or disability is low or manageable, including for future pregnancies.[1, p. 47]

17.6.4 The Informed Consent Process

The capacity of pregnant women to make decisions regarding clinical trial participation will be supported by providing adequate counseling and an opportunity to discuss risks and benefits.[10] The informed consent process should explain the nature of the study as maternal–fetal intervention, the purpose of the study, its clinical benefits and risks, what participation entails and the role of the pregnant subject, and the right to discontinue participation. Some pregnant women may have a strong interest in participation, which they may or may not express. It is therefore essential that the informed consent process emphasize that the study is an experiment: its outcome cannot be reliably predicted. The goal of this emphasis is to prevent what is called "therapeutic misconception." This originally meant the risk that research subjects would assume that all aspects of the study are chosen based on clinical judgment and thus fail to appreciate that some aspects, e.g., stepped-up dosage during the course of a Phase I trial or randomization in a Phase III trial, are chosen solely for research purposes.[12] Its meaning has been expanded to include conflation of standard clinical management with investigational clinical intervention.[13] Pregnant women with a strong interest in participation are at understandable – but preventable – risk of making this conflation. Finally, the informed consent process should emphasize that, because the study is an experiment and not standard care, the pregnant woman is free to refuse to enroll. Her decision to enroll should be voluntary, in the sense that it is free of controlling external and internal influences.

17.7 Research with Pregnant Patients with Mental Illnesses and Disorders

The clinical care of women with mental illnesses and disorders is especially challenging for obstetricians.[14] These challenges originate in and focus in the impaired decision-making capacity of these patients.[15,16] This impairment may be compounded by concomitant nicotine, alcohol, and other drug use.[17] Pregnant women with mental illnesses and disorders, especially poorly managed illnesses and disorders, may present to obstetricians with a history of physical or sexual abuse.[18–22] In addition, obstetric complications are slightly elevated in those with major mental disorders.[23–27]

A mainstay of appropriate treatment for nonpregnant patients is pharmacologic management. Unfortunately, obstetricians are often hard pressed to design and implement an appropriate plan of care for pregnant patients, because of the paucity of research on the safety and efficacy of pharmacologic therapy for this population of patients.[16,28]

Pregnant women with mental disorders and illnesses pose particularly vexing ethical challenges for clinical investigators seeking to improve their obstetric and psychiatric care. There are concerns about possible teratogenic and other effects of psychiatric medications but also concerns about adverse effects on pregnant, fetal, and neonatal patients of inadequately treated mental illnesses and disorders during and after pregnancy. There is a compelling need for improved pharmacologic management of mental illnesses and disorders during pregnancy that ethically justified research can create.

17.7.1 Guidance from the Council for International Organizations of Medical Societies

The Council for International Organizations of Medical Societies (CIOMS) has provided general ethical guidance for research involving pregnant women: "Research in this population should be performed only if it is relevant to the particular health needs of a pregnant woman or her fetus, or to the health needs of pregnant women in general, and, when appropriate, if it is supported by reliable evidence from animal experiments, particularly as to risks of teratogenicity and mutagenicity.[29] The ethical principle of beneficence in professional ethics in obstetrics becomes the basis for ethical reasoning about the balance among clinical benefits and risks to the pregnant patient, clinical benefits and risks to the fetal patient, and clinical benefits and risks to the neonatal patient and future child.[1,30,31] (See Chapter 3.)

17.7.1.1 Balance of Benefits and Risks to the Pregnant Patient

Medications confer clinical benefit on pregnant women by treating symptoms of mental illnesses and disorders.[30,31] Pregnant women with mental illnesses and disorders may be less likely to present for, receive, and cooperate with prenatal care. For example, patients with depression value treatment less and become less motivated to come in for prenatal care. Psychotic patients, for example, may deny the existence of pregnancy.[32] These complications increase the risk of unassisted delivery with its maternal complications, such as eclampsia or uncontrolled hemorrhage, and precipitous delivery with its maternal complications such as emergency cesarean section that might otherwise might have been prevented. Lack of prenatal care combined with nontreatment leaves the pregnant patient vulnerable to challenges of decision making about intrapartum management. These can be anticipated and addressed during prenatal care.[33,34] Lack of prenatal care is not psychosocially benign for new mothers, who, perhaps because of the lost opportunity for developing parenting skills and other factors, risk having their newborn child given up for others to raise.[35] On the other hand, use of some medications during pregnancy is associated with an increased risk of gestational diabetes,[36,37] and cesarean delivery.[37] However, one study found no difference in selected maternal medical outcomes when comparing antipsychotic and non-antipsychotic users during pregnancy.[27] Pharmacologic management can be reliably expected to relieve symptoms that could interfere with self-care during pregnancy and adherence to the schedule of prenatal visits, but there are significant risks to the pregnant woman.

In beneficence-based deliberative clinical judgment pharmacologic management should be considered on balance superior to nonmanagement for the pregnant patient. With respect to the pregnant patient pharmacologic research on psychosis during pregnancy is ethically permissible and therefore not ruled out ethically.

17.7.1.2 Balance of Benefits and Risks to the Fetal Patient

Pharmacologic management of mental illnesses and disorders improves prenatal and intrapartum care, creating clinical benefit for the fetal patient. In general, as noted earlier, adverse pregnancy outcomes are increased in this population,[24–27] although confounders and underlying psychiatric pathology may contribute to risks.[24–27,38–40] Fetal death and stillbirths in the offspring of women with psychotic disorders are also increased.[26]

The absence of RCTs makes it is very difficult to know how much weight to assign to pharmacologic interventions or to maternal morbidity. In the case of depression during pregnancy, for example, antidepressant exposure is associated with an elevated risk of preterm births,[41] spontaneous abortions,[42] persistent pulmonary hypertension in the newborn,[43] and autism in the offspring.[44] The risk of autism in the offspring, however, is almost completely offset by adjusting for confounding and maternal mental illness.[44]

Treatment with atypical antipsychotic therapy has been associated with a higher proportion of low birth weight babies compared to a matched group of women not exposed to neuroleptic agents.[38] One study comparing women with and women without schizophrenia reported increased fetal risk for restricted growth and stillbirth among women with schizophrenia.[39] Another study found that pregnant women who receive treatment with typical antipsychotics compared to those not receiving antipsychotics were at a slightly higher risk of preterm birth.[45]

A major concern for fetal risk is teratogenicity of drugs used to treat psychosis. The general evidence-based consensus is that these medications have not been documented to constitute a clinically significant teratogenic risk.[14,39,46-50] There are theoretical teratogenic risks. However, in beneficence-based clinical judgment, theoretical risks do not count against a form of treatment but are matters for investigation.

The fetal patient will likely benefit from better management of pregnancy. However, there remain unknown and incompletely understood risks. In beneficence-based deliberative clinical judgment pharmacologic management appears on balance to be superior to nonmanagement for the fetal patient because of improved outcomes from improved maternal health. Pharmacologic research on psychosis during pregnancy for fetal benefit is ethically permissible.

17.7.1.3 Balance of Benefits and Risks to the Neonatal and the Pediatric Patient

There is a paucity of studies to guide beneficence-based reasoning about the outcomes for the neonatal and pediatric patient of pharmacologic management of psychosis during pregnancy. One review found that both bipolar disorder and schizophrenia were linked to slightly increased risks for the newborn although data on drug exposure during pregnancy was not given in the majority of included studies.[27] In one study rates of special care nursery admission were elevated in neonates of women with severe mental illness taking psychotropic medications.[51] In another,[52] the risks of adverse child outcomes of women who continued antipsychotic use in pregnancy was not greater than of those who discontinued use before pregnancy.

Lack of prenatal care from untreated psychosis is not psychosocially benign for newborns and children as they grow and develop, because of the lost opportunity for these women to develop parenting skills. There is a report of longer-term neuromotor impairments associated with neuroleptic medication,[53] although there is no information about whether these are correctable. This is an association that is also difficult to distinguish from the effects of maternal illness.

The neonatal and pediatric patient may benefit from pharmacologic management of mental illnesses and disorders during pregnancy. There may, however, be unknown or incompletely understood short-term and long-term developmental risks. The benefit to the neonatal and pediatric patient from the pharmacologic management of psychosis during pregnancy is uncertain. In beneficence-based deliberative clinical judgment pharmacologic management is not ruled out ethically and therefore is ethically permissible.

17.7.1.4 Overall Ethical Evaluation

Beneficence-based ethical reasoning about outcomes reported in the pertinent literature supports the conclusion that pharmacologic management of mental illnesses and disorders during pregnancy can have acceptable outcomes for the pregnant, fetal, or neonatal patient. Obstetricians, reasonably, take seriously theoretical risks to the fetal, neonatal, and pediatric patient. However, in beneficence-based reasoning theoretical risks do not automatically prohibit clinical practice or research. The task of research is to study theoretical risks, to determine whether theoretical risks actually occur and, if they do, assess them in relationship to benefits that occur. Any claim that research on the pharmacologic management of mental illnesses and disorders during pregnancy is ethically impermissible because of unacceptable harm to pregnant, fetal, neonatal, or pediatric patients cannot be supported.[15,16,30,31] Such claims should not influence investigators, IRBs and RECs, funding agencies, sponsoring organizations, or referring physicians.

Research on the pharmacologic management of psychosis during pregnancy is therefore ethically permissible. The next ethical question becomes, What ethical considerations should guide study design?

17.7.2 Ethically Justified Study Design

Selection criteria should not be based on abortion preference.[30] As explained in Chapter 9, the decision about whether to elect induced abortion before viability is governed by the ethical principle of respect for autonomy in obstetrics.

17.7.2.1 Phase of Study

For some forms of pharmacologic management of mental illnesses and disorders, evidence-based equipoise for treatment versus no treatment of psychosis during pregnancy does not exist. These forms of pharmacologic management should therefore be considered for innovation or Phase I safety and efficacy trials only if they meet the following criteria. We emphasize that the ethical concept of the fetus as a patient requires that criteria for innovation and research for maternal benefit must be based on *both* beneficence-based ethical obligations to the pregnant patient and beneficence-based ethical obligations to the fetus because they are both patients who have become research subjects. As required by the ethical concept of the fetus as a patient, these criteria originate in the obstetrician's prima facie beneficence-based ethical obligations to the pregnant patient and to the fetal patient.

Ethically Justified Criteria for Innovation and Early Phase Research for Maternal Benefit

1. The medical or surgical intervention should be reliably expected to be efficacious in managing the pregnant woman's diagnosis: there is a reasonable expectation of prevention of serious, far-reaching, and irreversible clinical sequelae of her diagnosis. The evidence base for this clinical judgment should include all previous animal and human studies. Medications or surgeries with an evidence base that supports reasonable expectation of efficacy should receive priority for preliminary investigation with pregnant women. Medications or surgeries without such an evidence base should not receive priority for clinical investigation.
2. There should be no documented mortality or documented serious, far-reaching, and irreversible injury to the fetal patient, especially to the central nervous system, sensory system, or other major organ system from use of the medication or performance of the surgery.
3. There should be no or very low documented risk of less serious injury to the fetal patient.[1, p. 45]

When evidence-based equipoise does exist, RCTs may be considered but only when they meet the following criteria. We emphasize that the ethical concept of the fetus as a patient requires that criteria for innovation and research for maternal benefit must be based on *both* beneficence-based ethical obligations to the pregnant patient and beneficence-based ethical obligations to the fetus because they are both patients who have become research subjects.

Ethically Justified Criteria for Randomized Controlled Trials for Maternal Benefit

1. In preliminary studies, such as Phase I and II or cohort studies, the medication or surgery has demonstrated efficacy in preventing serious, far-reaching, and irreversible clinical sequelae of the pregnant woman's diagnosis.
2. In these preliminary studies there have been no documented cases, attributable to the investigational drug or surgery, of mortality or of serious, far-reaching, and irreversible injury to the fetal patient, especially to the central nervous system, sensory system, or other major organ system.
3. There should be no or only rare documented occurrences of less serious injury to the fetal patient.[1, p. 45]

These studies should be prospectively monitored by a Data and Safety Monitoring Board. Its recommendations to continue a trial should be based on an assessment that its criteria continue to be satisfied.

17.7.2.2 The Informed Consent Process

The informed consent process should explain the nature of the study as maternal–fetal intervention, the purpose of the study, its clinical benefits and risks, what participation entails and the role of the pregnant subject, and the right to discontinue participation. Some pregnant women may have a strong interest in participation, which they may or may not express. It is therefore essential that the informed consent process emphasize that the study is an experiment: its outcome cannot be reliably predicted. The goal of this emphasis is to prevent what is called "therapeutic misconception." This originally meant the risk that research subjects would assume that all aspects of the study are chosen based on clinical judgment and thus fail to appreciate that some aspects, e.g., stepped-up dosage during the course of a Phase I trial or randomization in a Phase III trial, are chosen solely for research purposes.[12] Its meaning has been expanded to include conflation of standard clinical management with investigational clinical intervention.[13] Pregnant women with a strong interest in participation are at understandable – but preventable – risk of making this conflation. Finally, the informed consent process should emphasize that, because the study is an experiment and not standard care, the pregnant woman is free to refuse to enroll. Her decision to enroll should be voluntary, in the sense that it is free of controlling external and internal influences.

The presence of a mental illness or disorder that is not responding sufficiently to pharmacologic management raises legitimate concerns about decision-making capacity. Study design should therefore include routine assessment of decision-making capacity, by evaluating its components (Table 17.2. See also Chapter 3) adapted to this clinical context.

It is ethically justified in study design to exclude from participation potential subjects who are reliably judged to have impaired decision-making capacity. Participation in clinical research that requires self-administration of medication, self-monitoring, attending follow up, reporting potentially adverse events, and discontinuing enrollment under adequate clinical supervision are cognitively and affectively demanding. Patients with impaired decision-making capacity should be considered at increased risk of noncooperation with these demands of being a research subject. They are at increased risk of discontinuation. This could jeopardize completion of the study and also may put such subjects, as well as fetal and neonatal patients, at preventable risk from unsupervised discontinuation.

Pregnant women whose mental illnesses or disorders become well managed in the course of a trial have the decision-making capacity to decide whether to remain pregnant. This decision is not primarily a medical decision but, instead, is primarily a personal decision. (See Chapter 9.) Moreover, pregnant women whose psychiatric conditions are well managed do elect termination of pregnancy and women with schizophrenia have higher abortion rates compared to those without schizophrenia.[54] There is no ethical justification to restrict subjects' autonomy about

Table 17.2 Seven components of decision-making capacity.

Attention	The patient pays attention to the information that is provided.
Information intake and use	The patient absorbs, retains, and recalls this information as needed in subsequent components.
Cognitive understanding	The patient can reason from present events (clinical management) to their future likely consequences (clinical outcomes).
Appreciation	The patient believes that these consequences could happen to her (in gynecology) or to her or her fetus or her future child should the pregnancy continue to delivery (in obstetrics).
Evaluative understanding	The patient assesses these consequences on the basis of her values and beliefs.
Explicit authorization	The patient explicitly authorizes clinical management that has been offered or recommended or refuses to do so in a voluntary fashion, i.e., free of control by external factors (other people, including family and healthcare team members) or internal factors (such as unreasoning fear or auditory hallucination).
Communicating reasons	The patient can, when requested, explain her authorization or refusal of authorization on the basis of her cognitive and evaluative understanding.

continuation of pregnancy. Pregnant subjects have the same right to decide about the continuation of pregnancy that all pregnant patients have. This should be made clear in the informed consent process and informed consent form.

Sample size estimation will need to account for the possibility that some subjects will elect termination of pregnancy, which should be an endpoint in the trial. Multicenter trials may be needed to accomplish timely completion of enrollment and data collection.

The informed consent process should be clear that subjects have the right to discontinue enrollment in a clinical trial. When doing so creates clinical risk, this should be made clear in the informed consent process.[30]

References

1. Chervenak FA, McCullough LB. An ethically justified framework for clinical investigation to benefit pregnant and fetal patients. Am J Bioeth 2011; 11: 39–49.
2. North American Fetal Therapy Network. Available at NAFTNET.org (accessed January 14, 2019).
3. Sala P, Prefumo F, Pastorino D, Buffi D, et al. Fetal surgery: an overview. Obstet Gynecol Surv 2014; 69: 218–228.
4. American College of Obstetricians and Gynecologists. Committee on Ethics; American Academy of Pediatrics, Committee on Bioethics. Committee Opinion No. 501: Maternal-fetal intervention and fetal care centers. Obstet Gynecol 2011; 118: 405–410.
5. Moise K. The history of fetal therapy. Am J Perinatol 2014; 31: 557–566.
6. Biffl WL, Spain DA, Rietsma AM, et al. Responsible development and application of surgical innovations: a position statement of the Society of University Surgeons. J Am Coll Surg 2008; 206: 1204–1209.
7. Chervenak FA, McCullough LB. The ethics of maternal-fetal surgery. Semin Fetal Neonatal Med 2018; 23: 64–67.
8. Adzick NS, Thom EA, Spong CY, et al. MOMS Investigators. A randomized trial of prenatal versus postnatal repair of myelomeningocele. N Engl J Med 2011; 364: 993–1004.
9. Brody BA. The Ethics of Biomedical Research: An International Perspective. New York: Oxford University Press, 1998.
10. Heyrana K, Myers B, Stratton P. Increasing the participation of pregnant women in clinical trials. JAMA 2018; 320: 2077–2078.
11. Brody BA, McCullough LB, Sharp R. Consensus and controversy in research ethics. JAMA 2005; 294: 1411–1414.
12. Appelbaum PS, Roth LH, Lidz C. The therapeutic misconception: informed consent in psychiatric research. Int J Law Psychiatry 1982; 5: 319–239.
13. Lidz CW, Appelbaum PS, Grisso T, Renaud M. Therapeutic misconception and the appreciation of risks in clinical trials. Soc Sci Med 2004; 58: 1689–1697.
14. American College of Obstetricians and Gynecologists. ACOG Committee on Practice Bulletins – Obstetrics. ACOG Practice Bulletin: Clinical management guidelines for obstetrician-gynecologists number 92, April 2008. Use of psychiatric medications during pregnancy and lactation. Obstet Gynecol 2008; 111: 1001–1020.
15. McCullough LB, Coverdale J, Chervenak F. Ethical challenges of decision making with pregnant patients who have schizophrenia. Am J Obstet Gynecol 2002; 187: 696–700.
16. Coverdale J, McCullough LB, Chervenak FA. The ethics of randomized placebo-controlled trials of antidepressants with pregnant women. A systematic review. Obstet Gynecol 2008; 112: 1361–1368.
17. Hartz SM, Pato CN, Medeiros H, Cavazos-Rehg P, et al. Comorbidity of severe psychotic disorders with measures of substance use. JAMA Psychiatry 2014; 71: 248–254.
18. Coverdale J, Turbott SH. Sexual and physical abuse of chronically ill psychiatric outpatients compared to men with a matched sample of medical outpatients. J Nerv Ment Dis 2000; 188: 440–445.
19. Kamperman AM, Henrichs J, Bogaerts S, Lesaffee EM, et al. Criminal victimization in people with severe mental illness: a multi-site prevalence and incidence survey in the Netherlands. PLoS ONE 2014, March 7; 9(3): e90129.
20. Khalifeh H, Oram S, Osborn D, Howard LM, Johnson S. Recent physical and sexual violence against adults with severe mental illness: a systematic review and meta-analysis. Int Rev Psychiatry 2016; 28(5): 433–451.
21. Oram S, Trevillion K, Feder G, Howard LM. Prevalence of experiences of domestic violence among psychiatric patients: a systematic review. Br J Psychiatry 2013; 202: 94–99.
22. Teplin LA, McClelland GM, Abram KM, Weiner DA. Crime victimization in adults with severe mental illness: comparison with the National Crime Victimization Survey. Arch Gen Psychiatry 2005; 62: 911–921.
23. Coughlin CG, Blackwell KA, Bartley C, Hay M, Yonkers KA, Bloch MH. Obstetric and neonatal outcomes after antipsychotic medication exposure in pregnancy. Obstet Gynecol 2015; 125: 1224–1235.
24. Jablensky AV, Morgan V, Zubrick SR, Bower C, Yellachich L-A. Pregnancy, delivery, and neonatal complications in a population cohort of women with schizophrenia and major affective disorders. Am J Psychiatry 2005; 162: 79–91.
25. Schneid-Kofman N, Sheiner E, Levy A. Psychiatric illness and adverse pregnancy outcome. Int J Gynaecol Obstet 2008; 101: 53–56.
26. Webb R, Abel K, Pickles A, Appleby L. Mortality in offspring of patients with psychotic disorders: a critical review and meta-analysis. Am J Psychiatry 2005; 162: 1045–1056.
27. Tosato S, Albert U, Tomassi S, Lasevoli F, Carmassi C, Nanni MG, et al. A systematized review of atypical antipsychotics in pregnant women: balancing between risks of untreated illness and risks of drug-related adverse effects. J Clin Psychiatry 2017; 78: e477–e489.
28. Webb RT, Howard L, Abel KM. Antipsychotic drugs for non-affective psychosis during pregnancy and postpartum. Cochrane Database Syst Rev 2004; 2: CD004411.

29. Council for the International Organization of Medical Societies (CIOMS), in conjunction with the World Medical Association (WMA). International Guidelines for Biomedical Research Involving Human Subjects. Geneva: CIOMS, 2002. Available at www.cioms.ch/publications/layout_guide2002.pdf (accessed March 1, 2019).

30. McCullough LB, Coverdale J, Chervenak FA. A comprehensive ethical framework for responsibly designing and conducting pharmacologic research that involves pregnant women. Am J Obstet Gynecol 2005; 193: 901–907.

31. McCullough LB, Chervenak FA, Coverdale J. An ethical framework for conducting research on pregnant, opioid-dependent women. Addiction 2013; 108: 248–249.

32. Miller LJ. Psychotic denial of pregnancy: phenomenology and clinical management. Hosp Comm Psychiatry 1990; 41: 1233–1237.

33. Babbitt KE, Bailey KJ, Coverdale J, Chervenak FA, McCullough LB. Professionally responsible intrapartum management of patients with major mental disorders. Am J Obstet Gynecol 2014; 210: 27–31.

34. McCullough LB, Chervenak FA, Coverdale J. Managing care of an intrapartum patient with agitation and psychosis: ethical and legal implications. AMA J Ethics 2016; 18: 209–214.

35. Coverdale J, Turbott SH, Roberts H. Family planning needs and STD risk behaviors of female psychiatric outpatients. Br J Psychiatry 1997; 171: 69–72.

36. Boden R, Lundgren M, Brandt L, Reutfors J, Kieler H. Antipsychotics during pregnancy; relation to fetal and maternal metabolic effects. Arch Gen Psychiatry 2012; 69: 715–721.

37. Reis M, Kallen B. Maternal use of antipsychotics in early pregnancy and delivery outcome. J Clin Psychopharmacol 2008; 28: 279–288.

38. McKenna K, Koren G, Tetelbaum M, Wilton L, Shakir S, Diav-Citrin O, et al. Pregnancy outcome of women using atypical antipsychotic drugs: a prospective comparative study. J Clin Psychiatry 2005; 66: 444–449.

39. Nilsson E, Lichtenstein P, Cnattingius S, Murray RM, Hultman CM. Women with schizophrenia: pregnancy outcome and infant death among their offspring. Schizophrenia Research 2002; 58: 221–229.

40. Newham JJ, Thomas SH, MacRitchie K, McElhatton PR, McAllister-Williams RH. Birth weights of infants after maternal exposure to typical and atypical antipsychotics; prospective comparison study. Br J Psychiatry 2008; 192: 333–337.

41. Eke AC, Saccone G, Berghella V. Selective serotonin reuptake inhibitor (SSRI) use during pregnancy and risk of preterm birth: a systematic review and meta-analysis. BJOG 2016; 123: 1900–1907.

42. Hemels ME, Einarson A, Koren G, Lanctot KL, Einarson TR. Antidepressant use during pregnancy and the rates or spontaneous abortions: a meta-analysis. Am Pharmacother 2005; 39: 803–809.

43. Masarwa R, Bar-Oz B, Gorelik E, Reif S, Perlman A, Matok I. Prenatal exposure to selective serotonin reuptake inhibitors and serotonin norepinephrine reuptake inhibitors and risk for pulmonary hypertension of the newborn: a systematic review, meta-analysis, and network meta-analysis. Am J Obstet Gynecol 2019; 220: 57.e1–57.

44. Andrade C. Antidepressant exposure during pregnancy and risk of autism in the offspring, 1. Meta-review of meta-analyses. J Clin Psychiatry 2017; 78: e1047–e1051.

45. Lin HC, Chen IJ, Chen YH, Lee HC, Wu FJ. Maternal schizophrenia and pregnancy outcome: does the use of antipsychotics make a difference? Schizophr Res 2010; 116: 55–60.

46. Altshuler LL, Cohen L, Szuba MP, Burt VK, Gitlin M, Mintz J. Pharmacologic management of psychiatric illness during pregnancy: dilemmas and guidelines. Am J Psychiatry 1996; 153: 592–606.

47. Diav-Citrin O, Shechtman S, Ornoy S, Amon J, Schaefer C, et al. Safety of haloperidol and penfluridol in pregnancy: a multicenter, prospective, controlled study. J Clin Psychiatry 2005; 66: 317–322.

48. Gentile S. Antipsychotic therapy during early and late pregnancy. A systematic review. Schizophr Bull 2010; 36: 518–544.

49. Habermann F, Fritzsche J, Fuhlbruck F, Wacker E, Alignol A, et al. Atypical antipsychotic drugs and pregnancy outcome: a prospective, cohort study. J Clin Psychopharmacol 2013; 33: 453–462.

50. Huybrechts KF, Hernandez-Diaz S, Patorno E, et al. Antipsychotic use in pregnancy and the risk for congenital malformations. JAMA Psychiatry 2016; 73: 938–946.

51. Frayne J, Nguyen T, Bennett K, Allen S, Hauck Y, Liira H. The effects of gestational use of antidepressants and antipsychotics on neonatal outcomes for women with severe mental illness. Aust NZ J Obstet Gynecol 2017; 57: 526–532.

52. Petersen I, McCrea RL, Sammon CJ, et al. Risks and benefits of psychotropic medications in pregnancy: cohort studies based on UK electronic primary health records. Health Technol Assess 2016; 20: 1–176.

53. Johnson KC, LaPrairie JL, Brennan PA, Stowe ZN, Newport J. Prenatal antipsychotic exposure and neuromotor performance during infancy. Arch Gen Psychiatry 2012; 69: 787–794.

54. Brown HK, Dennis C-L, Kurdyak P, Vigod SN. A population-based study of the frequency and predictors of induced abortion among women with schizophrenia. Br J Psychiatry 2018; DOI:10.1192/bjp.2018.262.

Section 6 Professionally Responsible Health Policy and Advocacy

Chapter 18

Health Policy and Advocacy

GOAL
This chapter provides an ethical framework for the role of obstetrician-gynecologists in advocating for pregnant, fetal, and neonatal patients.

OBJECTIVES
On completing study of this chapter, the reader will:
- Specify the general ethical principle of justice to healthcare justice in professional ethics in obstetrics and gynecology
- Identify challenges to substantive justice in healthcare for female, pregnant, fetal, and neonatal patients
- Identify challenges to procedural justice in healthcare for female, pregnant, fetal, and neonatal patients
- Describe an antidote to cynicism about the ethical principle of healthcare justice
- Apply the ethical framework for the role of obstetrician-gynecologists in advocating for pregnant, fetal, and neonatal patients in clinical practice

TOPICS

18.1 Healthcare Justice, Health Policy, and Advocacy	216
18.2 Advocacy: Women and Children First	217
18.2.1 Healthcare-Justice–Based Ethical Framework	217
18.2.2 Challenges to Justice in the Allocation of Healthcare Resources to Women and Children	218
18.2.2.1 Challenges to Substantive Justice	218
Self-Interests of Adults	218
Age Bias	218
Bias against the Medically Indigent	219
Economic Bias against Obstetrics in Hospitals	219
Professional Liability Insurance	220
Trumping Power of Economic Values	220
18.2.2.2 Challenges to Procedural Justice	220
Bias in Favor of Persons	220
Bias against Those Who Cannot Speak for Themselves	221
18.3 Antidote to Cynicism about the Ethical Principle of Healthcare Justice	221
18.3.1 Identifying and Addressing Social Conditions that Impede Healthcare Justice	221
18.3.2 The Impact of Climate Change on the Life and Health of Female, Pregnant, and Neonatal Patients	222
18.4 "Women and Children First – or Last?" The New York Declaration of the International Academy of Perinatal Medicine	222

Section 6: Professionally Responsible Health Policy and Advocacy

The Ethical Principle of Justice and the Responsible Allocation of Healthcare Resources	222
Justice-Based Responses to Ethical Challenges in Allocating Perinatal Healthcare Resources	222
Implications for Health Policy Leaders	223

> **Key Concepts**
>
> Ethical ideal
> Ethical obligation
> Ethical principle of beneficence in professional ethics in gynecology
> Ethical principle of beneficence in professional ethics in obstetrics
> Ethical principle of healthcare justice in professional ethics in obstetrics and gynecology
> Ethical principle of justice in medical ethics and bioethics
> Prima facie ethical obligation
> Procedural justice
> Substantive justice

18.1 Healthcare Justice, Health Policy, and Advocacy

Healthcare justice is the specification of the general ethical principle of justice. Justice applies to populations of individuals and is thus the basis of public policy because public policy concerns how state power should be used to protect and promote the interests of various populations of individuals. (See Chapter 2.) For example, policy concerning criminal justice aims to protect and promote the interests, welfare, and rights of alleged victims and those subject to criminal arrest, indictment or criminal charges, trial, imprisonment, and parole.

The general ethical principle of justice applies to populations of individuals and requires that they be treated equally fairly. This general concept of justice originates in the moral and political philosophy of Aristotle[1] (384 BCE–322 BCE).

"Equally" and "fairly" are highly abstract terms and thus provide no guidance for public policy. To become applicable "equally" and "fairly" must be specified to a population of individuals who share a common trait. (See Chapters 1 and 2.) Individuals who have become patients share the common trait of being under the protection of a physician who has become a professional by committing to the ethical concept of medicine as a profession. (See Chapters 1 and 2.) All individuals in a population defined by this trait are equally patients. Thus "equally" in the general ethical principle of justice has been specified. Physicians have the ethical obligation, originating in the ethical concept of medicine as a profession, to see to it that all patients receive clinical management that is supported in deliberative clinical judgment as medically reasonable. Thus, "equally" and "fairly" in the general ethical principle of justice have been specified to healthcare.

The specification of healthcare justice to obstetrics and gynecology can now be stated: Every obstetrician-gynecologist has the prima facie ethical obligation to see to it that each female patient, pregnant, fetal, and neonatal patient is provided medically reasonable clinical management of his or her condition. The phrase "see to it" does not mean that each obstetrician-gynecologist is required to provide such clinical management because such a requirement is impossible to satisfy. Instead, obstetrician-gynecologists fulfill the prima facie ethical obligation of healthcare justice by advocating for the organizational and societal resources needed to provide every female, pregnant, fetal, and neonatal patient with medically reasonable clinical management.[2]

Advocacy based on healthcare justice prevents advocacy for organizational and societal resources from being based on self-interest, especially the group self-interest of physicians. This is known as guild self-interest,[3] against which Thomas Percival (1740–1804), one of the inventors of the ethical concept of medicine as a profession, warned when he called for the profession of medicine to be understood by physicians and society as a "public trust."[4] (See Chapters 1 and 16.) Healthcare justice gives this phrase its meaning in professional ethics in obstetrics and gynecology.

The public trust is protected when every pregnant, fetal, and neonatal patient receives medically reasonable clinical management of his or her condition. In well-resourced countries and clinical settings, the ethical concept of obstetrics and gynecology as a public trust creates ethical obligations to provide such clinical management. Advocacy should be for the resources needed to do so. In less-well-resourced countries and clinical settings the ethical concept of obstetrics and gynecology public trust functions as an ideal by setting a long-term goal toward which incremental progress is ethically obligatory. (See Chapter 1.) Advocacy should be for incremental increase in resources to improve patient care and its outcomes with the long-term goal of seeing to it that every patient is provided medically reasonable clinical management for her condition or diagnosis.

18.2 Advocacy: Women and Children First

"Women and children first" is a familiar phrase the origin of which is less well known. In 1852 the HMS *Birkenhead*, carrying more than 600 sailors and troops, was evacuating the civilians from Cape Town, South Africa during the Cape Frontier War (1850–1853). At 2 a.m. on the morning of February 26 she struck uncharted rocks near Danger Point and began to take on water and sink. The number of lifeboats was insufficient to convey all safely off the doomed ship.

Many of the troops on board drowned in their berths as the ship foundered. The remaining men and officers of the 74th Regiment of Foot were mustered on deck by their commanding officer, Lt. Colonel Seton. He realized the nature of the situation and ordered his men to stand fast while the women and children were boarded onto the lifeboats. His soldiers obeyed and many went down with the ship.[5] While it is not known whether Lt. Colonel Seton used the phrase, "women and children first," he is credited with being among the first to put it into practice. His heroism and that of his men allowed the women and children on board to be saved.

The *Birkenhead* incident occurred during a period of British imperialism and colonialism. Any incident from such a time would seem to be out of place as an exemplar for medical ethics and health policy today. We think otherwise: from the perspective of professional ethics in obstetrics and gynecology "women and children first" was a defining moment in the history of world civilizations and therefore has direct relevance for healthcare today.

The sad reality is that women and children are not first in our world; indeed, they are often last. This is especially the case in low-income regions, which often do not provide adequate healthcare for women and children, as reflected in perinatal mortality rates.[6] International organizations, such as UNICEF,[6] the World Health Organization,[7] and the World Bank,[8] and international associations of physicians, such as the International Federation of Gynecology and Obstetrics (FIGO),[9] Matres Mundi,[10] and the World Association of Perinatal Medicine,[11] have led major efforts to identify problems in obstetric and neonatal care in low-income regions and have advocated for improvement. The International Academy of Perinatal Medicine has added its voice to these advocacy efforts, with its "New York Declaration" on "Woman and Children First – or Last?" which was presented at the United Nations on July 7, 2008. (See Section 18.4.) The Declaration defined sources of bias against the just allocation of healthcare resources for women and children in the developing world.[12]

The lack of prioritization for healthcare for women and children is not confined to low-income countries. This can also be a problem in the United States and other high-income countries. The ethical principle of healthcare justice in professional ethics in obstetrics and gynecology provides obstetrician-gynecologists with effective tools to advocate for the just allocation of healthcare resources for women and children. This advocacy should be for the priority of women and children in a world that has been largely dominated by politics and, at times, by injustice.

18.2.1 Healthcare-Justice–Based Ethical Framework

Like the general ethical principle of justice, healthcare justice emphasizes both substantive and procedural justice. Substantive justice concerns who gets what or the outcomes of allocation of resources.[13,14] Substantive justice requires that the reasons for setting priorities among competing interests of stakeholders, which determine the outcome of the decision-making process, be persuasive. There are competing accounts in ethical theory about which reasons should count as persuasive and therefore about which actual allocations of scarce resources are fair. In the course of our analysis of challenges to substantive justice in the allocation of healthcare for women and children in healthcare policy, we will identify and justify the reasons that should be invoked to guide responses to these challenges.

Procedural justice concerns the process or procedure for allocating scarce resources.[13,14] Procedural justice requires that interests of every individual and organization affected by the allocation of scarce resources should have his, her, or its interests identified and taken into account in the decision-making process. In the course of our analysis of challenges to procedural justice in the allocation of healthcare for women and children in healthcare policy, we will identify how the interests of pregnant, fetal, and neonatal patients should be taken into account as the basis for responding to these challenges.

18.2.2 Challenges to Justice in the Allocation of Healthcare Resources to Women and Children

Challenges to justice in the allocation of healthcare resources to women and children in the United States arise for both substantive and procedural justice. We address each set of challenges in turn.

18.2.2.1 Challenges to Substantive Justice

Challenges to substantive justice include the self-interest of adults, age bias, and economic bias. There can be two kinds of economic bias: against pregnant, fetal, and neonatal patients; and against obstetric services.

Self-Interests of Adults

The first challenge to substantive justice in the allocation of healthcare resources to women and children arises from the self-interest of adults. Adults will never again be fetal or neonatal patients but virtually all will be patients at some time(s) in their lives, especially as they age and, for many, also experience chronic disease and disability. In a society with a lower replacement birth rate among some subpopulations than in the past, such as the United States, the self-interest of adults who have not or will not have children may be another source of self-interest in having healthcare resources allocated to themselves. These sources of self-interest create a major challenge to substantive justice in the allocation of healthcare resources to women and children.

The response to this challenge draws on professional ethics in obstetrics and gynecology, which creates the prima facie ethical obligation of physicians to protect and promote the health-related interests of patients. (See Chapter 2.) By their very nature, these beneficence-based ethical obligations to patients are not a function of the patient's age or interest in having children but of what should be considered medically reasonable. It follows that, for physicians, the healthcare interests of one population of patients should not be neglected in order to advance the healthcare interests of another population of patients. Allocating healthcare resources based on the self-interest of one population of patients when doing so results in inadequate resources for another population of patients is not compatible with professional ethics in medicine. Physicians should therefore identify and expose such inadequate allocations of healthcare resources as violations of substantive justice based on professional ethical considerations.

Age Bias

A closely related challenge is age bias. In the United States public funding of healthcare favors the elderly, in the form of Medicare, which enjoys broad and enduring political support. In 1965, when Medicare was enacted, millions of elderly Americans had been plunged into poverty or near-poverty by major illness requiring hospitalization. President Johnson argued that this was not acceptable, because of the sacrifices that the older generation had made, especially during the Great Depression, and that aging cohorts had made in World War II. This was sound ethical reasoning, because it appealed to reciprocal justice: those who have sacrificed for society's good have a legitimate claim on society's resources. The commitment to prevent medically induced poverty among the elderly remains sound ethical reasoning.

The response to this ethical challenge is not to argue against Medicare and other public support for the elderly, because substantive justice does not support such a response. Instead, obstetrician-gynecologists should invoke the life-cycle principle to argue for increased priority for healthcare resources for children.[15] This ethical principle holds that everyone should have an opportunity to live and develop through all stages of life. The younger one is, the more years one is expected to live. This creates a priority for allocating healthcare resources to the youngest, fetal and neonatal patients, and, by necessity, pregnant women. The resources that fulfilling such a priority requires, while substantial, are not of the same scale as Medicare. Allocating healthcare resources to women and children may be cost-saving, e.g., from improved outcomes of pregnancy. In addition, healthier children are more likely to become productive members of society and repay the investment in their healthcare many times over economically, socially, and other important ways.

A second variant of substantive justice is also relevant, i.e., the investment refinement principle, which has direct implications for substantive justice in the allocation of healthcare resources to pregnant women. This ethical principle "emphasizes gradations within a life span. It gives priority to people between early adolescence and middle age on the basis of the amount the person invested in his or her life balanced by the amount left to live."[15] Pregnant women are in this category and have an enormous biopsychosocial investment in pregnancies being taken to term and the lives of their future children. With comprehensive obstetric and other general and specialty care, pregnant women can be expected to live for many years and their children even longer. The investment refinement principle is therefore abundantly satisfied and creates a powerful response to the challenge of age bias by justifying allocation of healthcare resources to pregnant women.

Bias against the Medically Indigent

We are not alone in believing that there is a general bias against the medically indigent in the United States. Medicare's justification was and remains reciprocal justice: to those who have sacrificed much for others and society, much is owed. It can be argued that poverty or near-poverty resulting from major illness is not the fault of the elderly and so such poverty is undeserved. In an older discourse from eighteenth-century Britain, which came to the North American British colonies, the elderly poor were considered the worthy poor. This contrasts with the eighteenth-century concept of the unworthy poor, those who are able but unwilling to work and support themselves and therefore have no justice-based claim of reciprocity on society.[16]

The phrases "worthy poor" and "unworthy poor" are no longer in use, but the concepts may continue to shape healthcare policy in the United States. Medicaid, a state–federal program of healthcare for the medically indigent, is not adequately funded, unlike Medicare. Medicaid also has much lower reimbursement schedules than Medicare. The precarious funding of Medicaid, compared to Medicare, may reflect the historical and disturbing distinction between the unworthy and worthy poor, a form of economic bias.

This bias becomes especially vicious and therefore egregiously unacceptable when it is applied to children of poverty and fetuses being carried by pregnant women of poverty. This is because impoverished fetal and neonatal patients and many impoverished pregnant women are not able to work and support themselves and are therefore not responsible for their poverty.

A powerful response to economic bias comes from the application of the ethical theory of justice of John Rawls (1921–2002), arguably the most important American political philosopher of the last century. Rawls' concern was that allocation of resources can seriously disadvantage the economically vulnerable, the "least well off," in his nomenclature. A utilitarian public policy would allocate resources to maximize the benefits to the greatest number, but this could leave the situation of the least well off unchanged or even worse. Rawls sought to modify utilitarian substantive justice by arguing that such a policy is ethically permissible only if it also improves the economic and social circumstances of the least well off. He called this the "maximin" principle.[17] Failure to constrain the utilitarian impulse by the maximin principle violates justice because unconstrained utilitarianism perpetuates exploitation, i.e., a situation in which some are benefited and many others are burdened with no or very limited opportunity to experience offsetting benefit.

The least well off in healthcare justice can be understood in terms of vulnerability to not receiving medically reasonable clinical management for one's condition. Fetal and neonatal patients are certainly among the most vulnerable patients, as are pregnant women who are socially or politically disadvantaged. The substantive justice-based maximin principle is therefore justifiably invoked to make allocation of resources to fetal, neonatal, and impoverished pregnant patients a healthcare priority.

Economic Bias against Obstetrics in Hospitals

Unlike neonatal services, which are usually profit centers in modern hospitals, there can also be economic bias against obstetric services in healthcare organizations. This bias results from what can be called the "trumping power" of economic values, which is distinct from economic bias against the poor. By "trumping power" we mean the tendency in public policy and therefore in healthcare organizations for economic concerns to override or even eliminate all other ethical considerations. This trumping power becomes more pronounced when economies experience stagnant growth or contraction, as is currently the case.

It is certainly a legitimate interest of healthcare organizations to have a fiscally sound business model. This is succinctly stated: "No margin, no mission." To protect this legitimate interest, it is ethically permissible for healthcare organizations to emphasize higher-margin clinical services, such as cardiovascular surgery, orthopedics, or oncology, and the profits they generate from high-quality patient care. Ethical concern arises when other clinical services that may not be profitable may be cut back or eliminated, such as inpatient pediatrics. As a consequence, some patient populations come to be viewed as less valuable and therefore less important than other patient populations, an organizational attitude that threatens professional integrity.[18]

Professional Liability Insurance

The cost of professional liability insurance has hit obstetrics especially hard in many parts of the United States.[19] As a consequence, obstetrics' cost profile can be markedly different from that of other specialties. The high cost of professional liability insurance for obstetrics in many states means that economic values gain trumping power at the level of healthcare organization leadership. The result is that obstetrics often comes to be seen exclusively as a cost center. This means that obstetrics can be viewed as a problem rather than a mission-vital clinical service. This can be manifest by a low prioritization for obstetrics in organizational philanthropic endeavors.

The response of obstetrician-gynecologists should be based on professional ethics in obstetrics and gynecology, as explicated in Chapter 2: no group of patients, grouped by specialties and their economic value to healthcare organizations, should count in deliberative clinical judgment for less than any other group of patients. All groups of patients are equally patients in professional medical ethics, whether or not one group of patients happens to generate more net revenues than another. Before making the case for organizational resources based on the equal importance of pregnant, fetal, and neonatal patients, leaders in obstetrics need to get their financial houses in order, i.e., run obstetrics on a sound business basis.[14] Otherwise, legitimate advocacy will be subjected to unnecessary vulnerability.

Trumping Power of Economic Values

There is a tendency in all healthcare systems for economic values to trump or automatically override all other considerations, especially including professional integrity. As the great American folk singer and philosopher, Bob Dylan, once put it, "While money doesn't talk, it swears."[20] By getting their own financial houses in order, and advocating for the equal importance of pregnant, fetal, and neonatal patients, obstetrician-gynecologists will be in a position to talk back, countering the trumping power of economic considerations with advocacy for obstetric services as mission vital.

18.2.2.2 Challenges to Procedural Justice

There are also challenges to procedural justice. The first is bias in favor of persons and the second is bias against those who cannot speak for themselves.

Bias in Favor of Persons

Persons in the ethics literature are understood to be human beings with independent moral status and autonomy. (See Chapter 2.) Personhood comes into existence only after birth and, on some accounts, not until the acquisition of language and social identity some time after birth. Personhood is a self-generated moral status, usually expressed in the language of rights.[13] The interests of stakeholders with personhood-based rights obviously have to be taken into account in order to meet the requirements of procedural justice.

Any claim that fetuses are also persons and therefore have rights is highly controversial in both philosophical ethics and theological ethics. (See Chapter 2.) As a consequence, fetuses are put at a competitive disadvantage in decision-making processes about allocation of resources, because their very status as stakeholders is in doubt, especially for those who think that only persons can be stakeholders. The result is a bias in procedural justice in favor of persons, because it assumes that only the interests of persons need to be taken into account.

Professional ethics in obstetrics and gynecology provides a powerful antidote: the generation of interests from a human being's status as a patient, rather than as a person. (See Chapter 2.) All patients have an interest in the protection and improvement of their health. Patients have this interest in virtue of being presented to a physician or other healthcare profession and the existence of clinical interventions that can protect and improve health. The genius of the ethical concept of the fetus as a patient is that it goes beyond the binomial of being a person or not and therefore undercuts the biases generated by this categorization.

The way to take the interests of all patients into account is to recognize that all patients have an interest in being treated according to accepted standards of care. This applies to fetal patients, who are not yet persons, as well as to pregnant patients, who clearly are persons. Obstetricians should therefore point out that procedural justice requires that the interests of all patients be taken into account by those responsible for making and implementing healthcare policy. In particular, obstetrician-gynecologists should advocate that healthcare resources be made available to ensure that all patients – pregnant, fetal, and neonatal patients included – are treated according to accepted standards of care.

Bias against Those Who Cannot Speak for Themselves

Fetal and neonatal patients cannot speak for themselves in the policymaking process. In many cultures, pregnant women struggle to have their interests recognized and taken into account in setting healthcare priorities. As a consequence, the health-related interests of fetal, neonatal, and pregnant patients may not be routinely taken into account in forming and implementing healthcare policy, which violates procedural justice.

Obstetrician-gynecologists are in a unique position to assume an advocacy role because they have expert scientific and clinical knowledge about how to identify and protect the health-related interests of pregnant, fetal, and neonatalpatients. On this basis, obstetrician-gynecologists should advocate for healthcare priorities that create resources to support the development and global implementation of evidence-based medical care for pregnant, fetal, and neonatalpatients, so that their interests are taken into account in a scientific, unbiased fashion. The goal should be the elimination, to the greatest extent possible, of national and wide area variation in the processes and outcomes of obstetric care. Ideally, where a patient lives should not make a difference in the quality of medical care that an individual receives.

18.3 Antidote to Cynicism about the Ethical Principle of Healthcare Justice

Obstetrician-gynecologists can be cynical about the ethical principle of justice because it appears abstract and therefore to lack clinical application. This cynicism can be reinforced by their experience with the professional liability crisis.[19] The antidote to this understandable cynicism and therefore to effective advocacy is to distinguish substantive and procedural justice; explicitly identify biases that distort organizational culture and healthcare policy; and use relevant concepts of justice to advocate for fetal, neonatal, and pregnant patients whose healthcare otherwise is at risk of unacceptable compromise. By focusing on the interests of patients and keeping their own individual and group self-interests secondary, obstetrician-gynecologists can advocate for their patients from the moral high ground of making women and children first as a matter of justice and professional integrity.

18.3.1 Identifying and Addressing Social Conditions that Impede Healthcare Justice

A major social impediment to healthcare justice for female, pregnant, fetal, and neonatal patients is social invisibility concerning such matters as trafficking in girls and young women; female genital mutilation; history of childhood sexual abuse; sexual violence, including intimate-partner violence; forced or early marriage; and forcing use or nonuse of contraception for male sexual partners.[21-23] Social movements, such as #MeToo and those concerned with climate change and its effects on health, have begun the long process of increasing social awareness of these and other violations of human rights, respect for autonomy, beneficence, and nonmaleficence. The ethical principle of healthcare justice creates a prima facie ethical obligation of obstetrician-gynecologists to lay the foundations for successful social advocacy by documenting and reporting these abuses and crimes.

The first step in addressing this matter in clinical practice is becoming aware of the possibility of one's own discomfort that might subtly discourage one from initiating awkward conversation. One should be mindful of these feelings, as a first step toward preventing them from influencing the taking of a comprehensive history. The professional virtue of self-effacement requires not being influenced by differences in social and experiential backgrounds, in which it is difficult to imagine oneself living. The professional virtue of self-sacrifice requires one to discipline one's discomfort by taking a comprehensive history. As this becomes routine, the discomfort will abate.

The American College of Obstetricians and Gynecologists has provided a step-wise, clinically practical approach to counseling women about intimate-partner violence, including a focus on the patient's sense of her own safety and need for support to deal with an unsafe domestic setting. The goal is to invite female and pregnant patients to begin the process of communicating with their obstetrician-gynecologist about biopsychosocial risk.[24] Other screening questions may include "Can you come and go as you please?" and "Have you been physically harmed in any way?" and "Is anyone forcing you to do anything physically or sexually that you do not want to do?"[23] Physical examination should be thorough with respect to being alert to physical signs of abuse, violence, sexually transmitted infections, and genital mutilation. By incorporating this approach, the obstetrician-gynecologist can prevent cynicism about healthcare justice and the sometimes glacial pace changes. Practicing obstetrician-gynecologists should respond positively to invitations to participate in research to identify and optimally manage the biopsychosocial conditions, diseases, and injuries of abuse of women, so that they become increasingly visible, which is the key to health policy change.

18.3.2 The Impact of Climate Change on the Life and Health of Female, Pregnant, and Neonatal Patients

Climate change can have deleterious health effects on many populations, including female, pregnant, and neonatal patients.[25] Chronic conditions such as drought can have an adverse impact on the supply of food and potable water. Climate change can also lead to mass relocation, putting already vulnerable female, pregnant, fetal, and neonatal patients at increased risk of morbidity, mortality, and disability. Increasing ambient temperatures that appear to result from climate change are associated with increased violence against women. These health impacts of climate change are undeniably "in the wheelhouse" of the obstetrician-gynecologist. Obstetrician-gynecologists should support advocacy for research on effective responses at both the public health and clinical levels.

18.4 "Women and Children First – or Last?" The New York Declaration of the International Academy of Perinatal Medicine*

The Ethical Principle of Justice and the Responsible Allocation of Healthcare Resources

A major concern of public policy in all countries is the allocation of healthcare resources. Justice is the ethical principle that requires fairness in such allocation decisions. Without the principle of justice guiding healthcare allocation decisions, these decisions can be idiosyncratic and arbitrary and injure the interests of many. With the ethical principle of justice guiding healthcare allocation decisions, these decisions become reasoned and fair, by protecting and promoting the interests of all who are affected.

Substantive and Procedural Justice

The principle of justice has substantive and procedural components. Substantive justice requires that the outcomes of priority setting in the allocation of healthcare resources reasonably protect and promote the interests of all of those with a stake in the priorities that are actually set. Procedural justice requires that the interests of everyone with a stake in the outcomes of priority setting in the allocation of healthcare resources be taken into account in the decision-making process.

Justice-Based Responses to Ethical Challenges in Allocating Perinatal Healthcare Resources

The first ethical challenge in allocating resources for perinatal healthcare is economic and political bias. In many countries and cultures, women and children do not control economic resources and political power to the same extent as adult men. Allocation of healthcare

---

* Presented by The International Academy of Perinatal Medicine at the United Nations, New York, New York July 7, 2008. Available at https://www.ajog.org/article/S0002-9378(09)00772-8/pdf (accessed March 1, 2019).

resources that favors only those with economic and political power violates substantive justice. The response of justice is to emphasize that allocation of healthcare resources should also benefit those who are vulnerable as a result of being economically least well off or politically least powerful.

The second challenge is age bias. In many countries, there is a bias in allocation of healthcare resources toward adults. This reflects the fact that adults will never again be fetal or neonatal patients but will become patients themselves as they age and experience disability. Such bias can be stronger in societies with a low population-replacement rate. Age bias in the allocation of healthcare resources violates substantive justice. The response from justice is the life cycle principle that requires that all should have the opportunity to live and develop through all stages of life. Specifically, the younger one is, the more years one is expected to live, creating an increased priority of healthcare resources for fetal patients and children.

The third challenge is the bias in favor of persons. In the language of philosophical ethics, persons are human beings with independent moral status and autonomy, which occurs only after birth. In philosophical ethics, fetal patients are not persons. Bias in favor of persons violates procedural justice by not taking into account the interests of fetal patients, who undeniably have a stake in the allocation of healthcare resources. The response of justice derives from the ethical concept of the fetus as a patient. This concept is an accepted component of perinatal ethics, which emphasizes that a human being does not need to be a person in order to be a patient. Allocation of healthcare resources should take account of the needs of all patients, not just persons.

The fourth challenge is bias against those who cannot speak for themselves. Fetal patients and children have a stake in the allocation of healthcare resources but cannot speak for themselves in the political process. This is also true of women in some countries. If no one speaks for those who cannot speak for themselves, their interests may not be taken into account in healthcare allocation decisions. This violates procedural justice. The response of justice derives the professional, fiduciary role of perinatologists. They are clinicians and scientists with scientific and clinical expertise about the medical care of fetal, neonatal, and pregnant patients. As their fiduciaries, perinatologists should speak and advocate for the interests of fetal, neonatal, and pregnant patients in the process of making healthcare allocation decisions.

Implications for Health Policy Leaders

Health policy leaders should make decisions about allocation of healthcare resources for fetal, neonatal, and pregnant patients on the basis of the requirements of justice. The expert judgments of perinatologists constitute invaluable but sometimes underutilized resources in this process. Health policy leaders should also support the development and implementation of evidence-based perinatal medicine as the means for eliminating to the greatest extent possible national, regional, and international variation in the processes and outcomes of perinatal care. International collaborative research and global perinatal education are essential components of this effort.

References

1. Aristotle. Nicomachean Ethics. Translated with an introduction and notes by Martin Oswald. Indianapolis: Boos-Merrill, 1962.
2. Chervenak FA, McCullough LB. "Women and Children First:" transforming an historic defining moment into a contemporary ethical imperative. Am J Obstet Gynecol 2009; 201: 351.e1–5.
3. Chervenak FA, McCullough LB, Hale RW. Guild interests: an insidious threat to professionalism in obstetrics and gynecology. Am J Obstet Gynecol 2018; 219: 581–584.
4. Percival T. Medical Ethics; or, A Code of Institutes and Precepts, adapted to the Professional Conduct of Physicians and Surgeons. London: Johnson & Bickerstaff, 1803.
5. Historic UK.com. "Women and children first": the silent heroes of the Birkenhead. Available at www.historic-uk.com/CultureUK/WomenandChildrenFirst.htm (accessed March 1, 2019).
6. United Nations. UNICEF. www.unicef.org/ (accessed March 1, 2019).
7. World Health Organization. www.who.int/en/ (accessed March 1, 2019).
8. The World Bank. www.worldbank.org/ (accessed March 1, 2019).
9. International Federation of Gynecology and Obstetrics. www.figo.org/ (accessed March 1, 2019).
10. Matres Mundi. www.matres-mundi.org/ (accessed March 1, 2019).
11. World Association of Perinatal Medicine. www.wapm.info/ (accessed March 1, 2019).
12. Chervenak FA, McCullough LB. International Academy of Perinatal Medicine. Women and Children First or Last? New York Declaration. Am J Obstet Gynecol 2009; 201: 335.

13. Available at www.ajog.org/article/S0002-9378(09)00772-8/pdf (accessed March 1, 2019).
13. Beauchamp TL, Childress JF. Principles of Biomedical Ethics, 7th ed. New York: Oxford University Press, 2013.
14. Chervenak FA, McCullough LB. Professionalism and justice: ethical management guidelines for leaders of academic medical centers. Acad Med 2002; 77: 45–47.
15. Emanuel EJ, Wertheimer A. Who should get influenza vaccine when not all can? Science 2006; 312: 854–855.
16. McCullough LB. John Gregory and the Invention of Professional Medical Ethics and the Profession of Medicine. Dordrecht, the Netherlands: Kluwer Academic, 1998.
17. Rawls J. A Theory of Justice. Cambridge, MA: Belknap Press of Harvard University, 1971. Revised edition 1999.
18. Chervenak FA, McCullough LB. The diagnosis and management of progressive dysfunction of healthcare organizations. Obstet Gynecol 2005; 105: 882–887.
19. Chervenak FA, McCullough LB. Neglected ethical dimensions of the professional liability crisis. Am J Obstet Gynecol 2004; 190: 1198–1200.
20. Bob Dylan. It's all right ma, I'm only bleeding. Lyrics available at www.bobdylan.com/#/songs/its-alright-ma-im-only-bleeding (accessed March 1, 2019).
21. Garcia-Moreno C, Zimmerman C, Morris-Gehring A, et al. Violence against women and girls 5. Addressing violence against women: a call to action. The Lancet 2015; 385: 1685–1695.
22. Park J, Nordstrom SK, Weber KM, Irwin T. Reproductive coercion: uncloaking an imbalance of social power. Am J Obstet Gynecol 2016; 214: 74–78.
23. Tracy EA, Macias-Konstatopoulos W. Identifying and assisting sexually exploited and trafficked patients seeking women's health care services. Obstet Gynecol 2017; 130: 443–453.
24. American College of Obstetricians and Gynecologists. Committee on Healthcare for Undeserved Women. Committee Opinion 518. Intimate partner violence. *Obstet Gynecol* 2012; 119 (2 Pt 1): 412–417.
25. Kuehn L, McCormick S. Heat exposure and maternal mental health in the face of climate change. Int J Environ Res Pub Health 2017; 14(8) pii: E853. DOI:10.3390/ijerph14080853.

Glossary of Key Concepts

A

Abortion: The expulsion of the previable fetus from the uterus of a pregnant woman. Abortion can be spontaneous or it can be induced medically or surgically. "Abortion" is a general, nonspecific clinical term and therefore should be specified, to promote clear and effective communication with the patient and among members of the healthcare team.

Absolute ethical obligation: An ethical obligation that permits no exceptions; it must always be fulfilled.

Absolute ethical obligation of confidentiality: An ethical obligation, without exception, to prevent unauthorized access to information about the patient. Failure to prevent unauthorized access is ethically impermissible.

Absolute ethical principle: An ethical principle that permits no exceptions to the ethical obligations that it generates.

Advance directive: A written statement or (as permitted in applicable law) an oral declaration that projects the patient's decision-making authority into the future to make decisions about setting limits on life-sustaining treatment (Living Will or Directive to Physicians) or to appoint someone to make decisions for him or her, a surrogate decision maker (Medical Power of Attorney or Durable Power of Attorney for Health Care). The first type of advance directive takes effect when the patient has lost decision-making capacity and has a terminal or irreversible condition as defined in applicable law. The second type of advance directive takes effect when the patient has lost decision-making capacity. A court finding that the patient is incompetent is not required.

Anatomic futility: 97%–100% rate of failure to achieve the anatomic goal of maintaining or restoring adequate anatomy.

Argument-based ethical reasoning: The use of ethical analysis and ethical argument to make reasoned judgments about behavior or character that is ethically ideal, impermissible, obligatory, or permissible.

Assent: A process in which decision making for a patient with impaired decision-making capacity refractory to assisted decision making occurs *with* the patient but *by* others who should take into account the results of the assent process. The authority of the patient's preferences is a function of the patient's cognitive and affective developmental status.

Assisted decision making: A clinical response to impaired decision-making capacity that begins with a clinical assessment of the patient's decision-making capacity, identification of impaired components, and clinical management designed to reverse these impairments to an acceptable threshold so that the patient can exercise her autonomy in the informed consent process.

B

Beneficence-based clinical judgment: Clinical judgment based on the ethical principle of beneficence in professional ethics in medicine and in obstetrics and gynecology.

Beneficence-based ethical obligation: An ethical obligation, either absolute or prima facie, created by the ethical principle of beneficence.

Best interests of the child standard in professional ethics in pediatrics: A concept that forms part of the foundation of professional ethics in pediatrics, which creates the prima facie beneficence-based obligations of the pediatrician and other healthcare professionals to protect the health-related interests of the pediatric patient.

Best interests standard of *surrogate decision making*: A standard that should guide the surrogate decision maker when he or she is not able to reliably satisfy the substituted judgment standard. The surrogate decision maker should base his or her decisions on a considered judgment of which course of clinical management is reliably predicted to protect and promote the patient's health-related interests. This is a beneficence-based standard.

Bioethics: The disciplined study of the morality of healthcare professionals, patients, healthcare organizations, biomedical and clinical research, and healthcare policy with the aim of improving bioethical morality, drawing on such disciplines as philosophy, theology, law, and social science.

Biopsychosocial concept of health and disease: Health and disease have three components: a biomedical component that concerns anatomy and physiology; a psychological component that concerns psychological responses to changes in anatomy and physiology; and a social component that concerns social responses to changes in anatomy and physiology. This concept was invented by the psychiatrist George Engel (1913–1999) as an antidote to equating health and disease to the biomedical component, which Engel thought was scientifically and clinically inadequate. This is known as biomedical or biological reductionism.

Glossary of Key Concepts

C

Chronically and variably impaired autonomy: Impairment of one or more of the components of decision-making capacity over time and to various degrees.

Clinical gaze: A concept originating in the philosophy of medicine of the French philosopher, Michel Foucault (1926–1984): biomedical clinical judgment about diagnosis and clinical management of the patient's condition, with the potential to transform the experience of conditions, diseases, disabilities, and illnesses. The clinical gaze is at risk of leaving out the psychosocial components of the concepts of health and disease, an omission known as biomedical or biological reductionism.

Coercion: The use of force accompanied by a threat, used to take control of the patient's decision making and behavior.

"Common morality": Comprises "norms about right and wrong conduct that are so widely shared that they form a stable social compact." (Beauchamp and Childress, Principles of Biomedical Ethics, 7th ed., 2013: 2–3.)

Competence: A legal or clinical judgment that a patient has the capacities required for making decisions, caring for oneself, and managing one's personal and family matters.

Confidentiality: The ethical obligation of all physicians and other healthcare professionals involved in a patient's care to maintain, as inaccessible, information about the patient by preventing access to that information by those without authorization to have access to it. This can be an absolute ethical obligation (no exceptions) or a prima facie ethical obligation (there are justified exceptions).

Conflict of commitment: Exists when the physician's ethical obligations to patients or research subjects become incompatible with the physician's ethical obligations to other people in his or her life, especially family members.

Conflict of interest: Exists when fulfilling ethical obligations to patients or research subjects become incompatible with legitimate self-interests.

Conscientious objection: Refusal by an obstetrician-gynecologist or other healthcare professional to fulfill ethical obligations to a female or pregnant patient, based on values, beliefs, and commitments other than the ethical concept of medicine as a profession.

Consequentialism: A general ethical theory that assesses the worth of character, behavior, organizations, and policy on the basis of consequences that are judged to be good. Utilitarianism is a subset of consequentialism.

Critical care as a trial of intervention: The initiation of critical care clinical management with the short-term goal of preventing imminent death and the long-term goal of survival with at least some interactive capacity.

Cynical organizational culture: An organizational culture that exhibits a deteriorating connection between organizational rhetoric and reality and a defensive posture of leadership in response to criticism.

D

Decision-making capacity: A clinical judgment that a patient can complete the components of decision-making capacity: pay attention to the information that is provided to her; absorb, retain, and recall this information as needed in subsequent components; possess cognitive understanding, appreciation, and evaluative understanding; explicitly authorize or refuse to authorize clinical management; when requested, she can explain her authorization or refusal of authorization on the basis of her cognitive and evaluative understanding.

Deliberative clinical judgment: Clinical judgment that is evidence-based (an appeal to the best available, critically appraised evidence), rigorous (especially in the effort to identify and reduce the influence of bias), transparent (the physician can explain the judgment to other clinicians, especially team members and the patient), and accountable (to meet an essential component of patient safety and quality).

Dependent moral status: Moral status that originates in a social role created by human beings, especially to protect human beings vulnerable to the power of others over them.

Descriptive ethics: The use of empirical methods of the social sciences to obtain data that describe the actual ethical judgments, practices, and policies of healthcare professionals and organizations, of patients and their families, and of the larger society.

Direct referral: The referring obstetrician-gynecologist sees to it that the patient will be seen by a colleague competent and willing to provide clinical management supported in deliberative clinical judgment.

Directive counseling: Making recommendations about clinical management. Making recommendations is ethically justified in two clinical circumstances: there is in deliberative clinical judgment only one medically reasonable alternative for the clinical management of the patient's condition or diagnosis; or there are two or more medically reasonable alternatives for the clinical management of the patient's condition or diagnosis and in deliberative clinical judgment one is clinically superior to the others.

Discipline of ethical reasoning: Going where ethical reasoning, ethical analysis and argument, take one and nowhere else.

Distress: The experience of disruption of one's behavioral repertoire.

Double effect: A concept created in Roman Catholic moral theology to deal with situations in which an intrinsically good act, e.g., cancer treatment during pregnancy, has both a good effect (treatment of the cancer with subsequent health-related benefits for the woman) and a bad or evil effect (the death of the fetus). The bad effect is permitted so long as it is not the cause of the good effect and the proportionate good outweighs the harm. When this causal condition is met, the bad effect is not intended as the causal means to the good effect. Sometimes, a variant of the concept of double effect detaches intent from the causal relationship between the bad and good effects.

E

Enlightened self-interest: The self-interests of the physician that align with the health-related interests of the patient. These become legitimate self-interests of the physician.

Enthusiasm: Beliefs that lack an evidence base.

Ethical analysis: Clearly expressing ethical concepts.

Ethical argument: Identifying the implications of clearly expressed ethical concepts.

Ethical concept of the fetus as a patient: A fetus becomes a patient when the fetus is presented to a physician or other healthcare professional and there exist forms of clinical management that in deliberative clinical judgment are predicted to result in net clinical benefit.

Ethical concept of medicine as a profession: Requires physicians to make three commitments: to become and remain scientifically and clinically competent, by submitting to the discipline of deliberative clinical judgment and clinical practice and research based on it; to make protection and promotion of the patient's health-related interests one's primary concern and motivation, keeping individual self-interest systematically secondary; and to make protection and promotion of the patient's health-related interests one's primary concern and motivation, keeping group or guild self-interest systematically secondary.

Ethical ideal: A valued goal worth pursuing, knowing that one might fall short. An ethical ideal creates a prima facie ethical obligation to make incremental progress in pursuit of the goal.

Ethical judgment: The use of ethical reasoning to classify character, behavior, or health policy as ethically ideal, ethically impermissible, ethically obligatory, or ethically permissible.

Ethical obligation: A form of behavior, character, or health policy that should occur.

Ethical principle: A guide to ethical judgment and behavior based on it.

Ethical principle of beneficence in medical ethics and bioethics: An ethical principle that creates the prima facie ethical obligation to act in a way that results in a net balance of good over harmful consequences for those affected by one's behavior, with good consequences and harmful consequences specified variously.

Ethical principle of beneficence in professional ethics in gynecology: An ethical principle that creates the prima facie ethical obligation of the gynecologist to provide clinical management that in deliberative clinical judgment is predicted to result in net clinical benefit for the female patient and therefore protect and promote her health-related interests.

Ethical principle of beneficence in professional ethics in medicine: An ethical principle creates the prima facie ethical obligation of the physician to provide clinical management that in deliberative clinical judgment is predicted to result in net clinical benefit for the patient and therefore protect and promote the patient's health-related interests.

Ethical principle of beneficence in professional ethics in obstetrics: An ethical principle that creates the prima facie ethical obligation of the obstetrician to provide clinical management that in deliberative clinical judgment is predicted to result in net clinical benefit for the pregnant and fetal patient (when the fetus is a patient) and to the future neonatal patient and therefore protect and promote their health-related interests.

Ethical principle of healthcare justice in professional ethics in gynecology: An ethical principle that applies to populations of female patients and creates the prima facie ethical obligation of the gynecologist to see to it that each female patient is provided medically reasonable clinical management of her condition or diagnosis.

Ethical principle of healthcare justice in professional ethics in medicine: An ethical principle that applies to populations of patients and creates the prima facie ethical obligation of the physician to see to it that each patient is treated equally or fairly as "equally" and "fairly" are understood clinically: each patient is to be provided medically reasonable clinical management of her or his condition or diagnosis.

Ethical principle of healthcare justice in professional ethics in obstetrics: An ethical principle that applies to populations of pregnant, fetal, and neonatal patients and creates the prima facie ethical obligation of the obstetrician to see to it that each pregnant, fetal, and neonatal patient is provided medically reasonable clinical management of her or his condition or diagnosis.

Ethical principle of justice in medical ethics and bioethics: An ethical principle that creates the prima facie ethical obligation to treat groups of individuals equally or with fairness, with "equally" and "fairness" specified variously, depending on which theory of justice is adopted. There is no agreement in the history of philosophy about which theory of justice should be accepted as the best theory of justice. The ethical concept of healthcare justice is not used in medical ethics and bioethics.

Ethical principle of nonmaleficence in medical ethics and bioethics: An ethical principle that creates the prima facie ethical obligation to act in a way that prevents or does not cause a net balance of harmful over good consequences for those affected by one's behavior, with good consequences and harmful consequences specified variously.

Ethical principle of nonmaleficence in professional ethics in medicine: An ethical principle that sets the limiting condition on the ethical principle of beneficence: When in deliberative clinical judgment the evidence for a medically reasonable alternative becomes weak, the physician must become alert to the increasing strength of the prediction that net clinical harm could be the outcome for the patient. There is a nonmaleficience-based *prima facie* ethical obligation to prevent such an outcome.

Ethical principle of nonmaleficence in professional ethics in obstetrics and gynecology: An ethical principle that sets the limiting condition on the ethical principle of beneficence. When the evidence for a medically reasonable alternative becomes weak, the obstetrician-gynecologist must become alert to the decreasing strength of the prediction that net clinical harm could be the outcome for the female, pregnant, fetal, or neonatal patient. There is a prima facie nonmaleficence-based ethical obligation to prevent the net harmful outcomes of overtreatment, i.e., treatment that does not result in net balance of clinical good over harms but a net balance of clinical harms over clinical goods. This is especially the case when the net harm is serious, far-reaching, and irreversible.

Ethical principle of respect for autonomy in medical ethics and bioethics: An ethical principle that is described by Beauchamp and Childress (Principles of Biomedical Ethics, 7th ed., 2013: 106) as the *prima facie ethical obligation*: "To respect autonomous agents is to acknowledge their right to hold views, to make choices, and to take actions based on their values and beliefs."

Ethical principle of respect for autonomy in professional ethics in gynecology: An ethical principle that creates the prima facie ethical obligation to empower the female patient to make informed and voluntary decisions about the management of her clinical condition or diagnosis by providing her with information about the medically reasonable alternatives for its clinical management.

Ethical principle of respect for autonomy in professional ethics in medicine: An ethical principle that creates the prima facie ethical obligation to empower the patient to make informed and voluntary decisions about the management of her clinical condition by providing her with information about the medically reasonable alternatives for its clinical management.

Ethical principle of respect for autonomy in professional ethics in obstetrics: An ethical principle that creates the prima facie ethical obligation to empower the pregnant patient to make informed and voluntary decisions about the management of her pregnancy by providing her with information about the medically reasonable alternatives for its clinical management.

Ethical reasoning: An intellectual and practical process of deploying ethical analysis and ethical argument to reach argument-based ethical judgments about what is ethically ideal, ethically impermissible, or ethically obligatory.

Ethically ideal: Always striving for the goal of a perfect outcome even while knowing that one may fall short. It is ethically impermissible not to attempt incremental progress toward the goal of a perfect outcome.

Ethically impermissible: A form of behavior, character, or health policy that should not occur.

Ethically obligatory: A form of behavior, character, of health policy that should occur.

Ethically permissible: A form of behavior, character, organizational culture, or health policy that may occur in circumstances in which there are multiple forms of behavior, character, or health policy supported by ethical reasoning.

Ethics: The disciplined study of morality with the goal of incrementally improving it, based on reasoned ethical judgments produced by ethical reasoning.

Evidence-based equipoise: In deliberative clinical judgment, a comprehensive, evidence-based evaluation of the outcomes of animal-model research (when it has been reported) and early phase investigation requires the physician to become uncertain about the relative clinical benefit of the maternal–fetal intervention versus expectant obstetric management and neonatal intervention. Evidence-based equipoise is required for the initiation of randomized controlled trials.

Experiment: A clinical intervention the outcome of which cannot be reliably predicted in deliberative clinical judgment.

F

Female patient: A living human being becomes a female patient when she is presented to a gynecologist (or other healthcare professional) and there exist forms of clinical management that are reliably predicted to result in net clinical benefit for her.

Fertility: A clinical condition, not a disease and not a disability. The biologic concept of fertility has at least two biological meanings. One meaning of "fertility" applies to both males and females of the human species: the capacity to produce gametes capable of fusing with gametes from the other sex to become zygotes. Another meaning of "fertility" applies only to females of the human species: the capacity to produce ova that can fuse with spermatozoa to become zygotes that can embed in the uterine wall and initiate pregnancy.

Fetal analysis: Interpreting information about the fetus' condition, including auscultation, chromosome analysis, genome sequencing, imaging, heart function tracings, and tissue samples (cells, blood).

Feticide: The killing of the fetus, independently of gestational age and of whether the uterus is emptied.

Fetus as a patient: A living human fetus becomes a patient when that the fetus is presented to a physician or other healthcare professional and there exist forms of clinical management that in deliberative clinical judgment are predicted to result in net clinical benefit for the fetus. The previable fetus becoming a patient is a function of the pregnant woman's autonomy. The pregnant woman is free to confer, withhold, or having once conferred withdraw, the moral status of being a patient on or from her fetus before viability. The viable fetus becomes a patient when a pregnant woman is presented to an obstetrician or other healthcare professional.

"First do no harm:" A misreading of the Hippocratic texts which states that the physician should "first help, or at least do no harm." "First do no harm" should not be used. The ethical principle of nonmaleficence in professional ethics in medicine should be used and functions as a limiting condition on the ethical principle of beneficence in professional ethics in medicine.

Force: The use of psychological or physical pressure to control the patient's decision-making and behavior.

Futility: A general clinical concept, meaning that a form of clinical management becomes futile when in deliberative clinical judgment it is predicted to have a high rate of failure in achieving the goal for which it was created. To be clinically applicable this general ethical concept must be specified as anatomic futility, imminent demise futility, interactive capacity futility, physiologic futility, or quality-of-life futility.

G

Geriatric assent: The assent process with geriatric patients.
Groningen Protocol: A clinical guide to the decision-making about infant euthanasia, i.e., killing neonatal patients. The protocol has two parts. The first addresses "requirements that must be fulfilled," including diagnosis and prognosis that are "certain," presence of "hopeless and unbearable suffering," and confirmation of the diagnosis and prognosis by an independent physician. The second addresses "information needed to support and clarify the decision about euthanasia" that covers five domains: diagnosis and prognosis; "euthanasia decision"; consultation; implementation; and "steps taken after death." The Protocol also presents a medical and legal justification for the protocol and clinical practice based on it.
Guild: The organization of physicians into groups to protect group self-interest as the primary concern and motivation of members and leaders. In medieval and Renaissance Europe physician guilds were formed to protect the economic, political, and social interests of physicians, not their professionalism.
Guild self-interest: The group self-interests of physicians who have organized into practice groups.

H

Harm principle: A beneficence-based and nonmaleficence-based ethical judgment that holds that no one is free to put others at risk of serious, far-reaching, and potentially irreversible harm without sufficient reason. A more expansive version invokes prevention of harm without qualification.
Hope: The desire for a future state of affairs that has a probability <1 and >0.
Humility: The habit of recognizing the limits of one's ethical judgments and working persistently to improve them.

I

Imminent demise futility: Critical care intervention will be physiologically effective for a short period of time (days to weeks) but then result in death (in the critical care unit) with a 97%–100% rate and without any interactive capacity before death occurs.
Impaired autonomy: Occurs when one or more of the seven components of decision making are reduced. Chronic impairment is long term. There are four variants of chronically impaired autonomy: chronic and variable impairment of autonomy, chronic and invariable impairment of autonomy, chronic and progressive impairment of autonomy, and chronic but decreasing impairment of autonomy.
Independent moral status: Moral status that originates in properties of an entity that it possesses independently of all other entities and that create the ethical obligation to protect and promote its interests.
Indirect referral: The obstetrician-gynecologist provides information to pregnant patient about clinics or agencies, such as Planned Parenthood in the United States, that provide competent and safe induced abortion or feticide.
Induced abortion: The use of medications or surgery to remove the fetus from a pregnant woman's uterus before viability. If the fetus is alive, induced abortion causes the death of the fetus. If the fetus is already dead, induced abortion does not cause the death of the fetus.
Informed consent process: A process that requires the obstetrician to present to the patient a description of the patient's condition or diagnosis, the medically reasonable alternatives for its clinical management, the clinical benefits and risks of each medically reasonable alternative and to support the patient in her completion of the seven components of decision-making capacity.
Informed refusal process: A process to be implemented when a patient refuses to authorize offered or recommended clinical management. There is a strict legal obligation to inform the patient about the clinical risks she is taking and document this disclosure. There is an ethical obligation to respond with respectful persuasion. If that fails, there is an ethical obligation to assure the patient that she can return for clinical care at any time and to inform her about signs and symptoms that would justify returning for clinical care.
Innovation: A clinical experiment with an individual patient to benefit that patient clinically.
Institutional Animal Care and Use Committee: A multidisciplinary committee charged under federal law and regulations with responsibility for prospective review and oversight of all research involving animal subjects.
Institutional Review Board: A multidisciplinary committee charged under federal law and regulations with responsibility for prospective review and oversight of all research involving human subjects.
Interactive capacity futility: Critical care intervention will be physiologically effective, prevent imminent demise, but with a 97%–100% likelihood of resulting in irreversible loss of interactive capacity.
In vitro embryo: The fertilized ovum once the process of cell division has begun in a petri dish or other vessel in a reproductive endocrinology and infertility or other laboratory. This is the meaning used in in vitro fertilization.
In vivo embryo: The biological entity that comes into existence when the blastocyst implants in the uterine wall until the eighth week of development, after which it becomes a fetus. This is the meaning of "embryo" used in obstetrics and gynecology.
Invasive fetal analysis: Fetal analysis of results of methods that penetrate the maternal abdomen, uterus, or amniotic cavity. Even though the skin and vein are penetrated, a maternal blood draw is characterized as noninvasive, because it poses no risk of clinical harm to the fetus.

Glossary of Key Concepts

J

Judgment: The process of classifying an entity by applying clear, justified, and practical criteria.

K

Kafkaesque organizational culture: An organizational culture in which organizational rhetoric and reality become dissociative.

L

Libertarian justice: A theory of justice that places the highest value on human freedom, especially freedom from the state. Libertarian justice defines unfairness or inequity in terms of the processes of decision making and therefore emphasizes fairness of process. Fair processes of organizational decision making identify and address the obligations, rights, and interests of all stakeholders.

M

Machiavellian organizational culture: An organizational culture in which the appearance of professionalism masks the neglect or absence of professionalism.

Manipulation: The use of psychological or physical pressure to strongly influence the patient's decision-making process and behavior. Withholding information about medically reasonable alternatives to strongly influence the patient's decision-making process and behavior is a form of manipulation.

Maternal–fetal intervention: Invasive and noninvasive clinical management of the fetus in clinical treatment, innovation, and research. Both "maternal" and "fetal" are required by the ethical concept of the fetus as a patient.

Medical emergency: Exists when there is immediate threat to the patient's life or threat of serious, far-reaching, and irreversible loss of health entailing immediate clinical management of the patient's condition to prevent these outcomes. There is therefore no time for either the informed consent process or the informed refusal process.

Medical ethics: The disciplined study of the morality of physicians, patients, innovation and research, organizational culture, and healthcare policy and advocacy with the aim of improving medical morality, drawing on such disciplines as medicine, philosophy, theology, law, religion, and social sciences.

Medically reasonable alternative: A form of clinical management that in deliberative clinical judgment is both technically feasible and supported in beneficence-based clinical judgment.

Minimal risk: As defined in federal regulations of human subjects research: "*Minimal risk* means that the probability and magnitude of harm or discomfort anticipated in the research are not greater in and of themselves than those ordinarily encountered in daily life or during the performance of routine physical or psychological examinations or tests."

Minimized risk: The mortality and morbidity to human subjects of research is reduced to the minimum necessary to conduct a clinical innovation and research.

Monopoly power: The power of sellers with a dominant position in a market.

Monopsony power: The power of buyers with a dominant position in a market.

Moral philosophy: Ethical reasoning using secular ethical concepts that are either discovered in the quest for certainty or invented in the quest for reliability.

Moral risk: The unwelcome probability of having to confront a morally challenging or unwelcome decision, e.g., about selective feticide to reduce the risks of a multifetal pregnancy.

Moral science: The application of the scientific method to discover moral truths. David Hume (1711–1776) used moral science to discover the principle of sympathy, an innate process that inclines us to enter into the experience of others and be motivated to help them when they are in distress, pain, or suffering.

Moral status: An entity is such that others have an ethical obligation to protect and promote its interests. Moral status can originate in properties of an entity that it possesses independently of all other entities and that create the ethical obligation to protect and promote its interests. This is known as independent moral status. Moral status can also originate in a social role created by human beings, especially to protect human beings vulnerable to the power of others over them. This is known as dependent moral status because it depends on the creation and maintenance of social roles.

Moral theology: Ethical reasoning based on sources of moral authority in a specific faith community, including sacred texts and their history of interpretation and authoritative figures such as imams, priests, and rabbis, as well as tradition.

Morality: Actual beliefs of an individual or an identifiable group about behavior and character that is morally impermissible, morally permissible, morally obligatory, and morally ideal.

Morally ideal: Always striving for the goal of a perfect outcome even while knowing that one may fall short. It is morally impermissible not to attempt incremental progress toward the goal of a perfect outcome.

Morally impermissible: A form of character, behavior, organizational culture, or public policy that should not occur.

Morally obligatory: A form of character, behavior, organizational culture, or public policy that should occur.

Morally permissible: A form of character, behavior, organizational culture, or public policy that may occur in circumstances in which there are multiple forms of character, behavior, organizational culture, or public policy supported by ethical reasoning.

Glossary of Key Concepts

N

Nondirective counseling: Offering medically reasonable alternatives but making no recommendations among them. Nondirective counseling is ethically justified when there are two or more forms of medically reasonable clinical management of the patient's condition or diagnosis and in deliberative clinical judgment none is clinically superior. This is the precise meaning of shared decision making. Nondirective counseling should guide the obstetrician-gynecologist's role in decision making with a pregnant patient about the disposition of her pregnancy.

Noninvasive fetal analysis: Fetal analysis of results of methods that do not penetrate the maternal abdomen, uterus, or amniotic cavity. Even though the skin and vein are penetrated, a maternal blood draw is characterized as noninvasive because it poses no risk of clinical harm to the fetus.

Normative ethics: The use of ethical reasoning, e.g., in professional ethics in obstetrics and gynecology. Normative ethics asks what professional ethics in obstetrics and gynecology ought to be.

O

Obligation: Behavior that should occur, either always (an absolute obligation) or with justified limits (a prima facie obligation).

Opportunity cost: A clinical circumstance in which the use of a limited resource, e.g., a critical care bed, blocks access to that resource by other patients. The concept of an opportunity cost is not the same as the financial costs of a patient's care; it is about resource use and its effects on other patients, not about financial cost.

Organizational culture: The expressed mission statement and values of an organization, what it values and disvalues, what it rewards and discourages, what it tolerates and does not tolerate, and, especially, what it tolerates that should not be tolerated.

P

Pain: The report in the central nervous system of tissue damage (some add threat of tissue damage) accompanied by awareness.

Patient: A living human being who is presented to a physician or other healthcare professional and there exist forms of clinical management that are reliably predicted to result in net clinical benefit for that human being.

Patients' rights: The negative and positive rights of patients in the clinical setting, usually originating in the ethical principle of respect for autonomy in professional ethics in medicine and therefore in professional ethics in obstetrics and gynecology.

Pediatric assent: The assent process with pediatric patients.

Perinatal Innovation Review Committee: A committee charged by departments of obstetrics and gynecology and of pediatrics with prospective review and oversight of maternal–fetal innovation.

Physiologic futility: 97%–100% failure rate to achieve the physiologic goal of a clinical intervention.

Postmodern organizational culture: An organizational culture in which the connection between organizational rhetoric and reality, as well as the response of leaders to criticism, becomes incoherent and unpredictable in its variation.

Power: The ability to form one's will and then put it into effect, directly oneself or through others.

Pregnant patient: A living adolescent or adult human woman who is pregnant becomes a pregnant patient when she is presented to an obstetrician (or other healthcare professional) and there exist forms of clinical management that are reliably predicted to result in net clinical benefit for her and for the fetal patient, when the fetus is a patient.

Presumption of decision-making capacity in adult patients: All patients who have attained the age of becoming a legal adult (18 in the United States) or adolescents who have had "the disabilities of minority" removed by a court are presumed in health law and professional ethics in obstetrics and gynecology to have the intellectual and affective capacity to participate in decision making about the clinical management of their condition and about participation in clinical innovation and research.

Preventive ethics: The use of the informed consent process to anticipate and prevent ethical conflict between the female or pregnant patient and her obstetrician-gynecologist.

Prima facie ethical obligation: An ethical obligation that permits exceptions; it should be fulfilled unless ethical reasoning shows that there is an overriding ethical obligation.

Prima facie ethical obligation of confidentiality: Ethical obligation that permits exceptions when they are ethically justified exceptions. The burden of proof is on establishing an exception. Unauthorized access to information by the patient is sometimes ethically permissible.

Prima facie ethical principle: An ethical principle that allows for exceptions to the ethical obligations that it creates when in ethical reasoning there is an overriding ethical principle.

Privacy: A zone of decision making (alone or with others) and behavior into which others, especially the state, should not intrude without ethical justification, e.g., to protect others from serious, far-reaching, and irreversible harm.

Procedural justice: An approach to justice that focuses on a fair process for deciding on the allocation of limited resources.

Profession of medicine as a public trust: The phrase "public trust" was used by Thomas Percival (1740–1804) as an antidote to the idea and reality, in his day, of medicine as a guild that protects group interests in social and political power. The concept of a public trust means that medicine is a profession that serves patients and society and that physicians hold the current fund of knowledge and clinical skills in trust for future physicians, their patients, and society.

Glossary of Key Concepts

Professional autonomy: The independence of physicians from state power, based on the commitment to the ethical concept of medicine as a profession.

Professional community standard: In the informed consent process the obstetrician-gynecologist should disclose to the patient clinical information that any experienced and qualified obstetrician-gynecologist would provide.

Professional ethics in gynecology: The disciplined study of the morality of physicians and female patients in clinical practice, innovation and research, organizational culture, and health policy and advocacy, based on the ethical concept of medicine as a profession.

Professional ethics in medicine: The disciplined study of the implications of the ethical concept of medicine as a profession for improving the morality of physicians and patients in clinical practice, organizational culture, innovation and research, and health policy and advocacy with the aim of improving them, based on the ethical concept of medicine as a profession.

Professional ethics in obstetrics: The disciplined study of the morality of physicians and pregnant and fetal patients in clinical practice, innovation and research, organizational culture, and health policy and advocacy, based on the ethical concept of medicine as a profession and the ethical concepts of the pregnant, fetal, and neonatal patients.

Professional ethics in obstetrics and gynecology: The disciplined study of the morality of physicians and female, pregnant, and fetal patients in clinical practice, innovation and research, organizational culture, and health policy and advocacy, based on the ethical concept of medicine as a profession and the ethical concepts of the pregnant, fetal, and neonatal patients.

Professional ethics in pediatrics: The discipline study of the morality of physicians and pediatric patients in clinical practice, innovation and research, organizational culture, and health policy and advocacy, based on the ethical concept of medicine as a profession, the best interests of the child standard, pediatric assent, and parental permission.

Professional ethics in perinatal medicine: The disciplined study of the morality of physicians in caring for pregnant, fetal, and neonatal patients in clinical practice, innovation and research, organizational culture, and health policy and advocacy, based on the ethical concept of medicine as a profession, the ethical concept of the fetus as a patient from professional ethics in obstetrics, and the best interests of the child standard from professional ethics in pediatrics.

Professional virtue of compassion: The habit of recognizing when one's patient experiences pain, distress, or suffering or is at risk for doing so and acting to prevent and effectively manage pain, distress, or suffering,

Professional virtue of humility: The habit of recognizing the limits of one's ethical judgments and working persistently to improve them.

Professional virtue of integrity: The habit of living by and not compromising the intellectual and moral commitment to the ethical concept of medicine as a profession.

Professional virtue of self-effacement: The habit of identifying and then minimizing the influences on one's clinical judgment and clinical management of features of the patient that are irrelevant in clinical judgment and put clinical judgment at preventable risk of bias.

Professional virtue of self-sacrifice: The habit of taking reasonable risks of harm to one's legitimate self-interest in patient care, research, and advocacy.

Public trust: Based on the professional medical ethics of Thomas Percival (1740–1804), the ethical concept that the fund of knowledge and clinical skills of medicine, and their improvement, are held by physicians in trust for current patients and for future obstetrician-gynecologists and their patients.

Q

Quality of life: Engaging in valued life tasks and deriving satisfaction from doing so. Which life tasks should be valued and how much satisfaction is worth pursuing and having is a function of each individual's autonomy, based on her values and beliefs.

Quality-of-life futility: Critical care intervention will be physiologically effective, prevent imminent demise, and preserve at least interactive capacity but the patient considers the resulting quality of life unacceptable from the patient's – and *only* from the patient's – perspective.

Quest for certainty: Aims for certainty of ethical judgment deriving from foundations that are beyond doubt.

Quest for reliability: Aims for ethical judgments that are reliable, in the sense that we can act on them with confidence that we have good reasons, which always remain open to revision and improvement.

R

Reasonable person standard: In the informed consent process the obstetrician-gynecologist should provide clinical information to the patient that any patient in her clinical circumstances needs to know. As a general rule, if clinical information should be regarded by the obstetrician-gynecologist as clinically significant, it should be provided to the patient.

Research: A clinical experiment with a group of patients, who become research subjects, to create generalizable knowledge.

Respectful persuasion: In response to a patient's refusal of offered or recommended clinical management, the obstetrician-gynecologist should elicit what is important to the patient and support the patient to make a decision based on her expressed beliefs and values.

Resuscitation as a trial of intervention: The initiation of resuscitation with the short-term goal of preventing imminent death by restoring spontaneous circulation.

Right: An ethically justified claim to be treated by others in a specified way. A negative right is a claim against interference in one's decision making and behavior by others. A positive right is a claim against others to their time, energy, and resources to advance one's own interests. A right can be claimed without exceptions, known as an absolute right. A limited right can be claimed, known as a prima facie right.

Right to privacy: An ethically justified negative right against interference with decision making (alone or with others) and behavior by others, especially the state.

Right to reproductive privacy: An ethically justified negative right against interference with decision making (alone or with the patient's obstetrician-gynecologist) and behavior about reproduction by others, especially the state.

S

Safety: Reduction of risk of morbidity and mortality to a minimum by reduction of uncontrolled variation in the processes of patient care when doing so improves outcomes.

Secular ethical reasoning: Ethical reasoning that makes no reference to deity, transcendent reality, sacred texts, or religious tradition for their authority. Nor is secular ethical reasoning necessarily hostile to religion and faith communities, such as secular reasoning in professional ethics in medicine, obstetrics and gynecology, and pediatrics. By contrast, some forms of secular reasoning in bioethics are hostile to religion and faith communities.

Severe fetal anomaly: There is a certain or near certain diagnosis of an anomaly that is reliably expected either to result in death, even with aggressive obstetric and neonatal intervention, or short-term survival with severe and irreversible deficit of cognitive developmental capacity

Shared decision making: Synonymous with nondirective counseling or offering medically reasonable alternatives but making no recommendations among them. Nondirective counseling is ethically justified when there are two or more forms of medically reasonable clinical management of the patient's condition or diagnosis and in deliberative clinical judgment none is clinically superior. In such clinical circumstances the patient's values and beliefs justifiably become the controlling consideration in evaluating which medically reasonable alternative is superior. Shared decision making should guide the obstetrician-gynecologist's role in decision making with a pregnant patient about the disposition of her pregnancy. Shared decision making is not a universal model for decision making with and by patients.

Simple consent: The patient has agreed to clinical management that has been offered or recommended.

Specification: The process of transforming abstract ethical concepts, such as ethical principles and virtues, into practical, clinically applicable guides to ethical judgment and behavior based on it.

Speculation: Made-up beliefs that do not pass muster as plausible hypotheses.

Substantive justice: An approach to justice that focuses on who gets what, or the fair outcomes of allocation of limited resources.

Substituted judgment standard of *surrogate decision making*: The surrogate decision maker should make a decision for the patient that is reliably based on the patient's values and beliefs. This is an autonomy-based standard.

Suffering: The experience of one's aims and intentions for current or future well-being becoming blocked or impeded to some degree.

Surrogate decision making: Decision making by the legally designated individual for a patient who has lost decision-making capacity and for whom assisted consent and assent cannot be employed. Surrogate decision making is guided, in priority order, by the substituted judgment standard and the best interests standard.

T

Tarasoff v. Regents of the University of California: A 1976 decision of the Supreme Court of the state of California that created a legal duty to warn third parties endangered by a patient: "the protective privilege ends where the public peril begins." This duty to warn is sometimes called the "Tarasoff rule." Some states by statute have rejected the Tarasoff rule.

Termination of pregnancy: The use of medication or surgery to end gestation, independently of gestational age. Before viability, fetal demise, feticide, and induced abortion are forms of termination of pregnancy. After viability, fetal demise, feticide, induced vaginal delivery, spontaneous vaginal delivery, and cesarean delivery are forms of termination of pregnancy. "Induced abortion" is not a synonym for "termination of pregnancy."

Therapeutic misconception: Originally introduced to mean the risk that patients who are clinical research subjects would assume that all aspects of the study are chosen based on clinical judgment and thus fail to appreciate that some aspects, e.g., stepped-up dosage during the course of a Phase I trial or randomization in a Phase III trial, are chosen solely for research purposes. Its meaning has been expanded to include conflation of standard clinical management with investigational clinical intervention.

Trial of intervention: The initiation of clinical management with the short-term goal of preventing imminent death and the long-term goal of survival with at least some interactive capacity.

U

Unacceptable opportunity cost: A clinical circumstance in which the use of limited clinical resources for a patient is reliably predicted not to clinically benefit the patient from that use and in which this use blocks access to those limited clinical resources by a patient reliably predicted to benefit from the use of those resources. This concept is independent of the financial costs of using the limited resource.

Undue influence: The use of intense psychological pressure or withholding information about medically reasonable alternatives to reduce the autonomy of the patient to elect the option preferred by the physician.

Utilitarian justice: A consequentialist theory of justice that calls for the maximization of valued consequences. Utilitarian justice in a healthcare organization endorses policies and practices that advance the organization's mission.

V

Virtues: Traits of character or habits of character that are judged to be worth cultivating because they reliably guide ethical judgment and behavior based on it.

Vitalism: The view that medicine is committed to the preservation of human life without qualification.

Voluntary: A decision-making process and behavior based on it that is free from internal or external controlling influences.

W

Wonderland organizational culture: An organizational culture in which organizational rhetoric becomes self-deceptive when used by leaders, who expect subordinates to embrace self-deception.

Index

AAN. *See* American Academy of Neurology
abandonment, of incurable patients, 179–180
abortion, 124. *See also* induced abortion
absolute ethical obligation, 36–37. *See also* ethical obligation
absolute ethical obligation of confidentiality, 71–72
absolute ethical principle, 9
access
  to clinical management of fertility, 113
  to termination of pregnancy services, 130
accountability
  Gregory's and Percival's call for, 101–102
  milestones in, 104
  organizational culture of, 102
  prevention of drift from, 101–103
  preventive ethics response to reduced, 103–105
Accreditation Council for Graduate Medical Education (ACGME)
  accreditation process of, 105
  professionalism as core competency of, 101
achondroplasia, 125–126
ACOG. *See* American College of Obstetricians and Gynecologists
advance directive. *See* directive, advance
advocacy
  healthcare justice and, 216–217
  for healthcare resources for women and children, 217–221, 222–223
  New York Declaration of International Academy of Perinatal Medicine on, 217, 222–223
  in pregnancy prevention, 113–114
  social, 221–222
Adzick, N. Scott, 33
age bias, 218–219, 223
alobar holoprosencephaly, 151–152
AMA. *See* American Medical Association

American Academy of Neurology (AAN), 157
American Academy of Pediatrics, 60
American College of Human Genetics, 75–76
American College of Obstetricians and Gynecologists (ACOG)
  on conflicts of interest, 83
  Consensus Statement on periviable birth from, 142–143
  on counseling women about intimate partner violence, 222
  embryo transfer guidelines of, 119
  failed critique of ethical concept of fetus as a patient adopted by, 40–41
  fetal analysis information provided by, 137
  on free fetal DNA analysis, 138
  pregnancy prevention methods identified by, 109
  on romantic and sexual relationships with patients, 88
American College of Occupational and Environment Medicine, 74
American Medical Association (AMA) Code of Medical Ethics, 101
  confidentiality limits identified by, 71–72
American Psychiatric Association, 88
American Society for Reproductive Medicine (ASRM), 119
Americans with Disabilities Act, 74
anatomic futility, 182
anesthesia
  disclosure to family members during and after, 73
  fetal, 34
animal models, in maternal–fetal intervention, 203
Annas, George, 39, 153
antepartum refusal, of cesarean delivery, 153
appreciation, in decision-making process, 48–49
argument-based ethical reasoning, 6
  critical appraisal of, 6, 95
  teaching of, 95–96

Aristotle
  on ethical principle of justice, 10–11, 216
  Nicomachean Ethics by, 7
  quest for reliability originating in moral philosophy of, 7
The Art (Hippocrates), 169–170
ASRM. *See* American Society for Reproductive Medicine
assent
  geriatric, 59–61, 63
  meaning of, 50
  mental disorders and, 157
  pediatric, 59–61, 112
assisted decision making
  assessment of decision-making capacity for, 58
  in fertility management, 111–112
  for impairment of decision-making capacity, 59
  in induced abortion and feticide, 128–129
  major mental disorders and, 111–112, 155
  meaning of, 50
  task-specific decision-making capacity in, 58–59
  time-specific decision-making capacity in, 59
  Ulysses contract in, 59
assisted reproduction
  ethical concept of moral status in, 117–120
  in vitro, 117–120
  moral risk anticipation in, 121
  obstetrician-gynecologist role in, 116
  self-regulation role in, 118–119
attending supervision, drift from professionalism with, 103
attention, in decision-making process, 48–49
Audi, Robert, 20
authorization, in decision-making process, 48–49
autonomy, 8. *See also* respect for autonomy
  of female patients, 26–27
  impairments of, 62–64

235

Index

autonomy (cont.)
　in informed consent process, 52, 53, 55
　negative, 39
　of pregnant patients, 36, 39
　professional, 113–114
　recommendations role in supporting, 160
autonomy-based clinical judgment, 109
autonomy-based ethical obligation
　indirect referral, 91
　for induced abortion or feticide before viability, 126–127
　in informed consent process, 52
　to pregnant patient, 36–37
　in surrogate decision making about pregnancy prevention, 64–65

baby pictures, perfect baby concept promoted by, 165
Bacon, Francis, 13, 14
Beauchamp, Tom L.
　on common morality, 19
　on ethical principle of beneficence, 9–10
　on ethical principle of respect for autonomy, 10
　on specification of ethical principles, 11
beneficence
　in fertility decision making, 109, 110–111
　history of, 10
　limits on life-sustaining treatment based on, 178–179
　in medical ethics and bioethics, 9–10
　in professional ethics in gynecology, 29
　in professional ethics in medicine, 17–18
　in professional ethics in obstetrics, 32, 90
beneficence-based clinical judgment, 109, 110–111
beneficence-based ethical obligation. *See also* ethical obligation
　direct referral, 90
　enforcement of, 37–38
　to fetal patient, 36–38
　for induced abortion or feticide before viability, 126
　in informed consent process, 51–52
　to patients with mental disorders, 157
　to pregnant patient, 36–37
　in surrogate decision making about pregnancy prevention, 64–65

beneficence-based ethical obligations, in cancer and pregnancy, 172–173, 174–176
best interests of the child standard, 41–42
　in periviable birth management, 141, 142
best interests standard of surrogate decision making, 62, 129
bias
　age, 218–219, 223
　economic, 219–220, 222–223
　in favor of persons, 220–221, 223
　against medically indigent, 219
　against patients who cannot speak for themselves, 221, 223
　political, 222–223
bioethics
　ethical principles in, 9–11
　field of, 8–9
　independent moral status dominance in, 34–35
　limitations of, 9
　professional ethics in medicine compared with, 8–9
　virtues in, 9
biological sex, 108
biopsychosocial concept of health and disease, 51
　fertility, 108–109
Birkenhead, HMS, 217
birth, 140. *See also* periviable birth
birth control pills, 89–90
birth defects
　fetal diagnosis of, 168–169
　obstetrician knowledge of, 167, 169
　patient knowledge of, 167–168, 169
"The Birthmark" (Hawthorne), 164–165, 169–170
Blackhall, Leslie, 180–181
Boerhaave, Herman, 13, 14
Brody, Baruch A., 205
Buchan, William, *Domestic Medicine* by, 13

cadaver, continuing pregnancy in, 157–158
cancer
　advance directives in, 176
　congruent beneficence-based ethical obligations to pregnant and fetal patient in, 172, 173, 174
　ethical challenges of pregnancy and, 172
　informed consent process in, 173–176
　noncongruent beneficence-based ethical obligations to pregnant and fetal patient in, 172–173, 174–176
candor, 16, 27, 30

capacity. *See* decision-making capacity
Cape Frontier War, 217
Cardozo, Benjamin, 50, 51
case-based teaching, 98–99
cephalocentesis, 151
　for hydrocephalus with associated anomalies, 152
　for hydrocephalus with severe associated abnormalities, 151–152
　for isolated fetal hydrocephalus, 151
certainty, quest for, 7
cesarean delivery, 142
　Consensus Statement from American College of Obstetricians and Gynecologists and Society for Maternal–Fetal Medicine on, 142–143
　court orders for forced, 154
　ethical principle of non-maleficence applied to, 32
　for fetal hydrocephalus, 151
　informed consent for, 149–151
　NICHD calculator for clinical judgments about, 143
　preventive ethics for, 149–151
　recommendations for, 150
　refusal of, 152–154
　requests for, 158
　vaginal delivery continuum with, 149, 150–151, 152
Childress, James F.
　on common morality, 19
　on ethical principle of beneficence, 9–10
　on ethical principle of respect for autonomy, 10
　on specification of ethical principles, 11
chorion villus sampling, 135, 166, 168–169
chronically and variably impaired autonomy, 62–63
CIOMS. *See* Council for International Organizations of Medical Societies
climate change, 222
clinical gaze, 165
clinical judgment
　attitudes distorting, 56–57
　fertility management using, 109, 110–111, 113–114
　limits of obstetric, 143
　meaning of, 4
　in periviable birth management, 140–141, 142–143, 144
clinical practice
　conflict of interest created by payment for, 83–84
　research transition into, 205, 206, 207

Index

retirement from, 82–83
clinical rounds, teaching ethics on, 99
Code of Medical Ethics. *See* American Medical Association
coercion
  involuntary requests due to, 158
  in pregnancy prevention, 112
cognitive understanding, in decision-making process, 48–49
colleagues, professional treatment of, 192–193
common law, on American life-sustaining treatment, 180
common morality, 19
Common Rule, 204
compassion
  in leadership, 192
  in professional ethics in gynecology, 27–28
  in professional ethics in medicine, 16
  in professional ethics in obstetrics, 30–31
competence, capacity compared with, 48
compliance demands, 196
confidentiality
  absolute ethical obligation of, 71–72
  disclosure to family during and after sedation or anesthesia as ethical challenge to, 73
  electronic communication as ethical challenge to, 77
  electronic medical records as ethical challenge to, 75
  employer inquiries as ethical challenge to, 74
  ethically justified limits on, 72–73
  genetic and genomic information as ethical challenge to, 75–76
  Gregory on, 70–71
  HIPAA as ethical challenge to, 76
  Hippocratic Oath treatment of, 69
  history of obligation of, 69–72
  Hoffmann's taciturn politic physician in history of, 69–70
  of induced abortion or feticide, 131
  insurance claims as ethical challenge to, 74
  medical emergencies as ethical challenge to, 73
  Percival on, 71
  as *prima facie* ethical obligation, 69, 71–72
  in professional ethics in obstetrics and gynecology, 69–72
  sexually transmitted disease as ethical challenge to, 76
  social media as ethical challenge to, 77
  teaching about, 94–95

conflict of commitment
  conflation of conflicts of interest with, 86
  conscientious objection as, 31, 89–92
  definition of, 85
  historical perspective on, 80
  management of, 85–86
  Percival on, 80, 85
  professional virtue of self-sacrifice in, 17, 28, 31
  teaching about, 95
conflict of interest
  conceptual confusion about, 83
  conflation of conflicts of commitment with, 86
  conscientious objection and, 31
  in cosmetic procedures, 84
  definition of, 81
  in entrepreneurial and professional relationships, 80–81
  Gregory on, 80, 81–82
  historical perspective on, 80
  in imaging use, 83
  management of, 83–85
  in payment for clinical practice, 83–84
  Percival on, 80, 82–83
  professional virtue of self-sacrifice in, 17, 28, 31
  in research, 84–85
  in romantic and sexual relationships with patients, 88–89
  teaching about, 95
Confucius, 7, 39
congenital malformations
  fetal diagnosis of, 168–169
  obstetrician knowledge of, 167, 169
  patient knowledge of, 167–168, 169
conscientious objection
  burden of proof in, 90
  as conflict of commitment, 31, 89–92
  to contraception, 89–90
  definition of, 89
  historical analogy of, 89
  to offers or recommendations of induced abortion or feticide, 129
  to performance of induced abortion or feticide, 130
  to referral for induced abortion and feticide, 90–92, 131
  in residency training, 89
consent. *See* informed consent; simple consent
consequentialism, 9–10
consumer rights movement, perfect baby concept promoted by, 166
contraception, conscientious objection to, 89–90
coping with loss, 145

cosmetic medicine, conflict of interest in, 84
Coulehan, Jack, 27
Council for International Organizations of Medical Societies (CIOMS), guidance for research involving pregnant women, 208
court orders, for forced cesarean delivery, 154
court-ordered clinical management, of fertility, 113–114
critical appraisal
  of argument-based ethical reasoning, 6, 95
  of ethical concept of fetus as a patient, 40–41
  formal assessment tool for, 96–98
  of organizational culture, 104
critical care. *See also* life-sustaining treatment
  of neonatal patient, 143
cynical organizational culture, 194

Darwin, Charles, 20
death
  in complete placenta previa or severe placental abruption, 153
  prevention of imminent, 178–179, 181
decision making. *See also* end-of-life decision making; informed consent
  advance directives in, 57–58
  assent, 50, 59–61, 155
  assisted, 50, 58–59, 111–112, 128–129
  by, with, and for patient, 47, 128–129, 154–157
  clinical ethical topics in, 62–64
  deliberative clinical judgment in, 4
  ethical principle of respect for autonomy in, 18, 29, 32
  about fertility management, 109–111
  fetal analysis in, 134
  impaired autonomy in, 62–64
  informed refusal, 55–56
  on limits of life-sustaining treatment, 181–184
  in medical emergencies, 66
  patient as ultimate decision maker in, 55
  preventive ethics in, 149
  shared, 53–54, 110, 127, 136
  simple consent, 49–51, 57
  surrogate, 50, 61–62, 64–66, 73, 112–113, 128–129, 155, 185–186
  teaching about, 94
  voluntary, 18, 29, 32, 53

237

Index

decision-making capacity, 47
  in adult patients, 47
  assessment of, 58, 155
  competence compared with, 48
  components of, 48–49
  impairment of, 59
  in minors with legal authority over themselves, 47–48
  of pregnant patients with mental illnesses and disorders, 211–212
  risk-adjusted assessment of, 58
  task-specific, 58–59
  time-specific, 59
deliberative clinical judgment, 4
  fertility management using, 109, 110–111, 113–114
  limits of obstetric, 143
  in periviable birth management, 140–141, 142–143, 144
delivery. *See also* intrapartum management
  multidisciplinary team approach to counseling before, 143–144
dependent moral status, 34, 38–39
  of embryo, 118
depression, decision making with, by, and for patients with, 128–129
descriptive ethics, 95–96
diagnosis, meaning of, 134–135
direct referral, 90, 91–92, 131. *See also* indirect referral
directive, advance
  in cancer and pregnancy, 176
  decision making using, 57–58
  limits of life-sustaining treatment set by, 182
  in medical emergencies, 66
directive counseling
  in fertility management, 109–110
  in induced abortion or feticide, 127
  in informed consent process, 53
Directive to Physicians, 57–58
discipline of ethical reasoning, 6
  precision of thought and speech in, 95
  teaching of, 95–96
disclosure, 52
  to family members during and after sedation or anesthesia, 73
  of genetic or genomic information, 74
  of sexually transmitted disease, 76
distress, 16, 27–28, 30–31
Domestic Medicine (Buchan), 13
double effect, 175
Down syndrome, 125–126
Drucker, Peter, 191
Durable Power of Attorney for Health Care, 57–58

dying patients. *See also* end-of-life decision making
  abandonment of, 179–180
Dylan, Bob, 220

economic bias, 219–220, 222–223
economic values, trumping power of, 220
effectiveness, of clinical management, 35
electronic communication, confidentiality challenges created by, 77
electronic medical records, confidentiality challenges created by, 75
emancipated minor, 47–48
embryo
  in vitro, 117–118, 119–120
  in vivo, 117
  manipulation of, 120
  moral status of, 116, 117–118
  pre-implantation analysis of, 119–120
embryo transfer
  number of, 118–119
  requests for high numbers of, 120
emergency medical care. *See* medical emergency
employer inquiries, confidentiality challenges created by, 74
encephalocele, 151, 152
end-of-life decision making
  advance directive law in, 182
  anatomic futility in, 182
  historical perspective on, 179–181
  imminent-demise futility in, 182
  inappropriate requests for treatment in, 185–186
  interactive-capacity futility in, 182–183
  obstetrician-gynecologist role in, 181–184
  physiologic futility in, 182
  preventive ethics in, 184–185
  quality-of-life futility in, 183
  unacceptable opportunity costs in, 183–184
Engel, George, 51, 108
enlightened self-interest, 12, 69–70, 87
enthusiasm
  in American life-sustaining treatment, 180
  ethical judgments avoiding, 4
entrepreneurial relationships, conflict of interest in, 80–81
Epidemics (Hippocrates), 10
equality, healthcare justice obtained through, 18–19

equipoise, evidence-based, 53–54, 150, 206
ESHRE. *See* European Society of Human Reproduction and Embryology
ethical analysis, 4–5
ethical argument
  meaning of, 4–5
  teaching of, 95–96
  validity of, 6
ethical concept of medicine as a profession
  commitments of, 14–15, 101–102
  conflicts of interest affecting, 80, 81–82, 83, 88
  conscientious objection and, 90
  invention of, 14–15, 101–102, 195–196
  in professional ethics in medicine, 11, 14–15, 19–21
  in professional ethics in obstetrics and gynecology, 26
  in professional ethics in perinatal medicine, 26
  reasons for physician commitment to, 19–21
  teaching of, 94
ethical concept of moral status. *See* moral status
ethical concept of the fetus as a patient. *See* fetus as a patient, ethical concept of
ethical ideal, 113
ethical judgment
  discipline of ethical reasoning achieved through, 6
  meaning of, 4
ethical obligation
  in cancer and pregnancy, 172–173, 174–176
  enforcement of, 37–38
  ethical principle of beneficence creating, 17–18, 29, 32, 90
  ethical principle of healthcare justice creating, 18–19, 29, 32–33, 216
  ethical principle of non-maleficence creating, 18, 29, 32
  ethical principle of respect for autonomy creating, 18, 29, 32, 90
  to female patient, 27
  to fetal patient, 33, 34, 35–38
  in informed consent process, 51–52
  to patients with mental disorders, 157
  to pregnant patient, 33, 34, 35–37
  professional virtue of compassion creating, 16, 27–28, 30–31
  professional virtue of integrity creating, 16, 27, 30

professional virtue of
    self-effacement creating, 16–17,
    28
professional virtue of self-sacrifice
    creating, 17, 28, 31
in surrogate decision making about
    pregnancy prevention, 64–65
ethical principle of beneficence
  in fertility decision making, 109,
    110–111
  history of, 10
  limits on life-sustaining treatment
    based on, 178–179
  in medical ethics and bioethics,
    9–10
  in professional ethics in gynecology,
    29
  in professional ethics in medicine,
    17–18
  in professional ethics in obstetrics,
    32, 90
ethical principle of healthcare justice
  advocacy for women and children
    based on, 217–221, 222–223
  antidote to cynicism about, 221–222
  in fertility management, 113–114
  health policy and advocacy and,
    216–217
  in professional ethics in gynecology,
    29
  in professional ethics in medicine,
    17, 18–19
  in professional ethics in obstetrics,
    32–33
ethical principle of justice
  healthcare justice as specification of,
    216–217
  in medical ethics and bioethics,
    10–11
  in professional ethics in gynecology,
    29
  in professional ethics in medicine,
    17, 18–19
  in professional ethics in obstetrics,
    32–33
ethical principle of non-maleficence
  distinct from non-malfeasance, 9–10
  history of, 10
  in medical ethics and bioethics,
    10
  in professional ethics in gynecology,
    29
  in professional ethics in medicine,
    17, 18
  in professional ethics in obstetrics,
    32
ethical principle of respect for
    autonomy
  in advance directives, 176
  in fertility decision making, 109

in informed consent process, 52, 53,
    54, 55
  limits on life-sustaining treatment
    based on, 178–179
  in medical ethics and bioethics, 10
  in professional ethics in gynecology,
    29
  in professional ethics in medicine,
    17, 18
  in professional ethics in obstetrics,
    32, 90
  recommendations role in
    supporting, 160
ethical principles
  absolute, 9
  in medical ethics and bioethics,
    9–11
  practice of, 11
  prima facie, 9
  in professional ethics in gynecology,
    29
  in professional ethics in medicine,
    15, 17–19
  in professional ethics in obstetrics,
    32–33
  teaching of, 94
ethical reasoning
  argument-based, 6, 95–96
  clinical judgment in, 4
  components of, 4–5
  creative literature in, 164–165
  critical appraisal of, 6, 95
  discipline of, 6, 95–96
  errors in, 5–6
  ethical judgment in, 4, 6
  of Gregory and Percival, 21
  principled, 21
  quest for certainty approach to, 7
  quest for reliability approach, 7
ethically ideal, 5
ethically impermissible, 5
ethically obligatory, 5
ethically permissible, 5
ethics, meaning of, 3–4
ethics work-up, case-based teaching
    using, 98–99
Eunice Kennedy Shriver National
    Institute of Child Health and
    Human Development, 140
European Society of Human
    Reproduction and Embryology
    (ESHRE), 119
euthanasia, in newborns, 184
evaluative understanding, in decision-
    making process, 48–49
evidence-based equipoise, 53–54, 150,
    206
evidence-based medicine, 13, 14
evolution, 20
experiment, 202

pregnancy in cadavers or patients in
    permanent vegetative state as,
    157–158
experimental maternal–fetal
    intervention, 169
explicit authorization, in decision-
    making process, 48–49
exploitation, 142

false hope, 145
family
  confidentiality challenges involving,
    73
  refusal of legally designated
    surrogate by, 65–66
fee-for-service, conflict of interest
    created by, 83–84
female patient
  advocacy for, 217–221, 222–223
  autonomy of, 26–27
  climate change effects on, 222
  as decision maker in gynecology and
    obstetrics clinical practice, 55
  decision making by, with, and for, 47
  decision-making capacity of adult,
    47
  decision-making capacity of minor,
    47–48
  Gregory on ethical obligations to,
    27
  presentation of, 26–27
fertility
  access to clinical management of,
    113
  assisted decision making in
    management of, 111–112
  autonomy-based clinical judgment
    in management of, 109
  beneficence-based deliberative
    clinical judgment in management
    of, 109, 110–111
  biologic concept of, 108
  biopsychosocial concept of, 108–109
  court-ordered clinical management
    of, 113–114
  decision making about management
    of, 109–111
  directive counseling in management
    of, 109–110
  healthcare-justice-based clinical
    judgment in management of,
    113–114
  organizational policy guiding
    management of, 113
  pediatric assent in management of,
    112
  preconception counseling in clinical
    management of, 116, 120–121
  shared decision making in
    management of, 110

239

Index

fertility (cont.)
  surrogate decision making in management of, 64–65, 112–113
fetal analysis
  communication among obstetricians about, 135
  communication with patients about, 135–136
  in decision making about obstetric management, 134
  election of invasive, 137
  election of noninvasive, 137–138
  informed consent for, 135–136
  nomenclature use in, 134–136
  nondirective counseling or shared decision making in, 136
  patient responses to, 136–138
  provision of clinical information about, 134–136
  refusal of, 137
  uncertainty about, 138
  use of results from, 138
fetal anesthesia, 34
Fetal Center, 202
fetal diagnosis, limits of, 168–169
fetal distress, refusal of cesarean delivery for, 154
fetal hydrocephalus, 151–152
fetal imaging
  discourse of fetal patient in, 34
  perfect baby concept promoted by, 165
fetal lung maturity, cancer treatment delay until, 175–176
fetal surgery, 203. *See also* maternal–fetal intervention
  discourse of fetal patient and, 34
feticide
  after-viability offers of, 125–126
  autonomy-based justifications for before-viability offers of, 126–127
  beneficence-based justifications for before-viability offers of, 126
  confidentiality in, 131
  conscientious objection to offers or recommendations of, 129
  conscientious objection to performance of, 130
  conscientious objection to referral for, 90–92, 131
  conscientious objection to residency training in, 89
  counseling pregnant women about, 124
  in patients with depression and psychoses, 128–129
  performance of, 129–130
  recommendations of, 127–128
  referrals for, 131
  thought and speech precision in, 124–125
  before viability, 125
fetus as a patient, ethical concept of, 30
  advantages of, 38–41
  advocacy for healthcare resources and, 217–221, 222–223
  bias in favor of persons and, 220–221, 223
  in cancer and pregnancy, 172–176
  discourse of, 33–34
  ethical concept of moral status as preliminary to, 34–35
  ethical obligations and, 33, 34, 35–38
  explanation of, 35–36
  failed critique of, 40–41
  independent moral status reductionism avoided by, 38–39
  in maternal–fetal intervention, 206–207
  obstetrician's *prima facie* beneficence-based obligations to fetal patients, 36–38
  periviability and, 36
  pregnancy threatening health or life of, 126, 127, 128
  presentation of fetal patients, 35
  previability and, 36, 125
  research benefits and risks and, 208–209
  right to life discourse avoided by, 38
  rights-based absolutism avoided by, 39–40
  after viability, 125–126
  viability and, 36
FIGO. *See* International Federation of Gynecology and Obstetrics
filial piety, 8
Filly, Roy, 33
"First do no harm." *See* ethical principle of nonmaleficence
Fletcher, John, 33
focused ethics question, in normative ethics literature, 96
force, in pregnancy prevention, 112
Foucault, Michel, 165
foundationalism, 7
free fetal DNA analysis, 137–138
futility, 180, 181
  anatomic, 182
  evaluation of neonatal patient for, 143
  imminent-demise, 182
  interactive-capacity, 182–183
  physiologic, 182
  quality-of-life, 183

gender, 108
genetic information
  confidentiality challenges created by, 75–76
  disclosure of, 74
  from pre-implantation analysis, 117, 119–120
Genetic Information Nondiscrimination Act (GINA), 74
genome sequencing, 168–169
genomic information
  confidentiality challenges created by, 75–76
  disclosure of, 74
  from pre-implantation analysis, 117, 119–120
geriatric assent, 59–61, 63
GINA. *See* Genetic Information Nondiscrimination Act
Golbus, Michael, 33
Goldie, John, 100
graduate medical education
  critical appraisal of organizational culture of, 104
  drift from professionalism in, 101–103
  preventive ethics response to reduced accountability in, 103–105
grand rounds presentation, 99–100
Gregory, John
  on commitment to ethical concept of medicine as a profession, 19, 20–21
  on confidentiality of patient's secrets, 70–71
  on conflicts of commitment, 80
  on conflicts of interest, 80, 81–82
  ethical concept of medicine as a profession invention of, 14–15, 101–102, 195–196
  on ethical obligations to female patient, 27
  ethical reasoning of, 21
  on humility, 16, 27, 30
  on leadership, 191–192
  Lectures on the Duties and Qualifications of a Physician by, 10, 13, 15, 27
  on organizational culture, 191, 192
  on patient's rights, 10
  professional ethics in medicine invention by, 13–14, 21
  reversal of abandonment of incurable patients by, 179–180
  on sexual relationships with patients, 87–88
  on wealth of patients, 16–17, 28, 31
Griswold v. Connecticut, 118–119

Index

Groningen Protocol, 184
guild, 11
guild self-interest, 13, 15, 81–83,
  195–197, 216–217
gynecologic cancer. *See* cancer

harm principle, 10
  as ethical justification for disclosure
    of sexually transmitted disease, 76
Harrison, Michael, 33
Hawthorne, Nathaniel,
  "The Birthmark" by, 164–165,
    169–170
Health Insurance Portability and
  Accountability Act (HIPAA), 76
health policy
  ethically ideal expression of, 5
  healthcare justice and, 216–217
  implications for leaders in, 223
  New York Declaration of
    International Academy of
    Perinatal Medicine on, 217,
    222–223
  resource allocation for women and
    children in, 217–221, 222–223
healthcare justice
  advocacy for women and children
    based on, 217–221, 222–223
  antidote to cynicism about, 221–222
  health policy and advocacy and,
    216–217
  in professional ethics in gynecology,
    29
  in professional ethics in medicine,
    17, 18–19
  in professional ethics in obstetrics,
    32–33
  social conditions impeding, 221–222
healthcare-justice–based clinical
  judgment, in fertility
  management, 113–114
HIPAA. *See* Health Insurance
  Portability and Accountability
  Act
Hippocrates
  abandonment of incurable patients
    by, 179
  medical ethics of, 11–12
Hippocratic Oath, 11–12
  confidentiality in, 69
  as guild oath, 195
  sexual relationships with patients in,
    86–87
Hobbes, Thomas, 193
Hoffmann, Friedrich
  politic physician concept of, 12,
    69–70, 87
  on sexual relationships with
    patients, 87
  on taciturnity, 69–70

home birth. *See* planned home birth
honor, obligation of confidentiality
  based on, 69
hope, 145
hospital policy, on life-sustaining
  treatment, 186
human biology
  belief in medicine's control over,
    164–166
  clinical and social conditions
    promoting belief in control over,
    165–166
  informed consent process in
    defusing expectation of control
    over, 166–169
  preventive ethics as antidote to belief
    in control over, 165
  quest for control over, 164
humanity, Hume's discovery of, 7, 14,
  19. *See also* sympathy
Hume, David, 7, 14, 19
humility
  in leadership, 192
  in professional ethics in gynecology,
    27
  in professional ethics in medicine, 16
  in professional ethics in obstetrics,
    30
  in quest for reliability, 7
hydranencephaly, 151
hydrocephalus, 151–152
hypoplastic distal phalanges, 152

imaging
  conflicts of interest in use of, 83
  perfect baby concept promoted by,
    165
imminent-demise futility, 182
impaired autonomy, 62
  chronic and decreasing, 63–64
  chronic and invariable, 63
  chronic and progressive, 63
  chronic and variable, 62–63
in vitro assisted reproduction, 117
  embryo manipulation in, 120
  embryo transfer in, 118–119,
    120
  ethical concept of moral status in,
    117–120
  pre-implantation analysis in,
    119–120
  seamless patient care in, 120
in vitro embryo, 117
  dependent moral status of,
    118
  independent moral status of,
    117–118
  manipulation of, 120
  pre-implantation analysis of,
    119–120

in vivo embryo, 117
incest, induced abortion or feticide in
  cases of, 126–127
incurable patients, abandonment of,
  179–180
independent moral status, 34
  of embryo, 117–118
  ethical concept of fetus as a patient
    and, 38–39
  medical ethics and bioethics
    dominance by, 34–35
  problems with, 35
indirect referral, 90, 91–92, 131. *See
  also* direct referral
induced abortion
  after-viability offers of, 125–126
  autonomy-based justifications for
    before-viability offers of,
    126–127
  beneficence-based justifications for
    before-viability offers of, 126
  confidentiality in, 131
  conscientious objection to offers or
    recommendations of, 129
  conscientious objection to
    performance of, 130
  conscientious objection to referral
    for, 90–92, 131
  conscientious objection to residency
    training in, 89
  counseling pregnant women about,
    124
  in patients with depression and
    psychoses, 128–129
  performance of, 129–130
  recommendations of, 127–128
  referrals for, 131
  thought and speech precision in,
    124–125
  before viability, 125
infertility, 116
  cancer treatment risk of, 174
informed consent
  attitudes distorting clinical
    judgment in, 56–57
  beneficence-based ethical
    obligations in, 51–52
  in cancer and pregnancy, 173–176
  for cesarean delivery, 149–151
  decision-making capacity and,
    47–49
  directive counseling role in, 53
  evaluation of information in,
    54
  for fetal analysis, 135–136
  healthcare team members qualified
    to obtain, 57
  information provided in, 52
  legal standards of disclosure satisfied
    in, 52

241

informed consent (cont.)
  for maternal–fetal innovation, 203, 207
  for maternal–fetal research, 203–204, 207, 210–212
  meaning of, 50
  outcomes of, 54
  patient as ultimate decision maker in, 55
  patient autonomy support in, 52, 53, 54, 55
  patient's role in, 54
  for patients with mental disorders, 155
  perfect baby expectation defused by, 166–169
  process of, 51–55
  recommendations made in, 54
  respectful persuasion in, 54–55
  shared decision making role in, 53–54
  simple consent compared with, 51
  voluntary decision making in, 53
informed decision making, ethical principle of respect for autonomy in, 18, 29, 32
informed refusal
  preventive ethics component of, 56
  strict legal obligation of, 55–56
initiation of pregnancy. See pregnancy initiation
innovation, clinical, 202
  ethically justified criteria for, 206, 210
  in vitro embryo manipulation in, 120
  informed consent for, 203, 207
  in maternal–fetal intervention, 203
Institutional Animal Care and Use Committee, 203
Institutional Review Board (IRB), 203–205
insurance claims, confidentiality challenges created by, 74
integrity
  in informed consent process, 56–57
  in professional ethics in gynecology, 27
  in professional ethics in medicine, 15–16
  in professional ethics in obstetrics, 30
  in professional ethics in obstetrics and gynecology, 152–153, 185
  in professional ethics in perinatal medicine, 185
intentional framing, 55
interactive capacity, life-sustaining treatment and, 180–181
interactive-capacity futility, 182–183

International Academy of Perinatal Medicine, 21, 33–34
  New York Declaration of, 217, 222–223
International Federation of Gynecology and Obstetrics (FIGO), 21, 217
International Society of the Fetus as a Patient, 33–34
intervention. See trial of intervention
intimate partner violence, 222
intrapartum management
  cephalocentesis, 151–152
  continuum of vaginal and cesarean delivery in, 149, 150–151, 152
  of patient in vegetative state, 157–158
  for patients with mental disorders and illnesses, 154–157
  in periviable birth, 142–143
  planned home birth, 158–160
  preventive ethics for cesarean delivery in, 149–151
  recommendations role in, 150
  refusal of cesarean delivery in, 152–154
  requests for cesarean delivery in, 158
intrapartum refusal, of cesarean delivery, 153
intuitions, 20
invasive fetal analysis, 135
  patient election of, 137
investment refinement principle, 219
involuntary requests, for cesarean delivery, 158
IRB. See Institutional Review Board
irreversible condition, 176, 182

James, William, 7, 21
Jehovah's Witnesses, 56
Johnson, President, 218
Jouanna, Jacques, 11–12
judgment. See also clinical judgment
  ethical, 4, 6
  meaning of, 4
justice. See also healthcare justice
  healthcare justice as specification of, 216–217
  libertarian, 193
  in medical ethics and bioethics, 10–11
  procedural, 217–218, 220–221, 222
  in professional ethics in gynecology, 29
  in professional ethics in medicine, 17, 18–19
  in professional ethics in obstetrics, 32–33
  substantive, 217–220, 222
  utilitarian, 193, 219

Kafka, Franz, 194
Kafkaesque organizational culture, 194
Kant, Immanuel
  categorical imperative of, 192–193
  on independent moral status, 34–35
  quest for certainty typified by, 7
karyotyping, 33, 166, 168–169
Kipling, Rudyard, 77

leadership. See also organizational culture
  Drucker on, 191
  ethical challenges in, 190
  Gregory and Percival on, 191–192
  guild self-interest management by, 195–197
  as navigation between Scylla and Charybdis, 197
  philosophy of, 190–192
  Plato on, 191
  professional virtues in, 191–192
Lectures on the Duties and Qualifications of a Physician (Gregory), 10, 13, 15, 27
legal standards for disclosure of information, 52
Leikin, Sanford, 60
liability insurance, 220
libertarian justice, 193
life-cycle principle, 218–219
life-sustaining treatment
  advance directive law in, 182
  anatomic futility in, 182
  beneficence-based and autonomy-based limits of, 178–179
  emerging consensus on limits of, 180
  goals of, 178
  Groningen Protocol and, 184
  historical perspective on limits of, 179–181
  hospital policy on, 186
  imminent-demise futility in, 182
  inappropriate requests for, 185–186
  interactive-capacity futility in, 182–183
  obstetrician-gynecologist role in decision making about limits of, 181–184
  physiologic futility in, 182
  preventive ethics approach to setting limits on, 184–185
  quality-of-life futility in, 183
  trends toward limits on, 183
  unacceptable opportunity costs in, 183–184
Liley, A.W., 33

Index

live birth, 140
Living Will. *See* directive, advance
Lombardo, Paul, 50
loss, coping with, 145
lung maturity, cancer treatment delay until, 175-176

Machiavelli, Nicolo, 194
Machiavellian organizational culture, 194
malignancy. *See* cancer
malpractice insurance. *See* professional liability insurance
Management of Myelomeningocele Study (MOMS), 205
manipulation, embryo, 120
man-midwife, 69-70, 87
maternal–fetal intervention, 202-203
  animal models of, 203
  ethically justified criteria for, 206-207, 210
  experimental, 169
  informed consent for, 203-204, 207, 210-212
  minimizing risk to fetal patient in, 205
  MOMS clinical trial as model for research in, 205
  oversight of clinical innovation in, 203
  oversight of clinical research in, 203-205
  in pregnant patients with mental illnesses and disorders, 207-212
  transition to clinical practice in, 205, 206, 207
Matres Mundi, 217
maximin principle, 219
Medicaid, 219
  professional virtue of self-effacement for patients covered by, 31
medical emergency
  confidentiality in, 73
  decision making in, 66
  induced abortion or feticide in, 130
medical ethics
  ethical principles in, 9-11
  Hippocratic, 11-12
  independent moral status dominance in, 34-35
  limitations of, 8
  philosophical, 7-8
  professional ethics in medicine compared with, 7-8
  tradition of, 7
  virtues in, 9
Medical Ethics (Percival), 10, 14, 21
Medical Power of Attorney, 57-58
medically indigent, bias against, 219

medically reasonable alternatives
  ethical principle of beneficence and, 17-18, 29, 32
  ethical principle of nonmaleficence and, 18
  for pregnancy prevention, 109
  vaginal and cesarean delivery as, 149, 150-151, 152
Medicare, 218-219
medicine as a profession, ethical concept of. *See* ethical concept of medicine as a profession
medicus politicus. See politic physician
men of interest, 13, 15, 81-82
mental disorders
  assent in, 157
  assessment of decision-making capacity in patients with, 155
  assisted decision making with patients with, 111-112, 155
  decision making with, by, and for patients with, 128-129, 154-157
  informed consent for patients with, 155
  intrapartum management for patients with, 154-157
  research with pregnant patients with, 207-212
  surrogate decision making in, 155
mental pain, 16, 27-28, 30-31. *See also* suffering
#MeToo, 86, 221
microcephaly, 151
minimal risk, 205
Minkoff, Howard, 153
minors, decision-making capacity of, 47-48
MOMS. *See* Management of Myelomeningocele Study
monopoly power, 193-194
monopsony power, 193-194
moral philosophy, 6
  philosophical medical ethics and differences in, 7-8
  quest for certainty in, 7
  quest for reliability in, 7
moral point of view, 8
moral risk
  in fetal analysis refusal, 137
  pre-conception counseling on, 120-121
moral science, 7, 14, 19
moral status, 34
  dominance of independent, 34-35
  of embryo, 116, 117-118
  ethical concept of fetus as a patient and, 38-39
  in in vitro assisted reproduction, 117-120

  as preliminary to ethical concept of fetus as a patient, 34-35
  of previable fetus, 36
  problems with independent, 35
moral theology, 145
morality, 3-4
morally ideal, 4
morally impermissible, 4
morally obligatory, 4
morally permissible, 4
multidisciplinary team, 143-144
multifetal pregnancy reduction, 124

National Academy of Medicine (NAM), on patient safety and care, 158
negative autonomy, 39
negative diagnosis, 135
negative right, 38, 152
neonatal patient, 30
  advocacy for, 217-221, 222-223
  climate change effects on, 222
  critical care of, 143
  euthanasia in, 184
  evaluation of, 143
  research benefits and risks to, 209
  resuscitation of, 143
New York Declaration of International Academy of Perinatal Medicine, 217, 222-223
NICHD calculator, 140, 142, 143
Nicomachean Ethics (Aristotle), 7
nondirective counseling
  in fetal analysis, 136
  on induced abortion or feticide, 127
noninvasive fetal analysis, 135
  free fetal DNA analysis, 137-138
  patient election of, 137-138
noninvasive prenatal diagnosis, 134
noninvasive prenatal screening, 134
noninvasive prenatal testing, 134
nonmaleficence
  history of, 10
  in medical ethics and bioethics, 10
  in professional ethics in gynecology, 29
  in professional ethics in medicine, 17, 18
  in professional ethics in obstetrics, 32
nonmaleficence-based ethical obligation, 37
normative ethics, 95-96
  formal assessment tool for, 96-98
  structured reviews of, 98
North American Fetal Therapy Network, 205
Norton, M.E., 138
Nutton, Vivian, 12

243

Index

obligation. *See* ethical obligation
obstetric management
    fetal analysis and, 134
    pre-conception counseling about, 121
obstetrics. *See also* professional ethics in obstetrics
    economic bias against, 219–220
    professional liability insurance for, 220
opinion, 96
opportunity cost, 183–184
Organ Procurement Organization, 145
organizational culture
    critical appraisal of, 104
    cynical, 194
    dysfunction of, 194–195
    Gregory and Percival on, 191, 192
    Kafkaesque, 194
    libertarian, 193
    Machiavellian, 194
    of patient safety and quality, 20
    post-modern, 194–195
    professional resource management in, 193
    professional treatment of colleagues in, 192–193
    professional use of power in, 193–194
    of professionalism, 102
    professionalism over guild interests in, 196–197
    utilitarian, 193
    Wonderland, 194
organizational leadership. *See* leadership
organizational policy
    in fertility management, 113
    on life-sustaining treatment, 186

pain, 16, 27–28, 30–31
palliative care, 179–180
Pap smear, 29, 55–56, 134
paternalism
    in assisted decision making, 111
    cesarean delivery and, 153
    respectful persuasion preventing, 54, 55
patient, 15. *See also* dying patients; female patient; fetus as a patient, ethical concept of; neonatal patient; pregnant patient
    decision making by, with, and for, 47, 128–129
    decision-making capacity of adult, 47
    decision-making capacity of minor, 47–48
    ethical concept of being, 19

Gregory's and Percival's concept of, 15
    romantic and sexual relationships with, 86–89
    teaching about, 94
    wealth of, 16–17, 28, 31
patient autonomy. *See* autonomy
patient care, in planned home birth, 158–159
patient quality
    ethical concept of medicine as a profession in, 20
    mastery of skillset of, 104–105
    thought and speech precision ensuring, 3, 95
patient safety
    ethical concept of medicine as a profession in, 20
    mastery of skillset of, 104–105
    in planned home birth, 158–159
    thought and speech precision ensuring, 3, 95
patients' rights, 10, 19
payments, conflict of interest created by, 83–84
pedagogical methods
    case-based teaching using ethics work-up, 98–99
    grand rounds presentation, 99–100
    of great teachers, 100–101
    teaching ethics on rounds, 99
pedagogical tools
    formal assessment tool for normative ethics literature, 96–98
    structured reviews of normative ethics literature, 98
pediatric assent, 59–61
    in fertility management, 112
pediatric patient, research benefits and risks to, 209
Percival, Thomas
    on beneficence, 10
    on commitment to ethical concept of medicine as a profession, 19, 21
    on confidentiality of patient's secrets, 71
    on conflicts of commitment, 80, 85
    on conflicts of interest, 80, 82–83
    ethical concept of medicine as a profession invention of, 14–15, 101–102, 195–196
    ethical reasoning of, 21
    on leadership, 191–192
    Medical Ethics by, 10, 14, 21
    on organizational culture, 191, 192
    on professional autonomy, 113–114
    professional ethics in medicine invention by, 13, 14, 21

    on public trust, 15, 82–83, 216–217
perfect baby
    belief in medicine's control over human biology in creating, 164–166
    cautionary tale from American literature on, 164–165
    clinical and social conditions promoting concept of, 165–166
    ethical reasoning and, 164–165
    inability to guarantee, 167
    informed consent process in defusing expectation of, 166–169
    pre-implantation analysis and, 119–120
    preventive ethics as antidote for pursuit of, 165
    unattainability of, 169–170
Perinatal Innovation Review Committee, 203
perinatal medicine. *See* professional ethics in perinatal medicine
perinatal team
    decision maker with, 143–144
    multidisciplinary, 144
periviability, fetal patient status and, 36
periviable birth, 140
    Consensus Statement from American College of Obstetricians and Gynecologists and Society for Maternal–Fetal Medicine on, 142–143
    deliberative clinical judgment in management of, 140–141, 142–143, 144
    evaluation of neonatal patient after, 143
    hope and coping with loss in, 145
    intrapartum management in, 142–143
    multidisciplinary team approach to counseling before, 143–144
    neonatal critical care after, 143
    requests to "do everything" in, 144–145
    resuscitation of neonatal patient after, 143
persons, bias in favor of, 220–221, 223
persuasion. *See* respectful persuasion
pharmacogenomics, 135
philosophical medical ethics, 7–8
Physician Charter, 101
physician-patient relationship, 15
    patient termination of, 152
    professional virtues and ethical principles guiding, 15
physiologic futility, 182
placenta accreta, 159
placenta previa, 153
placental abruption, 153

Index

placentophagy, 159
planned home birth
  implications for counseling women interested in, 159–160
  patient safety in, 158–159
  recommendations role in, 159–160
Planned Parenthood, 91, 131
Plato, 7
  on leadership, 191
  quest for certainty originating from moral philosophy of, 7
  on reasoned argument compared with opinion, 96
politic physician, Hoffmann's concept of, 12, 69–70, 87
political bias, 222–223
Porter, Dorothy, 13
Porter, Roy, 13
positive diagnosis, 135
positive right, 38, 152
post-modern organizational culture, 194–195
power
  Hobbes on, 193
  monopoly and monopsony, 193–194
  professional use of, 193–194
powerful responses, management of, 154–155
pragmatism, 7, 21
pre-conception counseling, 120–121
  moral risk anticipation in, 121
  about obstetric management, 121
  obstetrician-gynecologist role in, 116
pregnancy, biopsychosocial condition of, 51
pregnancy initiation
  assisted reproduction in, 116, 117–120, 121
  embryo manipulation and, 120
  obstetrician-gynecologist roles in, 116
  preconception counseling in, 116, 120–121
  self-regulation role in, 118–119
  thought and speech precision in, 117
pregnancy prevention
  access to, 113
  assisted decision making in, 111–112
  autonomy-based clinical judgment in, 109
  beneficence-based clinical judgment in, 109, 110–111
  biopsychosocial concept of fertility and, 108–109
  conscientious objection to, 89–90
  court-ordered, 113–114
  decision making about, 109–111
  directive counseling role in, 109–110
  healthcare-justice-based clinical judgment in, 113–114
  medically reasonable alternatives for, 109
  methods of, 109
  organizational policy guiding, 113
  pediatric assent in, 112
  shared decision making role in, 110
  surrogate decision making in, 64–65, 112–113
pregnancy termination. *See* termination of pregnancy
pregnant patient
  advocacy for, 217–221, 222–223
  autonomy of, 36, 39
  cancer treatment for, 172–173, 174–176
  climate change effects on, 222
  as decision maker in gynecology and obstetrics clinical practice, 55
  decision making by, with, and for, 47
  decision-making capacity of adult, 47
  decision-making capacity of minor, 47–48
  ethical obligations to, 33, 34, 35–37
  pregnancy threatening health or life of, 126, 127, 128
  presentation of, 30
  research benefits and risks to, 208
pre-implantation analysis, 117, 119–120
prenatal diagnosis, 134
  ethical concept of fetus as a patient and, 33
prenatal screening, 134
prenatal testing, 134
prepartum counseling, 143–144
presumption of decision-making capacity
  in adult patients, 47
  in minors with legal authority over themselves, 47–48
prevention of pregnancy. *See* pregnancy prevention
preventive ethics, 56
  as antidote for pursuit of perfection, 165
  for cesarean delivery, 149–151
  in decision making, 149
  goal of, 149
  informed consent process as, 150
  in limits on life-sustaining treatment, 184–185
  in periviable birth management, 140–141, 142, 144
  response to reduced accountability, 103–105
previability
  fetal patient status and, 36, 125
  in pregnant patient with cancer, 173, 174–175
Price, Richard, 14, 19
prima facie ethical obligation
  enforcement of, 37–38
  ethical principle of beneficence creating, 17–18, 29, 32, 90
  ethical principle of healthcare justice creating, 18–19, 29, 32–33, 216
  ethical principle of nonmaleficence creating, 18, 29, 32
  ethical principle of respect for autonomy creating, 18, 29, 32, 90
  to fetal patient, 33, 34, 35–38
  to pregnant patient, 33, 34, 35–37
  professional virtue of compassion creating, 16, 27–28, 30–31
  professional virtue of integrity creating, 16, 27, 30
  professional virtue of self-effacement creating, 16–17, 28
  professional virtue of self-sacrifice creating, 17, 28, 31
prima facie ethical obligation of confidentiality, 69, 72
  absolute ethical obligation shift to, 71–72
  disclosure to family during and after sedation or anesthesia as ethical challenge to, 73
  electronic communication as ethical challenge to, 77
  electronic medical records as ethical challenge to, 75
  employer inquiries as ethical challenge to, 74
  ethically justified limits on, 72–73
  genetic and genomic information as ethical challenge to, 75–76
  HIPAA as ethical challenge to, 76
  insurance claims as ethical challenge to, 74
  medical emergencies as ethical challenge to, 73
  sexually transmitted disease as ethical challenge to, 76
  social media as ethical challenge to, 77
prima facie ethical principles, 9
  teaching of, 94
privacy, right to, 71–72, 118–119
procedural justice, 217–218, 222
  challenges to, 220–221
productivity incentives, 196
profession of medicine, as public trust, 15, 82–83, 216–217
professional autonomy, in fertility management, 113–114
professional community standard, 52

Index

professional ethics in gynecology, 3
  critical appraisal of literature in, 6, 95
  ethical principles in, 29
  female patient in, 26–27
  professional virtues in, 27–28
  as quest for reliability, 7
  study of, 26
professional ethics in medicine, 3
  advantages of, 19
  bioethics compared with, 8–9
  ethical concept of medicine as a profession in, 11, 14–15, 19–21, 101–102
  ethical principles in, 15, 17–19
  Gregory's invention of, 13–14, 21
  Hippocratic medical ethics in invention of, 11–12
  Hoffmann's politic physician in invention of, 12
  invention of, 11–15, 101–102
  medical ethics compared with, 7–8
  Percival's invention of, 13, 14, 21
  professional virtues in, 15–17
  as quest for reliability, 7
  study of, 11
professional ethics in obstetrics, 3, 30
  beneficence-based and autonomy-based indications for referral in, 90
  critical appraisal of literature in, 6, 95
  ethical principles in, 32–33
  induced abortion and feticide before viability in, 125
  professional virtues in, 30–31
  as quest for reliability, 7
  right to life irrelevance in, 38
  study of, 26
professional ethics in obstetrics and gynecology. *See also* teaching professional ethics in obstetrics and gynecology
  basics of, 94–95
  confidentiality in, 69–72
  grand rounds presentation on, 99–100
  professional virtue of integrity in, 152–153, 185
  qualities of great teachers of, 100–101
  study of, 26
  viability in, 140
professional ethics in pediatrics, 41–42
professional ethics in perinatal medicine, 41–42, 140–141
  Groningen Protocol rejection in, 184
  obstetric component of, 141, 144

pediatric component of, 141–142, 144
professional virtue of integrity in, 185
study of, 26
professional liability, informed refusal in risk of, 56
professional liability insurance, 220
professional relationships, conflict of interest in, 80–81
professional resource management, 193
professional treatment, of colleagues, 192–193
professional virtue of compassion
  in leadership, 192
  in professional ethics in gynecology, 27–28
  in professional ethics in medicine, 16
  in professional ethics in obstetrics, 30–31
professional virtue of humility
  in leadership, 192
  in professional ethics in gynecology, 27
  in professional ethics in medicine, 16
  in professional ethics in obstetrics, 30
professional virtue of integrity
  in informed consent process, 56–57
  in leadership, 192
  in professional ethics in gynecology, 27
  in professional ethics in medicine, 15–16
  in professional ethics in obstetrics, 30
  in professional ethics in obstetrics and gynecology, 152–153, 185
  in professional ethics in perinatal medicine, 185
professional virtue of self-effacement
  in leadership, 191
  in professional ethics in gynecology, 28
  in professional ethics in medicine, 16–17
  in professional ethics in obstetrics, 31
professional virtue of self-sacrifice
  in leadership, 192
  in professional ethics in gynecology, 28
  in professional ethics in medicine, 16, 17
  in professional ethics in obstetrics, 31
professional virtues
  in leadership, 191–192
  in medical ethics and bioethics, 9

  in professional ethics in gynecology, 27–28
  in professional ethics in medicine, 15–17
  in professional ethics in obstetrics, 30–31
professionalism
  milestones in, 104
  organizational culture of, 102
  prevention of drift from, 101–103
  preventive ethics response to reduced, 103–105
prolapsed umbilical cord, 154
prudence
  in entrepreneurial relationships, 80–81
  Hoffmann's concept of, 12, 69–70, 87
psychoses, decision making with, by, and for patients with, 128–129
public policy. *See* health policy
public trust, profession of medicine as, 15, 82–83, 216–217

quality, patient. *See* patient quality
quality of life, 180–181
quality-of-life futility, 183
quest for certainty, 7
quest for reliability, 7
Quinlan, Karen Ann, 180

randomized controlled clinical trial (RCT), 206–207, 210
rape, induced abortion or feticide in cases of, 126–127
rationing, healthcare justice prohibiting, 18–19
Rawls, John, 219
RCT. *See* Randomized controlled clinical trial
reasonable person standard, 52
reasoning, ethical. *See* ethical reasoning
REC. *See* Research Ethics Committee
recommendations, in informed consent process, 54
refusal of treatment
  cesarean delivery, 152–154
  informed, 55–56
  life-sustaining, 179
regulatory demands, 196
reliability, quest for, 7
reproductive medicine
  assisted, 116, 117–120, 121
  clinical innovation and research in, 120
  in vitro meaning of embryo in, 117
  in vivo meaning of embryo in, 117

obstetrician-gynecologist roles in, 116
self-regulation role in, 118–119
reproductive privacy, 118–119
reproductive risks, 167
requests for clinical intervention, patients presenting with, 164
requests to "do everything"
 hope and coping with loss in, 145
 incomplete or inaccurate information in, 144–145
 in life-sustaining treatment, 185–186
 moral theological considerations in, 145
 preventive ethics approach to, 144
research, clinical, 202
 CIOMS guidance for, 208
 conflict of interest in, 84–85
 ethically justified criteria for, 206, 210
 in vitro embryo manipulation in, 120
 informed consent for, 203–204, 207, 210–212
 in maternal–fetal intervention, 203–205
 minimizing risk to fetal patient in, 205
 MOMS clinical trial as model for, 205
 with pregnant patients with mental illnesses and disorders, 207–212
 transition to clinical practice from, 205, 206, 207
Research Ethics Committee (REC), 203
residency training
 conscientious objection in, 89
 critical appraisal of organizational culture of, 104
 drift from professionalism in, 101–103
 preventive ethics response to reduced accountability in, 103–105
resource management, 193
respect for autonomy
 in advance directives, 176
 in fertility decision making, 109
 in informed consent process, 52, 53, 54, 55
 limits on life-sustaining treatment based on, 178–179
 in medical ethics and bioethics, 10
 in professional ethics in gynecology, 29

in professional ethics in medicine, 17, 18
in professional ethics in obstetrics, 32, 90
recommendations role in supporting, 160
respectful persuasion, 54–55
restricted duty hours, drift from professionalism with, 102–103
results of uncertain clinical significance, 135
resuscitation
 of neonatal patient, 143
 parental refusal of, 164
retirement from clinical practice, 82–83
right, patient, 10, 19
right to life, ethical concept of fetus as a patient and, 38
right to privacy, 71–72, 118–119
right to reproductive privacy, 118–119
rights-based absolutism, ethical concept of fetus as a patient and, 39–40
rights-based reductionism, 39
risk assessment, 135, 158
 non-invasive fetal analysis for, 137–138
risk-adjust assessment, of decision-making capacity, 58
Roe v. Wade, 140
romantic relationships with patients, 86
 contemporary perspective on, 88–89
 historical perspective on, 86–88
rounds, teaching ethics on, 99
Royal Infirmaries
 Gregory's professional ethics of medicine for, 13–14
 Percival's professional ethics of medicine for, 14, 191
Rush, Benjamin, 14

safety, of clinical management, 35
safety, patient. *See* patient safety
Sauer, Pieter J.J., 184
Schloendorff v. Society of New York Hospital, 49–51
screening, 134–135
sedation, disclosure to family members during and after, 73
selective feticide (selective reduction), 124, 126
self-effacement
 in leadership, 191
 in professional ethics in gynecology, 28
 in professional ethics in medicine, 16–17

in professional ethics in obstetrics, 31
self-interest
 of adults, 218
 enlightened, 12, 69–70, 87
 Gregory on, 81–82
 guild, 13, 15, 81–83, 195–197, 216–217
 Percival on, 82–83
 prioritization of, 81
self-physicking, 13
self-sacrifice
 in leadership, 192
 in professional ethics in gynecology, 28
 in professional ethics in medicine, 16, 17
 in professional ethics in obstetrics, 31
 reasonable limits on, 197
Seton, Lt. Colonel, 217
severe fetal anomaly
 feticide of fetuses with, 125–126, 128
 hydrocephalus with, 151–152
severe fetal distress, refusal of cesarean delivery for, 154
sex, biologic concept of, 108
sexual relationships with patients, 86
 contemporary perspective on, 88–89
 historical perspective on, 86–88
sexually transmitted disease, confidentiality challenges created by, 76
shared decision making
 in fertility management, 110
 in fetal analysis, 136
 in induced abortion or feticide, 127
 in informed consent process, 53–54
shift mentality, 103
simple consent
 decision-making capacity and, 47–49
 healthcare team members qualified to obtain, 57
 informed consent compared with, 51
 legal origin of, 49–51
 meaning of, 49–51
social advocacy, 221–222
social media, confidentiality challenges created by, 77
Society for Maternal–Fetal Medicine, Consensus Statement on periviable birth from, 142–143
Society of Critical Care Medicine, 184
Society of University Surgeons, 203
solidarity, 8
specification, of ethical principles, 11
speculation, ethical judgments avoiding, 4

Index

speech, precision of, 3, 95, 117, 124–125, 134
spina bifida, 184
strategic ambiguity, 195
strategic procrastination, 195
Strong, Carson, 38–39
structured reviews, of normative ethics literature, 98
study design, 210
subjective standard, 52
substantive justice, 217–218, 222
  challenges to, 218–220
substituted judgment standard of surrogate decision making, 61–62, 129
suffering, 16, 27–28, 30–31
  of worried well, 27
supervision by attending physicians, drift from professionalism with, 103
Surgical Innovation Committee, 203
surrogate decision making, 61
  best interests standard of, 62, 129
  confidentiality challenges in, 73
  family refusal to accept legally designated surrogate in, 65–66
  in induced abortion and feticide, 128–129
  meaning of, 50
  mental disorders and, 155
  prevention of pregnancy, 64–65, 112–113
  reliability of surrogate in, 65
  requests to "do everything" and, 185–186
  substituted judgment standard of, 61–62, 129
  termination of pregnancy, 64
Sutkin, Gary, 100
sympathy, Hume's discovery of, 7, 14, 19. *See also* humanity

taciturnity, 69–70
Talmud, 159
Tarasoff v. Regents of the University of California, 72
task-specific decision-making capacity, 58–59
Taylor, John, 19
teaching professional ethics in obstetrics and gynecology
  basics, 94–95
  discipline of ethical reasoning, 95–96
  pedagogical methods for, 98–101
  pedagogical tools for, 96–98

prevention of drift from professionalism, 101–103
preventive ethics response to reduced accountability, 103–105
terminal condition, 176, 182
termination of pregnancy, 124–125
  access to, 130
  performance of, 129–130
  surrogate decision making in, 64
testing, 134–135
thanatophoric dysplasia, 151–152
therapeutic misconception, 169, 207, 210–211
thought, precision of, 3, 95, 117, 124–125, 134
time-specific decision-making capacity, 59
TOLAC. *See* trial of labor after cesarean
trafficking, 72, 221
triage ethics, 16–17
trial of intervention
  neonatal critical care as, 143
  resuscitation as, 143
trial of labor after cesarean (TOLAC), 52, 149
trisomy 13, 128, 151–152
trisomy 21, 137
Truman v. Thomas, 55–56
twinning, 117–118

ultrasound, conflicts of interest in use of, 83
ultrasound diagnosis, 134
ultrasound screening, 134
ultrasound testing, 134
Ulysses contract, 59. *See also* informed consent
umbilical cord, prolapsed, 154
unacceptable opportunity cost, 183–184
undue influence, in pregnancy prevention, 112
UNICEF, 217
University of Edinburgh, professional ethics of medicine invention at, 13, 14
unworthy poor, 219
utilitarian justice, 193, 219

vaccination, 159, 167, 168
vaginal delivery, 142, 149, 150–151, 152
validity, of results in normative ethics literature, 97–98

vegetative state, continuing pregnancy in patient in, 157–158
verbal interventions, 155
Verhagen, Eduard, 184
Veterans Health Affairs, 61
viability
  fetal patient status and, 36
  induced abortion and feticide after, 125–126
  induced abortion and feticide before, 125, 126–127
  in pregnant patient with cancer, 173–176
  in professional ethics in obstetrics and gynecology, 140
violence against women, 222
virtues
  in informed consent process, 56–57
  in medical ethics and bioethics, 9
  in professional ethics in gynecology, 27–28
  in professional ethics in medicine, 15–17
  in professional ethics in obstetrics, 30–31
vitalism, 178
voluntary decision making
  ethical principle of respect for autonomy in, 18, 29, 32
  in informed consent process, 53

Warren, Mary Ann, 38
wealth, patient, 16–17, 28, 31
Williams Obstetrics, discourse of fetal patient in, 33–34
women and children first
  advocacy for healthcare resources based on, 217–221, 222–223
  New York Declaration of International Academy of Perinatal Medicine on, 217, 222–223
  origin of phrase, 217
Wonderland organizational culture, 194
work-life balance, 17, 28, 31
World Association of Perinatal Medicine, 21, 217
World Bank, 217
World Health Organization, 21, 140, 217
World Medical Association, 21, 71
worried well, 27
worthy poor, 219